Clinical
Examination
of the
Shoulder

Clinical Examination of the Shoulder

Todd S. Ellenbecker, MS, PT, SCS, OCS, CSCS

Clinic Director

Physiotherapy Associates Scottsdale Sports Clinic

Scottsdale, Arizona

with 170 illustrations

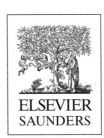

ELSEVIER
SAUNDERS

MT

ELSEVIER
SAUNDERS

11830 Westline Industrial Drive
St. Louis, Missouri 63146

CLINICAL EXAMINATION OF THE SHOULDER   0-7216-9807-7
Copyright © 2004, Elsevier, Inc. All rights reserved.

NOTICE

Physical Therapy is an ever-changing field. Standard safety precautions must be followed, but as new research and clinical experience broaden our knowledge, changes in treatment and drug therapy may become necessary or appropriate. Readers are advised to check the most current product information provided by the manufacturer of each drug to be administered to verify the recommended dose, the method and duration of administration, and contraindications. It is the responsibility of the licensed prescriber, relying on experience and knowledge of the patient, to determine dosages and the best treatment for each individual patient. Neither the publisher nor the editor assumes any liability for any injury and/or damage to persons or property arising from this publication.

Publisher

Library of Congress Cataloging in Publication Data

Ellenbecker, Todd S., 1962–
   Clinical examination of the shoulder / Todd
S. Ellenbecker.
   p. ; cm.
   Includes bibliographical references and index.
   ISBN 0-7216-9807-7
   1. Shoulder–Examination. 2. Shoulder–Wounds and injuries–Diagnosis. I. Title. [DNLM:
1. Shoulder Joint–injuries. 2. Shoulder Joint–physiopathology. 3. Diagnostic Techniques and
Procedures. 4. Shoulder–injuries. 5. Shoulder–physiopathology. WE 810 E45c 2004]
   RC939.E45 2004
   617.5'72044–dc22   2004046718

Acquisitions Editor: Marion Waldman
Developmental Editor: Jacquelyn Merrell
Publishing Services Manager: Linda McKinley
Project Manager: Jennifer Furey
Designer: Amy Buxton

Printed in the United States of America

Last digit is the print number: 9 8 7 6 5 4 3 2 1

3/1/06

To my wife and best friend—Gail

PREFACE

Advances in basic science and clinical research of the shoulder have significantly increased the understanding of the anatomy, biomechanics, and pathophysiology of the human shoulder. With these advances has come an influx of clinical tests and methods used to examine the patient with a musculoskeletal shoulder injury. The primary purpose of this book is to provide the reader with an overview of the available research substantiating or negating the use of many clinical tests for the patient presenting with shoulder dysfunction. In addition to simply providing a detailed description of these tests, each chapter provides an overview of the primary pathology for which these tests are used and summarizes the research performed on these tests to provide a level of understanding regarding their effectiveness.

The inclusion of research is not meant to confuse the reader, but rather to allow for a more scientific approach to the examination process. Repeated use of the terms *specificity* and *sensitivity* can be at times intimidating. However, these statistical values can assist the clinician in identifying clinical tests that are the most effective for patients with shoulder dysfunction. Two simple descrip-

tors can be used to better understand the seemingly complicated terms of *specificity* and *sensitivity*. These terms are *spin* and *snout*, and the use of these terms may make it easier to apply the concepts of specificity and sensitivity using these everyday terms. *Spin*, used for *specificity*, indicates that specificity refers to ruling "in" conditions, whereas *snout*, representing *sensitivity*, assists in ruling conditions "out." While oversimplified, these simple descriptors can be used while reading through the often detailed research on many clinical tests described in this text.

Finally, it is hoped that the practical information included in the latter portion of this text on strength testing, proprioception, and functional evaluation can be used to provide the most detailed clinical examination of the high-functioning shoulder. Understanding the clustering of signs and symptoms obtained during the clinical examination processes inherent in the "master" clinician's clinical behaviors is summarized in the final section of this book in the form of case studies. It is hoped that this book will provide a valuable clinical reference tool for the practicing clinician by consolidating practical and research-specific information in one place.

ACKNOWLEDGMENTS

While many individuals have provided guidance, both in this project and throughout my career, I would like to acknowledge the following, whom this book could not have been written without—George Davies, Janet Sobel, Kevin Wilk, Dr. Ben Kibler, and Dr. Robert Nirschl—for their excellence and guidance in teaching me shoulder examination and treatment.

I would also like to thank the physicians, therapists, tennis teaching professionals, and coaches for the daily opportunity to examine and treat their patients and athletes and allow me the privilege to focus on clinical practice and research of the shoulder.

CONTENTS

Clinical
Examination
of the
Shoulder

GENERAL OVERVIEW

Introduction to Clinical Examination of the Shoulder

HOW TO USE THIS BOOK

This book is designed to present the integral parts of the examination process, combined with clinical research identifying the effectiveness of the procedures and techniques used by clinicians, to evaluate the patient with shoulder dysfunction. The research provided in this text provides crucially important information for the clinician and contains specific terms, such as *specificity, sensitivity,* and *predictive value.* A discussion of these terms is warranted to improve the application of this research to the clinical evaluation process.

Definition of Key Terms

The use of terms such as *specificity, sensitivity,* and both *positive* and *negative predictive value* are commonly applied in research reporting the accuracy and effectiveness of examination techniques on patients. In many studies, patients are examined clinically and results are compared to determine the reliability of the clinical test both for one examiner on numerous occasions of testing (intrarater reliability) and among several examiners (interrater reliability). Clinical tests contained in this book are also often compared with the results of other diagnostic tests such as magnetic resonance imaging (MRI) or radiographs, as well as with intraoperative findings. The presence of injury or pathology at time of surgery confirms or negates the result of clinical testing and is a common research design presented in this book.

Sensitivity

The validity of a screening or evaluation test is measured in terms of its ability to accurately assess the presence or absence of the target condition (Portney & Watkins, 1993). *Sensitivity* can be defined as the ability of a test or evaluation maneuver to obtain a "positive" result when the condition the test is testing for is really present. In other words, sensitivity is the ability of the test to produce a true positive result when the patient being tested actually has the disorder for which the examiner is testing. Sensitivity is represented by the percentage of individuals who test positive for the condition out of all those individuals who

actually have the condition (Portney & Watkins, 1993). The sensitivity of a test increases as the number of persons who are correctly identified as having the condition increases. Another way of thinking of sensitivity is that it increases when fewer persons with the disorder are missed. Obviously, it is advantageous for a clinician to use tests that have high indexes of sensitivity.

Specificity

Specificity is the ability of a test to obtain a negative result when the condition the clinician is testing for is truly absent. Specificity is represented by the proportion of individuals who test negative for the condition out of all those who do not have the condition. According to Portney and Watkins (1993), a highly specific test will rarely test positive when a person does *not* have the disease or condition for which he or she is being tested.

Combining Sensitivity and Specificity

Obviously, using tests with high sensitivity and specificity enhances a clinician's ability to correctly identify pathology and arrive at the best possible clinical impression and subsequent treatment plan. As with many clinical scenarios, however, there are tradeoffs between the two characteristics. Tests that are designed to be highly sensitive have testing criteria that are typically less stringent; thus fewer cases are missed (Portney & Watkins, 1993). In this scenario, the chances of obtaining false-positive results increase (decreased specificity) because less stringent qualifying responses are used to render a test positive. Likewise, if the test criteria are made more stringent, such that only a narrow range of individuals with the criterion variable will test positive, a greater proportion of those who are normal will test negative (increasing specificity); however, a larger number of the true cases (individuals who have the condition) will be missed, which decreases sensitivity.

Sensitivity is most important when the risk associated with missing a diagnosis is high, such as identifying cancer or other life-threatening disease. Using the musculoskeletal tests mentioned in this book, including the clinical elimination maneuvers for the glenoid labrum, which may render a patient a candidate for a surgical procedure, would also carry a high risk, as an inaccurate diagnosis may subject a patient to an unnecessary surgical procedure. Specificity is more important when either the costs or risks involved with further intervention are substantial (Portney & Watkins, 1993). This book includes multiple tests in most areas to provide the clinician with a variety of clinical tests, so that the results of several examinations can be combined to minimize the tradeoffs between specificity and sensitivity.

Predictive Value

To determine whether the performance of a clinical test or series of clinical tests is feasible and an efficient use of both the examiner's and patient's time, the test's predictive value can be assessed. Positive predictive value (PPV) estimates the likelihood that a person who tests positive will actually have the condition for which he or she is being tested. PPV is the proportion of patients who test positive and who truly have the condition. A clinical test with a very high PPV provides a strong estimate of the number of patients who actually have the condition.

Likewise, negative predictive value (NPV) indicates the probability that a person who tests negative on a clinical test actually does not have the condition for which he or she is being assessed. Research by Itoi et al (1999) illustrates the concept of predictive value. They studied the effectiveness of the empty and full can clinical tests in identifying patients with full-thickness rotator cuff tears. By using the criterion of muscular weakness, the full can clinical test had a PPV of 49%. This finding tells clinicians that approximately one of every two patients who have substantial weakness during the performance of the full can rotator cuff test actually has a full-thickness rotator cuff tear. Likewise, one of every two patients who test positive during the full can test is actually normal.

Applying positive and negative predictive values to the clinical environment may at first seem overly scientific and academic. However, consider the ramifications of using a clinical test with a very low PPV during the evaluation of a patient who presents with symptoms consistent with a labral tear. If an individual were to test positive for a labral tear using a test with a very low PPV, considerable time and additional resources would be required to further determine whether that initial clinical test was actually correct. In some cases, the use of clinical tests with a very low PPV or NPV is not worth the potential discomfort and time required. Another potential problem with using tests with low predictive value is that alternative tests are often required to confirm the results of the first test. For example, use of a clunk test to identify labral pathology may place the patient in a more apprehensive clinical posture that does not allow further testing as a result of decreased relaxation. Therefore careful selection of the most important and clinically accurate tests is an important responsibility of the clinician when performing a clinical shoulder examination.

Prevalence

The concept of prevalence must be considered when applying and interpreting clinical tests. The term *prevalence* refers to the number of cases of a condition that exist in a certain population at any given time (Portney & Watkins, 1993). When the prevalence is high, the likelihood of identifying cases correctly using tests with a given sensitivity and specificity increases. Also, when prevalence is high, a test will tend to have a higher PPV. When prevalence is low, the chances of obtaining a false-positive result are much higher than when the prevalence of a particular condition is high. When using the empty or full can test to detect a full-thickness rotator cuff tear, knowledge regarding the prevalence of rotator cuff tears plays a considerable part in applying the results of the test. For example, when testing an 11-year-old elite junior tennis player with anterior shoulder pain, a positive empty or full can test is unlikely to indicate a full-thickness tear of the supraspinatus tendon, as full-thickness rotator cuff tears in that young population are less common and occur at a very low prevalence. In contrast, if the empty or full can test resulted in significant muscular weakness in a 79-year-old competitive tennis player with anterior shoulder pain, the likelihood that this finding would indicate a full-thickness tear is much greater because of the greater prevalence of full-thickness tears in older individuals.

Summary

This book provides detailed descriptions of clinical tests along with research reporting their sensitivity and specificity, as well as their positive and negative predictive value. This information provides a better indication of the actual effectiveness of a specific clinical test or group of clinical tests, as well as a better understanding of the role that an examination maneuver or group of maneuvers can play in the comprehensive evaluation of the patient with shoulder pathology.

COMPARISON OF CLINICAL EVALUATION FINDINGS WITH OTHER DIAGNOSTIC TESTS AND SURGICAL FINDINGS

One of the most common methods of determining the effectiveness of a group of clinical examinations of the shoulder is to compare the results with established diagnostic tests. Naredo et al (2002) compared the results of physical examination to ultrasound testing in 31 consecutive patients with a first episode of shoulder pain. Examinations were performed by two rheumatologists, with a third rheumatologist blinded to the results of the clinical examination performing the ultrasound. The clinical examination consisted of active and passive range of motion and 10 special examination maneuvers. Results of the comparison showed very low sensitivity in the clinical diagnosis of nearly all shoulder lesions, especially rotator cuff tears; however, specificity was high for rotator cuff tear, tendonitis of the subscapularis and infraspinatus, and acromioclavicular joint injury. Specificity was very low for supraspinatus tears, biceps tendonitis, and rotator cuff impingement. This study emphasized that pain elicited during impingement testing by placing the rotator cuff beneath the acromial arch can be diagnostic for many types of rotator cuff lesions, and the induced pain cannot be clearly diagnostic for one particular condition. The authors concluded that clinical assessment by experienced physician examiners of the patient with a first-time injured shoulder was often inaccurate and that ultrasonography should be used whenever possible to improve diagnostic accuracy.

Research results comparing MRI with clinical evaluation is also available. These studies are covered in greater detail in Chapter 13. MRI has been reported to have a high sensitivity (100%) and specificity (95%) for the diagnosis of rotator cuff tears (Ianotti et al, 1991) and can differentiate normal rotator cuff tendons from tendons with "tendonitis" (93% sensitivity, 87% specificity).

Liu et al (1996a) introduced the crank test for clinical identification of labral tears and reported a higher sensitivity of 90% compared with sensitivity of MRI (59%) and a specificity that equaled that of MRI (85%). This study found that a clinical test was more accurate than MRI in identifying labral tears in 62 patients who had an average of 3 months of shoulder symptoms that did not resolve with physical therapy.

Finally, comparison of clinical examination findings with arthroscopic shoulder surgery continues to be one of the more common means to measure the validity of clinical tests. Itoi et al (1999) used this approach to study the effectiveness of the empty and full can clinical test to identify supraspinatus tears. Magarey et al (1989) compared the results of a clinical examination of the shoulder by two physical therapists with findings obtained during arthroscopic surgery. The two therapists independently reached the same conclusion regarding the "tissue source" of the patient's pain 100% of the time. There was 72% agreement in their ability to place the patient into one of four diagnostic categories: impingement, tendonitis, tendon rupture, and instability. The use of arthroscopy to identify tissue source agreed with the clinical examination 51% of the time and with the diagnostic categories 80% of the time (Magarey et al, 1989). Further research on the use of diagnostic categories as well as continued comparison of clinical test results with arthroscopic evaluation will assist in determining accuracy and guide therapists in both the performance and especially the interpretation of clinical examination methods for the shoulder.

GENERAL CONCEPTS APPLIED DURING CLINICAL EXAMINATION OF THE SHOULDER

Several general concepts are important when performing clinical examination of the shoulder. These concepts are referred to throughout this book, but are described in detail here. They are essential to the successful examination of the patient with shoulder pathology.

Resting Position of the Glenohumeral Joint

The resting position of the human glenohumeral joint is generally considered to be the position of maximum range of motion and laxity, as a result of minimal tension or stress in the supportive structures surrounding the joint (Hsu et al, 2002). This position has been referred to as the *loose-pack* position of the joint. Kaltenborn (1989) and Magee (1997) have both reported that the resting position of the glenohumeral joint ranges between 55 and 70 degrees of abduction (trunk humeral angle) in the scapular plane (see definition of scapular plane in this chapter). This loose-pack position is generally considered to be in mid-range position, but only recently has been subjected to experimental testing.

Hsu et al (2002) measured maximal anteroposterior displacements and total rotation range of motion in cadaveric specimens, with different positions of glenohumeral joint elevation in the plane of the scapula. They identified the loose-pack position, where maximal anteroposterior humeral head excursion and maximal total rotation range of motion occurred within the proposed range of 55 to 70 degrees of humeral elevation in the scapular plane (trunk-humeral angle) at a mean trunk humeral angle of 39.33 degrees. This rate corresponded to 45% of the available range of motion of the cadaveric specimens. Anteroposterior humeral head translations and maximal total rotation ranges of motion were significantly less, at 0 degrees of abduction and near 90 degrees of abduction in the plane of the scapula, and were greatest near the experimentally measured resting position of the glenohumeral joint. This study provides key objective evidence for the clinician to obtain the maximal loose-pack position of the glenohumeral joint by using the plane of the

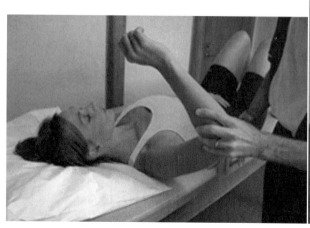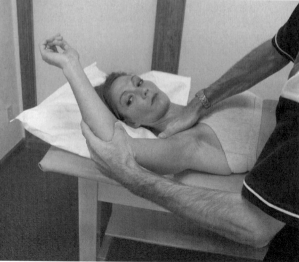

Figure 1-1 Balance point position allowing clinician to support the patient's extremity with one hand. Note the position of the hand near the epicondyles of the elbow.

scapula and approximately 40 degrees of abduction. This information is important to clinicians who wish to evaluate the glenohumeral joint in a position of maximal excursion or translation to determine the underlying accessory mobility of the joint.

This cadaveric research provides additional clinical guidance for identifying relative or percent of abduction range of motion where this position occurs. In patients with restrictions in humeral elevation resulting from capsular tightness, the loose-pack position occurs in less abduction than in individuals with full range of abduction range of motion. Clinicians should use this information during both evaluation and treatment of the human shoulder.

Scapular Plane Position

According to Saha (1983), the scapular plane is defined as being 30 degrees anterior to the coronal or frontal plane of the body. Placement of the glenohumeral joint in the scapular plane optimizes the osseous congruity between the humeral head and the glenoid and is widely recommended as an optimal position for performing both various evaluation techniques and many rehabilitation exercises (Saha, 1983; Ellenbecker, 1995). With the glenohumeral joint placed in the scapular plane, bony impingement of the greater tuberosity against the acromion does not occur because of the alignment of the tuberosity and acromion in this orientation (Saha, 1983). Also, no internal or external rotational movement is theo-

retically required to allow for full overhead elevation in the scapular plane (Inman et al, 1944). Throughout this book, the scapular plane position is used during specific evaluation techniques, including humeral head translation tests and impingement tests.

Balance Point Position of the Upper Extremity

The balance point position concept, used frequently in clinical tests to evaluate the glenohumeral joint, is not technically based on a calculated or measured balancing point for the human upper extremity. Rather, this concept refers to the position the clinician can use when grasping and supporting the patient's extremity with only one hand, allowing use of the other hand for additional stabilization or function.

Figure 1-1 shows the approximate position and grip that can be used to control or balance the patient's upper extremity. This position is referred to throughout this book as the *balance point* position. Note the location near the elbow and the use of the fingers and thumb to optimize contact on a rather wide area at the elbow. This position allows the clinician to influence humeral rotation, as well as move the glenohumeral joint in flexion, abduction, and circumduction. Care should be taken to avoid overly aggressive grasping of the patient's elbow, as this can lead to an increase in patient apprehension and unwanted muscular activation. Repetitive practice with both the clinical tests and patient contact enables the clinician to use optimal patient contacts throughout the upper extremity and ensures that an adequate amount of pressure is used to stabilize and handle the patient's extremity, while avoiding a painful or apprehensive response.

Extremity Examination Sequence

The sequence of actual tests used in shoulder evaluation varies based on several factors. Although each clinician or educator may prefer a specific sequence of elements when performing the shoulder examination, few objectively based criteria exist. One aspect of the examination process that is widely recommended and followed closely is the ordering of the initial extremity to be evaluated. It is recommended that the examiner perform clinical test procedures on the uninjured extremity first, followed by the involved extremity. Following this order promotes greater patient relaxation during examination of the involved extremity, which is often painful, and reduces the apprehension often encountered during the examination process because the patient may be unsure of which movements or maneuvers the examiner will be performing.

Examination: Patient History

INTRODUCTION

A thorough, organized history of the patient with shoulder dysfunction is required in the complete examination process. It is important to include both general questions with regard to shoulder pathology and specific questions based on the patient's sport or activity. Although there are many approaches to history taking, one example of a thorough history applicable for a patient with shoulder dysfunction is listed in Box 2-1. This chapter covers several areas of the patient history in greater detail.

IMMEDIATE HISTORY

One of the initial areas of focus on the subjective evaluation is the patient's immediate history, which typically includes the chief complaint. Although many types of questions can be asked, the following four questions summarize one approach to obtaining the immediate history:

1. What is the problematic area?
2. How did the problem occur?
3. When did the problem develop?
4. Where did the problem occur?

Although these questions may seem simplistic, they can effectively elicit the basic information required from the patient (Maughon & Andrews, 1994).

The description of the chief complaint or complaints typically involves pain, weakness, instability, sensory changes, and crepitus. Attempts by the examiner to quantify the degree, severity, and exact location of these factors via the patient's subjective responses involve sequential, organized dialogue between the patient and examiner. During the subjective evaluation of the shoulder, attempts should be directed toward delineating and localizing the symptoms to the injured segment or segments. Identification of radicular symptoms into the distal upper extremity, constant pain without change or relief, and the presence of headaches, low back or neck pain, and psychosocial stresses that may be influencing the patient's overall health provide rationales for further objective evaluation outside the upper extremity kinetic chain. For a more detailed discussion of differential diagnosis, the reader is referred to a summary of nonmusculoskeletal causes of shoulder region pain in Chapter 5. To perform a complete and thorough patient examination, careful analysis of subjective information provided in the patient's history is required to alert the examiner to the possible presence of nonmusculoskeletal causes. This information directs the clinician to a broader base of examination techniques and possible referral to specialists to rule out nonmusculoskeletal contribution of shoulder dysfunction.

PAST HISTORY

A thorough understanding of the patient's past history of shoulder injury and disability is essential to a successful subjective evaluation. Using the example of a patient with shoulder instability, it is important to delineate whether the patient has "one time" anterior dislocation from a traumatic event (TUBS classification of Matsen [*T*raumatic, *U*nidirectional, *B*ankart, *S*urgery]) or a repeated, chronic instability of the glenohumeral joint from repetitive stresses and an acquired atraumatic onset of injury (AMBRI classification of Matsen [*A*traumatic, *M*ultidirectional, *B*ilateral Laxity, *R*ehabilitation, *I*nferior Capsular Shift]). Knowledge of the patient's pertinent past shoulder history influences not only the sequence and inclusion of specific tests used in the evaluation but treatment procedures as well. Examination of a mature athlete with a rotator cuff injury from overhead activity is another example of the importance of obtaining a thorough history relating to shoulder pathology. Complete questioning often can reveal a fall onto the lateral aspect of the shoulder as long ago as 20 to 30 years or a shoulder separation in high school football that can shed light on the patient's impingement-type symptoms. Encroachment of the subacromial space as a result of degenerative changes in the acromioclavicular joint from previous injury has been reported as an etiologic factor in impingement lesions (Neer, 1983).

Specific questioning regarding previous treatment to the injured shoulder is also of interest to the rehabilitation specialist. Previous surgical procedures, steroid

- Chief complaint
- Nature of symptoms
- Behavior of symptoms
- Location of symptoms
- Onset of symptoms
- Course and duration of symptoms
- Effect of previous treatment
- Other related medical problems

Adapted from Saunders HD: Evaluation of a musculoskeletal disorder. In Gould JA, Davies GJ: *Orthopaedic and sports physical therapy*, St Louis, 1985, Mosby.

injections, therapeutic modalities, and exercise programs are relevant when formulating an evaluation-based treatment program.

LOCATION OF SYMPTOMS

Determining the location of symptoms is an important part of the subjective evaluation and is required to enhance the objective portion of the evaluation process. Isolating the area of discomfort is often difficult for the patient with an overuse injury to the rotator cuff because of the intimate association of the tendons of the rotator cuff to one another near their humeral insertion (Clark & Harryman, 1992). The splaying and interweaving of the rotator cuff, as well as an ensheathed biceps tendon by the subscapularis and supraspinatus tendon, may further complicate the isolation of a direct point of injury in these structures (Clark & Harryman, 1992). Identification of referral symptoms into the lateral aspect of the shoulder, or continuing into the elbow and distal upper extremity, indicates the need for further objective testing and specific joint clearing tests to rule out involvement of the cervical spine or elbow joints (Davies & DeCarlo, 1995). Confirmation of the location of patient symptoms is often achieved through the use of a body chart.

Gerber et al (1998) attempted to characterize pain patterns after an isolated injection of a hypertonic saline solution directly into the subacromial space and acromioclavicular joint. Figure 2-1 shows the pain patterns produced by the injections. Injection of the hypertonic saline into the acromioclavicular joint produced relatively isolated symptoms directly over the joint in all subjects. Pain was also reported over the anterolateral neck region and along the upper trapezius muscle, with extension distally to the anterolateral deltoid. This injection into the acromioclavicular joint produced palpable soreness over the joint, as well as tenderness over the coracoid in 87% of the subjects injected. Pain produced by cross-body abduction increased after injection in only 13% of the subjects.

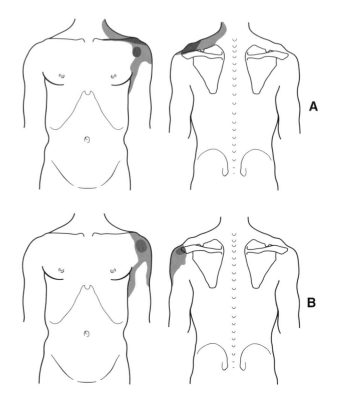

Figure 2-1 Pattern of pain presentation after localized injection into **A,** the acromioclavicular joint, and **B,** the subacromial space. (From Gerber C, Galantay RV, Hersche O: The pattern of pain produced by irritation of the acromioclavicular joint and the subacromial space, *J Shoulder Elbow Surg* 7(4):353, 1998.)

Injection into the subacromial space produced a characteristic pain pattern, which included mainly the region overlying the lateral aspect of the deltoid in 100% of the subjects injected (see Figure 2-1). All 10 subjects also had pain over the lateral border of the acromion. The acromioclavicular joint remained pain free in every case when injection was directed into the subacromial space.

This important study provided evidence regarding the typical pain patterns expected with irritation of either the subacromial space or acromioclavicular joint. It also characterized normal pain responses for irritation of these structures and identified the lack of posterior scapular and neck symptoms from isolated irritation of either the subacromial space or acromioclavicular joint (Gerber et al, 1998). One of the most common patterns of radicular pain that can be confused with shoulder dysfunction is the C6 radiculopathy. This pain is often referred to the shoulder, the anterosuperior aspect of the arm, the radial aspect of the forearm, and the thumb (Adams, 1977). This pattern is similar to the one described by Gerber et al (1998) for the acromioclavicular joint, except for the presence of posterior neck pain and exacerbation of the pain with movements of the cervical spine in cases of C6 radiculopathy. Weakness or abnormal C6 reflexes and a lack of tenderness directly over the acromioclavicular joint inherent in cases of C6 radiculopathy further assist the clinician in differentiating between acromioclavicular joint injury and C6 radiculopathy.

C7 nerve root compression affects the pectoral region, the medial axilla, the region of the scapula, and the triceps, as well as the dorsal aspect of the forearm and elbow and middle finger (Gerber et al, 1998). Tenderness is often most noted over the vertebral border of the scapula opposite vertebral segments T3 and T4 (Adams, 1977). This pattern is uniquely different from the patterns identified in the evidence-based research of Gerber et al (1998). Their study showed the importance of the history and physical examination in distinguishing pain arising in structures intimately associated with the glenohumeral joint versus more central pathology.

SEVERITY OF SYMPTOMS

The use of analog scales is typically recommended for quantification of the subjective response of pain severity. The patient's rating on a 10-point scale at rest and with activity or specific activities allows for comparison between visits and after treatment or activity trials. Using the analog scale involves asking the patient to rate the pain, with "0" being no pain and "10" being the worst pain ever encountered. Other scales are also used to quantify the patient's pain. These scales are generally used to evaluate the outcome of a specific surgical procedure or to determine the effectiveness of a treatment process. Refer to Chapter 15 for a complete discussion of subjective rating scales. The use of analog and subjective rating scales provides additional information for the subjective evaluation to complement the patient's report of pain.

GENERAL QUESTIONS

Additional questions specifically for the patient with shoulder pathology are recommended. One question involves the presence of night pain and sleeping position. In a magnetic resonance imaging study (Solem-Bertoft et al, 1993), the subacromial space was narrower in a position of scapular protraction as compared with scapular retraction. In a patient suffering from primary glenohumeral joint impingement, the side-lying position (i.e., lying on the involved side during sleeping) is not beneficial at rest

because of the possibility of encroachment of the subacromial space when the scapula is protracted.

An additional series of questions directed at the patient's sport or activity demands provides important information for the clinician. For example, establishing that a throwing or racquet sport athlete has pain when throwing or serving does not provide the appropriate level of information necessary to properly diagnose and formulate a treatment plan. Further questioning as to what stages of the throwing or serving motion produce the symptoms and after how many repetitions may provide insight into what structures are involved. Specific muscular activity patterns and joint kinematics inherent in each stage of the throwing motion and tennis serve can assist in identifying compressive disease or tensile-type injuries of the rotator cuff. The presence of instability of the glenohumeral joint, however subtle, during the cocking phase of overhead activities can produce impingement or compressive symptoms (Jobe & Bradley, 1989; Walch et al, 1992), whereas a feeling of instability or loss of control during the follow-through phase during predominant eccentric loading of the rotator cuff can indicate a tensile rotator cuff injury (Andrews & Alexander, 1995). Additional questions regarding a change in sport equipment, ergonomic environment, and training history/habits provide information that is imperative for understanding the stresses leading to the injury. Examples of additional specific questions used during the examination of a baseball or tennis player are provided in Boxes 2-2 and 2-3.

ACTIVITIES OF DAILY LIVING, VOCATIONAL, AND AVOCATIONAL GOALS

The individual's goals play an important part in the formulation of an evaluation-based treatment program. Knowledge of the patient's vocation and avocational activities and goals assists the clinician by allowing the use of more specific and functionally oriented evaluation and treatment methods. Testing the shoulder in positions required either in sport- or activity-specific movement patterns is required for each shoulder to completely evaluate the degree and level of injury and begin the formulation of a treatment program. The patient's symptoms can be more adequately elicited when specific positions, as well as mode and force-specific muscular contractions, are used in the evaluation process.

Box 2-2   Examination: History of the Throwing Shoulder

I. General Information
  A. Age
  B. Dominant Arm (Throwing)
  C. Bats (Left, Right, Switch)
  D. Years Throwing
    1. Years pitching
    2. Years in other positions
  E. Level of Competition
II. Medical Information
  A. Chronic or Acute Problem
  B. Review of Systems
  C. Preexisting or Recurrent Shoulder Problem
  D. Other Musculoskeletal Problems
    1. Acute
    2. Distant to shoulder (kinetic chain involvement)
III. Shoulder Complaints
  A. Symptoms (Specify Pitching Versus Throwing)
    1. Pain
    2. Weakness or fatigue
      a. Loss of velocity
      b. Loss of accuracy
    3. Instability/subluxation
    4. Stiffness (inability to get "loose")
    5. Catching/locking
  B. Injury Pattern
    1. Sudden onset or acute onset (pitching versus throwing)
    2. Gradual or chronic onset (pitching versus throwing)
    3. Traumatic onset—fall or blow to extremity
    4. Recurrent pattern
  C. Symptom Characteristics
    1. Location
    2. Character and severity
    3. Provocation
    4. Duration
    5. Paresthesias/referral pattern
    6. Phase of throwing or pitching
      a. Cocking phase
      b. Acceleration phase
      c. Deceleration phase
    7. Related activities/disability
  D. Related Symptoms
    1. Cervical
    2. Peripheral nerve
    3. Brachial plexus
    4. Entrapment

Adapted from Gillogly S, Andrews JR: In Andrews JR, Zarins B, Wilk KE, eds: *Injuries in baseball,* Philadelphia, 1998, Lippincott.

Box 2-3   Examination: History in the Tennis Player

I. Presence of Pain during Specific Stroke
  A. Forehand
    1. Preparation
    2. Acceleration
    3. Ball contact
    4. Deceleration/follow-through
  B. Backhand
    1. One-handed backhand
    2. Two-handed backhand
    3. Phase of pain development as in forehand above (I–IV)
  C. Serve/Overhead
    1. Cocking phase
    2. Acceleration phase
    3. Deceleration/follow-through phase
  D. Volleys
    1. Forehand
    2. Backhand
      a. One-handed versus two-handed volley
II. Specific Mechanism
  A. Single Stroke (Acute Onset)
  B. Overtraining (Gradual Onset)
  C. Able to Continue Playing
    1. Without stroke modification
    2. With stroke modification
III. Training History
  A. Change in Technique?
    1. Grip
    2. Stance
    3. Other
  B. Change in Coach
  C. Change in Training Program
    1. Surface
    2. On-court training
    3. Off-court training
IV. Equipment
  A. Racquet
    1. Type
    2. How long with current frame
    3. Modifications to current frame
      a. Weight
    4. Previous frame
  B. String
    1. Type
    2. Tension
    3. Change in tension/type?
V. Ability to Play Presently
  A. Certain Strokes Pain-Free
  B. Stroke Modification Required

Observation/Posture

INTRODUCTION

Evaluation of a patient's posture has been regarded as a crucial part of the comprehensive examination of a patient with spinal dysfunction. Gould stated, "the static and dynamic posture of the client can add insight to musculoskeletal problem solving," and the importance of a comprehensive evaluation of posture is no less important in the patient with shoulder dysfunction. Gould also stated, "the clinician should attempt to gain awareness not only of gross alterations in posture such as shoulder heights or iliac crest height, but also of subtle changes in muscle tone or subtle disruptions in rhythm" (Gould, 1985).

Evaluation of sitting and standing posture begins before the patient is aware of it. Observing the patient's seated posture in the waiting area can serve as an important initial finding. Common alterations in sitting are extreme variations in forward head posture, which include increases in cervical lordosis and thoracic kyphosis, as well as a protected posture that often includes shoulder girdle elevation with scapular protraction and placement of the arm across the stomach held closely against the body. As the patient ambulates to the evaluation room, careful observation of how the affected extremity moves during gait also provides valuable insight into the degree of protection the patient affords that extremity. The presence of this protective posture provides valuable insight into how approachable the patient may be with objective clinical tests. Approaching and handling the patient's extremity with both greater care and a softer touch are required if protected posturing is initially observed.

STANDING POSTURE EVALUATION

Evaluation of the patient in the standing position is indicated early in the evaluation process. A male patient should be evaluated with all shirts and undershirts removed to allow for full visualization of the shoulders and spine from the waist upward. When possible, observing the patient during removal of his shirt provides valuable insight into active movement capabilities and degree of hesitancy to initiate movement in various combinations. Females should be evaluated while wearing a gown or sports bra to preserve patient modesty. Clear visual inspection of the shoulder region and scapula is essential for a complete postural evaluation.

SHOULDER HEIGHT ASSESSMENT

The relative height of the shoulders should be assessed because this can provide significant information about the patient's muscular development, as well as the presence of any guarding through exaggerated use of the upper trapezius musculature. Typically, the dominant shoulder is lower than the nondominant shoulder in neutral, nonstressed standing postures. Although the exact reason for this phenomenon is unclear, increased mass in the dominant arm may cause the dominant shoulder to be lower secondary to the increased weight of the arm, as well as elongation of the periscapular musculature on the dominant or preferred side secondary to eccentric loading. In addition, stretching and elongation may occur from carrying heavy objects on the dominant side. Evaluation of the patient in the standing position should typically show the dominant shoulder to be slightly lower (no normative data currently exist in the scientific literature), or at least the shoulders should be level with each other.

ALTERATIONS IN SHOULDER HEIGHT

Visual observation of the patient's shoulders from the posterior and anterior views can identify alterations from the normal relationship described previously.

DOMINANT, INJURED SHOULDER HIGHER

Visual inspection of the dominant, injured shoulder often identifies this shoulder as higher than the uninjured, nondominant shoulder. This finding often indicates muscular guarding and lends insight to the examiner as to any exaggerated upper trapezius muscular activation that may require intervention (Figure 3-1). Objective data on the magnitude of dominant injured shoulder elevation are not

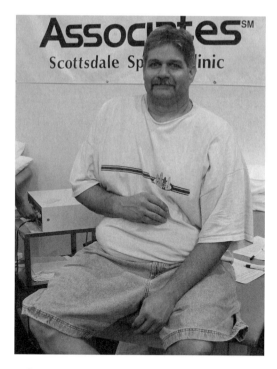

Figure **3-1** Patient with guarded right shoulder position demonstrating a higher dominant shoulder as seen after operative procedure.

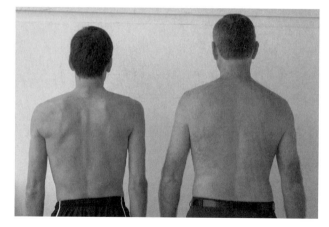

Figure **3-2** Characteristic postural deviations with regard to shoulder height of two elite level tennis players (player on *left* is left-handed; player on *right* is right-handed). Note the lowered dominant shoulder relative to the nondominant side.

available; however, it is recommended that this observational finding be noted.

TENNIS SHOULDER

"It is said that oarsman of ancient galleys developed a corporeal deformity when rowing only on one side of the ship, and that a favor the slave master could bestow upon an oarsman was to alternate him from one side of the ship to the other, allowing maintenance of symmetrical physique" (Priest & Nagel, 1976). The term *tennis shoulder* has been described by Priest and Nagel (1976) to describe a developmental characteristic in the dominant arm of tennis players, where the dominant shoulder droops inferiorly with an apparent scoliosis. The position of the shoulder girdle and scapula is one of depression, protraction, and often downward rotation. Tennis shoulder exists in unilaterally dominant athletes such as tennis players, baseball players, volleyball players, and individuals who ergonomically use one extremity without heavy or repeated exertion of the contralateral extremity (Priest & Nagel, 1976; Kibler, 1991, 1998a).

A total of 84 world class tennis players were initially examined by Priest and Nagel and found to have this drooping phenomenon of the dominant shoulder. Figure 3-2 shows this characteristic postural adaptation

in two elite level tennis players. Consequences of this depression on the dominant side included thoracic outlet syndrome, rotator cuff pathology from alteration of scapular positioning, and abutment of the rotator cuff on an altered acromial position, as well as spinal pathology (Priest & Nagel, 1976). Of particular importance is the finding of protraction and downward rotation of the dominant scapula. Solem-Bertoft et al (1993) used magnetic resonance imaging to demonstrate a narrowing of the subacromial space when shoulders were experimentally moved from positions of maximal retraction to protracted positions. This narrowing of the subacromial space can lead to glenohumeral joint impingement and alter normal scapulothoracic and glenohumeral joint arthrokinematics.

Downward rotation of the scapula can also lead to a change in the resting posture/position of the glenoid (Figure 3-3). Downward rotation secondary to postural alteration can lead to a more vertical glenoid position and change the angle of inclination. Changes in the angle of inclination of the scapula have been reported in patients with increases in inferior translation and multidirectional instability of the glenohumeral joint (Basmajian & Bazant, 1959).

HANDS-ON-HIPS POSITION

In the standing position, the clinician can observe the patient for symmetric muscle development and, more specifically, focal areas of muscle atrophy. One position that is recommended, in addition to observing the patient with the arms at the sides in a comfortable standing posture, is the "hands-on-hips position" (Figure 3-4). This position places the patient's shoulders in approximately 45

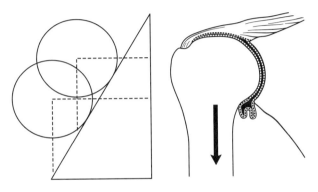

Figure 3-3 Angle of inclination of the glenoid. Note the upward tilt of the glenoid to prevent passive downward displacement of the humeral head. (From Basmajian JV, Bazant FL: Factors preventing downward dislocation of the adductor shoulder joint, *J Bone Joint Surg* 41A:1182, 1959.)

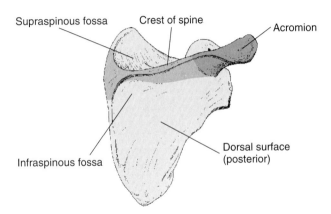

Figure 3-5 Scapular fossae and landmarks.

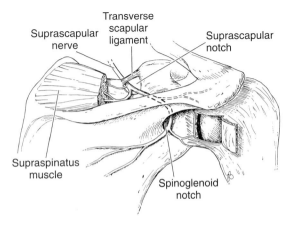

Figure 3-6 Posterior view of the scapula outlining the course of the suprascapular nerve.

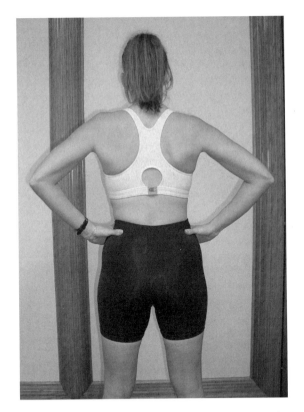

Figure 3-4 Hands-on-hips position in a right-handed patient.

to 50 degrees of abduction with slight internal rotation. The hands are placed on the iliac crests of the hips, with the thumbs pointed posteriorly. This position is also used during the Kibler lateral scapular slide test (see pages 22–25). Placement of the hands on the hips allows the patient to relax the arms and often enables the clinician to

observe focal pockets of atrophy along the scapular border, as well as more commonly over the infraspinous fossa of the scapula (Figure 3-5).

Thorough visual inspection using this position can often identify excessive scalloping over the infraspinous fossa present in patients with rotator cuff dysfunction, as well as in patients with severe atrophy who may have suprascapular nerve involvement. Impingement of the suprascapular nerve can occur at the suprascapular notch or spinoglenoid notch (Figure 3-6) and from paralabral cyst formation commonly found in patients with superior labral lesions (Piatt et al, 2002). Figure 3-7 shows the isolated atrophy present in the infraspinous fossa of a patient after arthroscopic labral repair. The patient stands in the hands-on-hips position, which exaggerates atrophy and assists the clinician in identifying this physical examination finding. Further examination of the patient with extreme wasting of the infraspinatus muscle is warranted

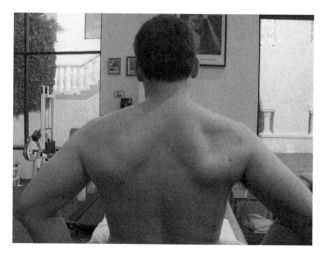

Figure 3-7 Patient with significant atrophy in the infraspinous fossa. Patient in hands-on-hips position after superior labral repair.

TABLE 3-1   Additional Postural Findings in Patients with Shoulder Pathology

PATIENT PRESENTATION	TYPICAL INDICATION OF POSTURE
Prominent acromion	Glenohumeral joint dislocation
Laterally depressed scapula Slightly abducted humerus	
"Stairstep" drop-off of the lateral aspect of the clavicle above the acromion	Acromioclavicular separation
"Popeye" biceps appearance	Biceps long head tendon rupture
Scapula grossly disassociated from the thoracic wall	Scapular winging from long thoracic nerve involvement

Adapted from Halbach JW, Tank RT: The shoulder. In Gould JA, Davies GJ, editors: *Orthopaedic and sports physical therapy*, St Louis, 1985, Mosby.

to rule out suprascapular nerve involvement. The use of nerve conduction tests, in addition to a detailed physical examination, can lead the clinician to the diagnosis of suprascapular nerve injury.

ADDITIONAL POSTURAL TESTS IN STANDING

Assessment of spinal position, in addition to shoulder height, is also important during this phase of the evaluation process. The spine should be inspected from posterior and lateral views to assess for the presence of the characteristic curvature of the spine in the sagittal plane and lack of curvature in the frontal plane. Although posture is individualized, with a wide variation in what can be thought of as "normal posture" among individuals, an "ideal" posture in the sagittal plane has been described (Davies & DeCarlo, 1995). This "ideal" lateral posture alignment has a plumb line traversing through the center or the external auditory meatus (ear), mid-acromial bisection of the scapula, greater trochanter of the femur, mid-lateral knee between the popliteal fossa and the patella, and just anterior to the lateral malleolus. Significant deviations from this alignment should be noted and ultimately will affect the overall treatment of the patient with shoulder pathology.

The incidence of scoliosis in unilaterally dominant athletes, even at very young developmental ages, has been reported secondary to asymmetric muscular development and sport-specific upper body loading patterns (Priest & Nagel, 1976). Methods of assessment for spinal curvature include solely visual observation, as well as visual observation with the assistance of a plumb line or posture grid (Davies & DeCarlo, 1995), in addition to radiographs. Evaluation of the patient using a maneuver known as the Adam's position (American Academy of Orthopaedic Surgeons, 1992; Grossman et al, 1995) involves placing the patient in a forward-flexed spinal posture between 45 and 60 degrees (approximate) to evaluate for the presence of a unilateral rib hump over the thoracic or lumbar spine. As a result of the rotation associated with lateral flexion of the spine characteristic in scoliosis, asymmetric rib protrusion exists and can be best identified by the clinician by placing the patient in the Adam's position and viewing the patient from a posterior position. Thorough evaluation of pelvic levels, as well as measurement of leg lengths, can also assist in the postural evaluation of the patient with shoulder pathology presenting with associated postural conditions such as scoliosis. Table 3-1 lists additional postural findings commonly encountered in patients with shoulder pathology.

Testing the Scapulothoracic Joint

INTRODUCTION

The importance of the scapulothoracic joint and its relationship to shoulder function and dysfunction have been extensively reported by Kibler (1991, 1998a). Although this important relationship is well understood and widely accepted, there are limited clinical tests to evaluate scapulothoracic function. Also, scapular position and movement have been most effectively documented in experimental research conditions and not in the clinical setting (Lukasiewicz et al, 1999).

DESCRIPTION OF NORMAL SCAPULAR RESTING POSITION

Although there are many variations in normal scapular positioning, Kibler (2003) described resting scapular orientation as being 30 degrees anteriorly rotated with respect to the frontal plane, as viewed from above. Also, the scapula is rotated approximately 3 degrees upward (superiorly), as viewed from the posterior orientation used during most clinical observations/examinations. Finally, the scapula is tilted anteriorly approximately 20 degrees when viewed from the direct lateral aspect of the body.

OVERVIEW OF SCAPULOTHORACIC MOTION

Scapulothoracic movement was initially described in clinical terms as "scapulo-humeral rhythm" by both Codman (1934) and Inman (1944). Inman stated that "the total range of scapular motion is not more than 60 degrees" and that the total contribution from the glenohumeral joint is not greater than 120 degrees. The scapulohumeral rhythm was described for the total arc of elevation of the shoulder joint to contain 2 degrees of glenohumeral motion for every degree of scapulothoracic motion (Inman et al, 1944).

In addition to this ratio of movement, Inman et al (1944) identified a "setting phase," which occurred during the first 30 to 60 degrees of shoulder elevation. They described this setting phase as when "the scapula seeks, in relationship to the humerus, a precise position of stability which it may obtain in one of several ways:" (1) the scapula may remain fixed with motion occurring solely at the glenohumeral joint until a stable position is reached, (2) the scapula moves laterally or medially on the chest wall, or (3) in rare instances the scapula oscillates until stabilization is achieved. After 30 degrees of abduction and 60 degrees of flexion have been reached, the relationship of scapulothoracic to glenohumeral joint motion remains remarkably constant.

Research using three-dimensional analysis and other laboratory-based methods has confirmed Inman's early descriptions of scapulohumeral rhythm (Doody et al, 1970; Bagg and Forrest, 1988). These studies have also provided more detailed descriptions of the exact contribution of the scapulothoracic and glenohumeral joint during arm elevation in the scapular plane. Doody et al (1970) found the ratio of glenohumeral to scapulothoracic motion to change from 7.29:1 in the first 30 degrees of elevation to 0.78:1 between 90 and 150 degrees. Bagg and Forrest (1988) found similar differences based on the range of motion. In the early phase of elevation, 4.29 degrees of glenohumeral joint motion occurred for every 1 degree of scapular motion, with 0.71 degrees of glenohumeral motion occurring for every 1 degree of scapular motion between the functional arc of 80 and 140 degrees.

Bagg and Forrest (1988) also identified the instantaneous center of rotation (ICR) of the scapulothoracic joint at various points in the range of motion. Figure 4-1 shows the ICR of the scapulothoracic joint at 20 degrees of elevation and Figure 4-2 at approximately 140 degrees of elevation. The ICR moves from the medial border of the spine of the scapula, with the shoulder at approximately 20 degrees of elevation near the side of the body, and migrates superolaterally to the region near the acromioclavicular joint at approximately 140 degrees. Bagg and Forrest also identified an increased muscular stabilization role of the lower trapezius and serratus anterior force couple at higher, more functional positions of elevation. Figures 4-1 and 4-2 also show the line of pull of

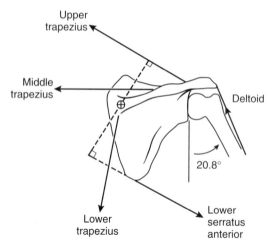

Figure 4-1 A biomechanical model of scapular rotation at 20.8 degrees of abduction. Note the position of the instantaneous center of rotation ICR and relative lengths of the lever arms of the scapular musculature. (Adapted from Bagg SD, Forrest WJ: A biomechanical analysis of scapular rotation during arm abduction in the scapular plane, *Arch Phys Med Rehabil* 67:243, 1988.)

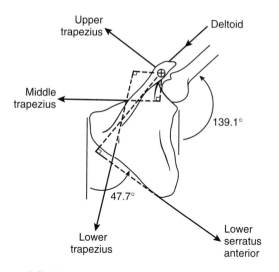

Figure 4-2 A biomechanical model of scapular rotation at 139.1 degrees of abduction. Note the position of the instantaneous center of rotation ICR and relative lengths of the lever arms of the scapular musculature. (Adapted from Bagg SD, Forrest WJ: A biomechanical analysis of scapular rotation during arm abduction in the scapular plane, *Arch Phys Med Rehabil* 67:243, 1988.)

the serratus anterior and trapezius muscles and the relative changes in the lever arm of each muscle in the two positions of glenohumeral joint elevation. This biomechanical information on the scapulothoracic joint is presented in this text as a precursor to the important evaluation methods and scapular dysfunction classification in the next section. Evaluating scapular position and scapulohumeral

rhythm and identifying unilateral alterations in normal scapular positioning are crucial in the complete evaluation of the patient with shoulder pathology (Kibler, 1991, 1998a).

OVERVIEW AND DESCRIPTION OF SCAPULAR MOTION

Typical movement of the scapula occurs in the coronal, sagittal, and transverse planes. Brief descriptions here provide a framework for the classification of scapular dysfunction and scapulothoracic joint testing sections presented later.

Upward/Downward Rotation

Movements of upward and downward rotation occur in the coronal or frontal plane. The angle typically used to describe the position of scapular rotation is formed between the spine and medial border of the scapula (Figure 4-3). Poppen and Walker (1978) reported normal elevation of the acromion at approximately 36 degrees from the neutral position to maximum abduction.

Anterior/Posterior Tilting

Sagittal plane motion of the scapula is referred to as *anterior/posterior tilting* (see Figure 4-3). The angle of scapular tilting is formed by a vector passing via C7 and T7 and a vector passing via the inferior angle of the scapula and the root of the spine of the scapula (Lukasiewicz et al, 1999).

Internal/External Rotation

Transverse plane movement of the scapula is referred to as *internal* and *external rotation* (see Figure 4-3). The angle used to describe internal/external rotation of the scapula is formed by the coronal (frontal) plane of the body and a vector passing via the transverse plane projection of the root of the spine of the scapula and the posterior angle of the scapula (Lukasiewicz et al, 1999). Abnormal increases in the internal rotation angle of the scapula lead to changes in the orientation of the glenoid. This altered position of the glenoid is referred to as "antetilting," and it allows for an opening up of the anterior half of the glenohumeral articulation (Kibler, 1991). The antetilting of the scapula has been shown by Saha (1983) to be a component of the subluxation/dislocation complex in patients with microtrauma-induced glenohumeral instability.

Protraction/Retraction

The movement of retraction and protraction occurs literally around the curvature of the thoracic wall (Kibler, 1998a). Retraction typically occurs in a curvilinear fashion

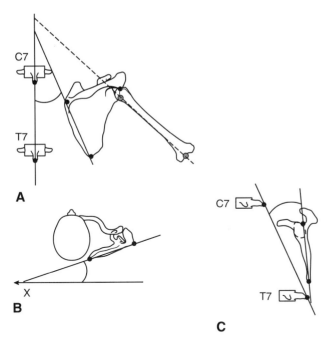

Figure 4-3 Definition of scapular position and orientation. **A,** Upward rotation angle. The scapulothoracic angle is between the medial border of the scapula (projected onto the frontal plane). Increasing values represent upward rotation. Total arm elevation is the angle between the spine and vector connecting the olecranon and a derived point 2 cm directly inferior to the posterior angle of the acromion. **B,** Scapular internal rotation angle. The angle between the frontal plane and a vector passing through the root of the spine of the scapula posterior angle of the acromion (projected onto the transverse lane). Increasing values represent internal rotation. **C,** Scapular posterior tilt angle. The angle between a vector passing through C7 and T7 and a vector passing through the inferior angle and the spine of the scapula (projected onto the sagittal plane). Increasing values represent posterior tilting. *C7,* Seventh cervical process; *T7,* seventh thoracic spinous process. (Adapted from Lukasiewicz AC et al: Comparison of 3-dimensional scapular position and orientation between subjects with and without shoulder impingement, *J Orthop Sports Phys Ther* 29(10):578, 1999.)

around the wall, whereas protraction may proceed in a slightly upward or downward motion, depending on the position of the humerus relative to the scapula (Kibler, 1998a). Depending on the size of the individual and the vigorousness of the activity, the translation of the human scapula during protraction and retraction can occur over distances of 15 to 18 cm (Kibler, 1993).

Elevation/Depression

The scapula can move in the coronal plane along the thoracic wall superiorly and inferiorly in movements typically called *elevation* and *depression,* respectively. Evaluation of the patient with rotator cuff weakness

often identifies excessive early scapular elevation as a compensatory movement to optimize humeral movement (Kibler, 1998a).

CLASSIFICATION OF SCAPULAR DYSFUNCTION

Before discussing specific tests for the scapulothoracic joint, it is appropriate to describe types of scapulothoracic pathology that can be identified by examination maneuvers.

The most widely described and overused term pertaining to scapular pathology is that of *scapular winging.* Scapular winging is used to describe gross dissociation of the scapula from the thoracic wall (Zeier, 1973). It is typically obvious to a trained observer when simply viewing a patient from the posterior and lateral orientation and becomes even more pronounced with active or resistive movements to the upper extremities. True scapular winging occurs secondary to involvement of the long thoracic nerve (Zeier, 1973). Isolated paralysis of the serratus anterior muscle with resultant "winged scapula" was first described by Velpeau in 1837. The cause of winged scapula is peripheral in origin and is ultimately derived from involvement of the fifth, sixth, and seventh spinal cord segments (Zeier, 1973). Isolated serratus anterior muscle weakness as a result of nerve palsy creates a prominent superior medial border of the scapula and depressed acromion, whereas isolated trapezius muscle weakness resulting from nerve palsy creates a protracted inferior border of the scapula and elevated acromion (Kibler, 1998).

Although it is possible that some patients with shoulder pathology may present with true scapular winging, most present with less obvious and less severe forms of scapular dysfunction. Clinicians have traditionally had little nomenclature or objective descriptions for scapular dysfunction, which has led to the use of numerous terms to describe nonoptimal or abnormal scapular positions and movement patterns (Kibler, 1998a).

Kibler Scapular Dysfunction Classification

Rubin and Kibler (2002) classified scapular dysfunction into two main types. When scapular dysfunction occurs proximal and posterior to the glenohumeral joint, the observed scapular dyskinesis is considered proximally derived and has been termed *proximally derived scapular dysfunction* (PDSD). PDSD is commonly associated with postural dysfunction such as forward head posture and lumbopelvic weakness, as well as injury to the long thoracic nerve or spinal accessory nerve, which leads to weakness of the serratus anterior and upper trapezius, respectively. When any of these types of pathology exist or combinations of pathology exist, they lead to a cascade of events that can result in glenohumeral joint dysfunction resulting from PDSD.

The second broad classification proposed by Rubin and Kibler (2002) is *distally derived scapular dysfunction* (DDSD). DDSD occurs from abnormality of the gleno-humeral joint, such as glenoid labrum tears and sub-acromial impingement. These abnormalities result in altered upper extremity movement patterns that lead to scapular muscle compensation and abnormal muscle recruitment and firing patterns. DDSD can be thought of as the result of a "recoil" or "kickback" from the gleno-humeral joint or link in the kinetic chain distal to the scapulothoracic joint. During the comprehensive evalua-tion of the patient with a shoulder injury, it is imperative to evaluate all factors relating to scapular dysfunction, both PDSD and DDSD, not only to identify the presence of scapular dysfunction, but also to better understand the derivation of the scapular dysfunction.

Kibler (1998a) and Kibler et al (2002) developed a more specific scapular classification system for clinical use that allows clinicians to categorize scapular dysfunction based on common clinical findings obtained via visual observation of both static posture and dynamic goal-directed upper extremity movements. Kibler identified three specific scapular dysfunctions or patterns—*inferior* or *type I, medial* or *type II,* and *superior* or *type III*—which are named for the area of the scapula that is visually prominent during clinical evaluation (Table 4-1). In the Kibler classification system, normal symmetric scapular motion characterized by symmetric scapular upward rota-tion "such that the inferior angles translate laterally away from the midline and the scapular medial border remains flush against the thoracic wall with the reverse occurring during arm lowering" (Kibler et al, 2002).

Inferior or Inferior Angle Dysfunction Type I

In this classification of scapular dysfunction, the primary external visual feature is the prominence of the inferior

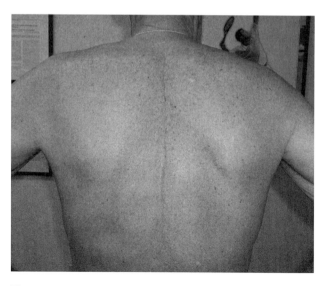

Figure 4-4 Kibler type I: Inferior angle scapular dysfunction. Note the prominence of the inferior angle of the scapula.

angle of the scapula (Figure 4-4). This pattern of dys-function involves anterior tilting of the scapula in the sagittal plane, which produces the prominent inferior angle of the scapula. No other abnormality is typically present with this dysfunction pattern; however, the prominence of the inferior angle of the scapula often increases in the hands-on-hips position, as well as during active goal-directed movements of the upper extremities. According to Kibler et al (2002), inferior angle dysfunc-tion or prominence is most commonly found in patients with rotator cuff dysfunction. The anterior tilting of the scapula places the acromion in a position closer to the rotator cuff and humeral head compromising the sub-acromial space.

Medial or Medial Border Dysfunction Type II

In this classification of scapular dysfunction, the primary external visual feature is the prominence of the entire medial border of the scapula (Figure 4-5). This pattern or

TABLE 4-1   Summary of Kibler Scapular Dysfunction Characteristics

Dysfunction	Primary Visual Feature	Dysfunction Pattern	Dysfunction Plane
Inferior/Inferior Angle Type I	Prominence of inferior angle	Anterior tilting	Sagittal
Medial/Medial Border Type II	Prominence of medial border	Internal rotation	Transverse
Superior Type III	Early, excessive superior elevation of scapula	Scapular elevation	Coronal (frontal)

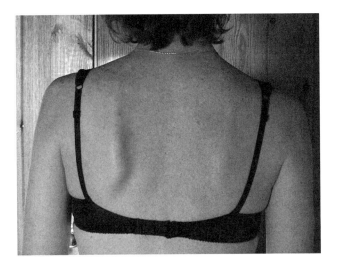

Figure 4-5 Kibler type II: Medial border scapular dysfunction. Note the prominence of the entire medial border of the scapula as opposed to only the inferior angle prominence in Figure 4-4.

dysfunction involves internal rotation of the scapula in the transverse plane. The internal rotation of the scapula produces a prominent medial border of the scapula. Similar to the inferior or inferior angle dysfunction, the medial or medial border dysfunction often increases in the hands-on-hips position, as well as during active goal-directed movements of the upper extremity. According to Kibler et al (2002) and Saha (1983), the medial border scapular dysfunction most often occurs in patients with instability or rotator cuff dysfunction secondary to glenohumeral joint instability. Earlier discussions in this chapter outlined the opening up of the anterior aspect of the glenoid that occurs with scapular antetilting, which is a characteristic of this medial border scapular dysfunction.

Superior Dysfunction Type III

This type of scapular dysfunction is characterized by excessive and early elevation of the scapula during arm elevation (Figure 4-6). This has been referred to as a *shoulder shrug* or "hiking" of the shoulder girdle by clinicians, and is most often present with rotator cuff dysfunction and deltoid-rotator cuff force couple imbalances (Inman, 1944). The superior movement of the scapula is thought to occur as a compensatory movement pattern to aid with arm elevation.

EVALUATION SEQUENCE FOR KIBLER SCAPULAR DYSFUNCTION

The specific sequence recommended for scapular evaluation includes both static and dynamic aspects. Both are crucial for obtaining the clinical cues that allow the

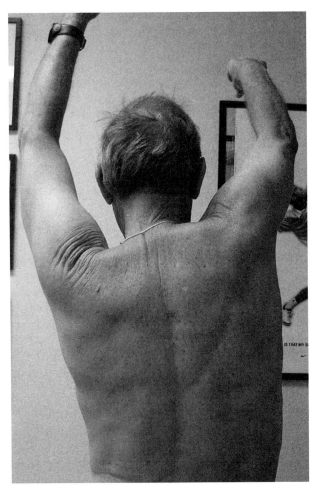

Figure 4-6 Kibler type III: Superior scapular dysfunction. Note the exaggerated superior movement of this patient's right scapula compared with the contralateral extremity with arm elevation.

clinician to determine the often subtle scapular dysfunction present in patients with shoulder pathology.

Static

As mentioned previously, evaluation of the patient occurs in the standing position with arms held comfortably against the sides of the body. The clinician should note the outline of the scapula and compare the scapulae bilaterally. Although many variations exist in standing posture, the clinician should be particularly discriminating when there are bilateral differences in scapular posture and, most notably, when greater prominence of the scapula is present on the involved side. Bilateral symmetry, with respect to scapular position and scapular prominence in the patient with unilateral shoulder dysfunction, is not necessarily an indicator of scapular dysfunction.

After examination of the patient with the arms in complete adduction at the sides of the body, the patient is then examined in the hands-on-hips position. This position creates slight internal rotation and abduction of the glenohumeral joint and often exaggerates the degree of prominence of the scapula (see hands-on-hips position, pages 14–15 for more detailed description).

Dynamic

After the static examination, the patient is asked to elevate the shoulders using a self-selected plane of elevation. The clinician should be directly behind the patient to best observe the movement of the scapula during concentric elevation and especially during eccentric lowering. Excessive superior movement of the scapula during concentric arm elevation, as well as inferior angle and medial border prominence during the eccentric phase are commonly encountered in patients with scapular dysfunction. Repeated arm elevation to confirm initial observations, as well as to determine the presence and location of symptoms (location in/on the shoulder as well as the range of motion where symptoms occur), is recommended. The effect of repeated movements is also crucial to assess the effects of fatigue on scapular stabilization.

TESTS FOR THE SCAPULOTHORACIC JOINT: KIBLER LATERAL SCAPULAR SLIDE TEST (LSST)

Indication

The LSST is the primary clinical test to measure scapular position.

About the Test

The LSST was developed by Kibler as a semidynamic test to evaluate scapular position and scapular stabilizer strength on the injured and noninjured sides, in relationship to a fixed point on the spine, as varying amounts or loads and movement are superimposed on the supporting musculature. The lateral scapular slide test is not a true dynamic test and relies on static positions to assess scapular muscle stabilization (Kibler, 1998a).

Starting Position

The patient is in a resting, standing position, with arms placed comfortably at the sides. The examiner is positioned behind the patient. To enhance the measurement and performance of this test, the patient should be tested without a shirt or undershirt (males) or in a gown (females) that allows for complete visualization of both scapulae and the thoracic spine. The examiner should

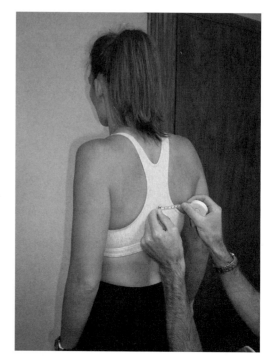

Figure 4-7 Kibler lateral scapular slide position 1.

have a standard tape measure that is capable of measuring in centimeters. The patient is measured in three positions (Figures 4-7 through 4-9):

Kibler Position 1: Standing position, with arms resting at the sides

Kibler Position 2: Hands-on-hips position, with hands placed on the iliac crests, such that the thumbs are pointing backward

Kibler Position 3: Ninety degrees of glenohumeral joint abduction in the coronal plane with full internal rotation

Action

In each of the three positions listed previously, the examiner measures between the inferior angle of each scapula to the corresponding vertebral spinous process. The corresponding vertebral spinous process can be defined as the spinous process in direct line (horizontally) with the inferior angle of the scapula. It should be noted that, in individuals with significant differences in shoulder heights or scoliosis, different vertebral spinous processes may be used for each side as a result of the discrepancy in shoulder/scapular height. The examiner records the distance in centimeters between the vertebral spinous process and the inferior angle of the scapula bilaterally before moving to the next testing position. Testing positions are typically started in Kibler position 1 and progress to Kibler positions 2 and 3.

What Constitutes a Positive Test?

In his original description of the Kibler LSST, Kibler wrote that, even in asymptomatic athletes, the original research with the LSST showed the function of the scapular stabilizing muscles to be symmetric, with less than 1 cm difference between sides in each of the three positions. Symptomatic individuals had differences of greater than 1 cm, and these differences were statistically associated with the presence of pain and decreased shoulder function (Kibler, 1991).

Further research on the LSST by Kibler (1998a) identified the typical range of difference between sides between 0.83 and 1.75 cm. For the purposes of clinical evaluation, Kibler now considers a positive finding with the LSST to be present when greater than a 1.5 cm difference between sides exists at any of the three testing positions. This 1.5 cm difference is the "threshold of abnormality," with differences in long-standing cases of shoulder and scapular pathology having a 2- to 3-cm difference between sides.

Kibler (1998a) also noted that subtle differences found between injured and uninjured sides in the resting positions of testing (Kibler position 1 and 2) may often decrease in Kibler position 3 as a result of the contraction of the musculature in patients exhibiting some degree of scapular muscle stabilization. This factor is important to analyze with this test in addition to determining whether the patient merely exceeds or does not exceed the 1.5 cm bilateral difference "threshold of abnormality."

Ramifications of a Positive Test

Patients with a positive Kibler LSST (bilateral difference of greater than 1.5 cm) have deficits in either dynamic scapular stabilization or have postural adaptations that produce significant differences in scapular positioning identified with this test. These patients are candidates for rehabilitative exercise to promote scapular stabilization.

Objective Evidence Regarding This Test

Electromyographic evaluation of the three positions used in the Kibler LSST shows that few muscles are working in Kibler position 1. The serratus anterior and lower trapezius muscles are working at low levels in position 2, and in Kibler position 3, the upper and lower trapezius, rhomboids, and serratus anterior are all working at about 40% of maximal levels.

The ability of the examiner to accurately reproduce and identify the inferior angle of the scapula has been tested

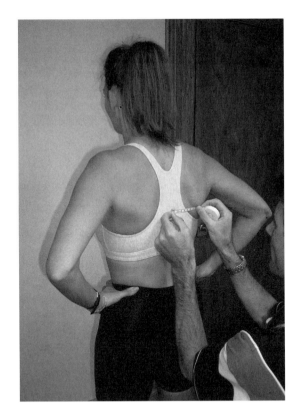

Figure 4-8 Kibler lateral scapular slide position 2.

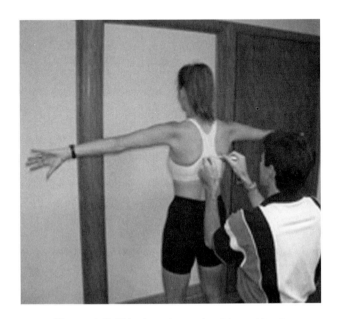

Figure 4-9 Kibler lateral scapular slide position 3.

using radiography. When the accuracy of marking the inferior angle of the scapula was compared with a radiographic evaluation of the same point when marked using a lead shot or "BB," there was a correlation of 0.91 with the three different positions (Kibler, 1998a). This finding confirms that the position selected by the examiner is likely closely associated with the actual inferior angle of the scapula during testing.

Test-Retest Reliability

Kibler (1998) performed a test-retest reliability investigation to assess both intratester and intertester reliability. Intraclass correlation coefficients (ICC) were between 0.84 and 0.88 for intratester reliability, with similar coefficients reported in all three positions of testing. Intertester reliability coefficients ranged from 0.77 to 0.85. These reliability coefficients indicate acceptable levels of reproducibility for the use of this clinical test (Portney & Watkins, 1993).

Additional studies have independently evaluated the Kibler LSST. Gibson et al (1995) reported intratester reliability of 0.81 to 0.94 and intertester reliability of 0.18 to 0.92. T'Jonck et al (1996) reported similar ICCs for intratester reliability (0.69 to 0.96) and ICCs for intertester reliability ranging between 0.72 and 0.90. In addition to the reliability coefficients reported, Gibson et al (1995) and T'Jonck et al (1996) identified lower intratester and intertester correlation coefficients with Kibler position 3. All of the researchers acknowledge the increased difficulty in palpating the inferior angle of the scapula in position 3 because of the greater contraction of the muscles surrounding the scapula itself (Kibler, 1998a; Gibson et al, 1995; T'Jonck et al, 1996).

Odem et al (2001) published a test-retest reliability study that conflicted with earlier studies of the Kibler LSST. The reliability research by Kibler (1998a), Gibson et al (1995), and T'Jonck et al (1996) all tested the distances between the inferior angle of the scapula and the vertebral spinous process. Odem et al (2001) tested the actual bilateral difference in subjects and found lower test-retest reliability coefficients ranging from 0.52 to 0.80 for intratester conditions and 0.43 to 0.79 for intertester conditions. They concluded that the Kibler test had compromised reliability and that caution should be used in interpretation of test results. This information is in contrast to the other reliability studies on the LSST.

Validity of the Kibler Lateral Scapular Slide Test

Litchfield et al (1998) tested 40 subjects, 20 of whom were diagnosed with unilateral glenohumeral joint impingement symptoms, using the Kibler LSST positions 1 and 2.

Significant differences in scapular symmetry were found between the subjects diagnosed with unilateral glenohumeral joint impingement and normal subjects for Kibler position 1. No difference was identified between groups in Kibler position 2. The authors concluded that the Kibler LSST is a valid test to identify patients with unilateral glenohumeral joint impingement.

Odem et al (2001) used a similar testing paradigm to determine the sensitivity and specificity based on the criterion of 1.5 cm bilateral difference in normal subjects and in patients diagnosed with shoulder impairments. The authors reported sensitivity values of 28%, 53%, and 50% at Kibler positions 1, 2, and 3, respectively, with specificity of 58%, 34%, and 52%, respectively at the three positions. In contrast to the findings of Litchfield et al (1998), Odem et al suggested the LSST should not be used to identify persons with shoulder pathology. Koslow et al (2003) measured the specificity of the LSST in asymptomatic competitive athletes. In all, 38 females and 33 male athletes were tested using the Kibler LSST. These athletes were involved in what the author classified as "one-arm dominant" sports: baseball, softball, tennis, volleyball, and basketball. A total of 51 of the 71 subjects displayed a difference of at least 1.5 cm or more in one of the three Kibler testing positions. Overall specificity of the test was 26.8%, and the authors concluded that scapular posture was extremely variable in this athletic asymmetric testing population. Specificity at each of the three Kibler testing positions was reported as 54.9%, 57.7%, and 35.2% for positions 1, 2, and 3, respectively. The authors concluded that these asymmetries do not necessarily identify or indicate dysfunction (Koslow et al, 2003). The low specificity of the LSST in this population led to the authors' recommendation not to use the LSST to determine shoulder dysfunction in one-arm dominant athletes. This finding agrees with the variable posture characteristics outlined in Chapter 3. Further, it supports the use of a complete evaluation of the scapulothoracic joint, coupled with a general posture evaluation and specific glenohumeral special tests, to more accurately identify shoulder pathology.

The presence of multiple classifications and types of scapular pathology identified by Kibler et al (2002) complicates the identification of individuals with scapular pathology with one test. Odem et al (2001) showed that although scapular pathology likely exists in their sample of patients with shoulder impairment, the Kibler LSST was not able to accurately identify those individuals based solely on scapular position. Alterations in the distance between the vertebral spinous process and the inferior angle of the scapula may be minimal in patients with internal rotation of the scapula (medial border prominence Kibler type II) or anterior tilting of the scapula (inferior angle prominence Kibler type I). Relying solely on the results from the Kibler LSST to identify scapular pathology is not recommended, and the results of Odem et al (2001), Koslow et al (2003), and Kibler (2002) supported the use of a complete scapular evaluation in addition to a glenohumeral and upper body musculoskeletal evaluation for patients with shoulder pathology.

ADDITIONAL TESTS TO ASSESS SCAPULAR POSITION

Lennie Test

Additional tests have been reported to assess static scapular position. A detailed scapular evaluation test called the *Lennie test* was published by Sobush et al (1996). This test consists of an extensive series of measurements of the scapula in standing, using a scoliometer and caliper. The examiner palpates and marks 12 landmarks along the medial aspect of the scapula and spinal midline, with the patient in the standing position with back exposed. The examiner then uses a caliper to measure the distance between the spinal midline and the scapular landmarks.

Sobush et al (1996) tested the reliability and validity of the Lennie test using three examiners and the scoliometer and caliper. Same-day radiographs were used to validate the scapular position identified using surface measurements. Results of the research by Sobush et al (1996) confirmed that the medial borders of the scapulae were parallel to the midline of the thoracic spine. The scapulae were, on average, 17.19 cm apart in the resting position at the level of the root of the scapular spine. The dominant scapula was 0.49 cm lower than the nondominant scapula in this population of normal healthy female subjects. ICCs for the surface measurements of scapular position ranged between 0.64 and 0.86. The authors concluded that the Lennie test can provide an accurate and reliable measurement of scapular position.

DiVeta Test

DiVeta et al (1990) described another test involving fewer measurements than those used for the Lennie test to estimate scapular position. The technique involves measuring the distance between the vertebral spinous process of the third thoracic vertebrae and the posterolateral corner of the acromion. The posterolateral corner of the acromion was referred to as the *inferior angle of the acromion* in their initial research. The linear distance (Figure 4-10) between the third thoracic vertebral spinous process and the posterolateral corner of the acromion was used to measure the amount of scapular abduction. To account for different

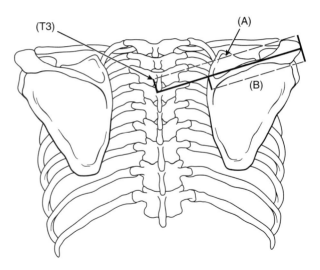

Figure **4-10** DiVeta scapular measurement technique. Measurement of scapular abduction was attained by measuring the distance A, from the spinous process of the third thoracic vertebrae (T3) to the inferior angle of the acromion. B, This measurement was normalized to scapular length, which was defined as the distance from the root of the spine of the scapula to the inferior angle of the acromion. (Adapted from DiVeta J, Walker ML, Skibinski B: Relationship between performance of selected scapular muscles and scapular abduction in standing subjects, *Phys Ther* 70(8):472, 1990.)

sizes of scapulae and to present the data from their scapular abduction measurement in a normalized format, DiVeta et al (1990) also measured the width of the scapula from the base or root of the spine of the scapula at the medial border to the posterolateral corner of the acromion (see Figure 4-10). This value was then divided into the initial measure from the T3 spinous process to the posterolateral corner of the acromion:

$$\frac{\text{Distance T3 thoracic vertebral spinous process to posterior lateral corner of the acromion}}{\text{Distance root of scapular spine to posterolateral measurement corner of the acromion}} = \text{DiVeta scapular abduction}$$

The unit of measure for the DiVeta test is centimeters. The authors believed that this test had greater relevance than other clinical measures of scapular position, as it was normalized to patient scapular size. For this reason their research used a scapular abduction measurement that was normalized to scapular length. An additional benefit of this technique is the use of the posterolateral corner of the acromion as a scapular landmark, instead of the inferior angle of the acromion. The posterolateral corner of the acromion is pointed and typically prominent, except in the most obese individuals.

The intrarater test-retest reliability for the measurement technique described by DiVeta et al (1990) was assessed using ICCs. The ICCs were 0.86 for scapular length and 0.94 for scapular distance from midline. Based on results, this test can be used in a reliable clinical format with a tape measure to quickly assess scapular position. Further research regarding bilateral symmetry and normalized scapular abduction ratios in different populations of athletes and in normal individuals is needed to assist in the application of this test in clinical formats.

Posterior Scapular Displacement Test—The Perry Tool Test

Although the tests reported by Kibler (1998a), Sobush et al (1996), and DiVeta et al (1990) all measure the position of the scapula relative to the midline of the body, they do not assess the degree of posterior scapular displacement such as those reported in both the Kibler scapular dysfunction classification (2002, 2003) and the description of true scapular winging (Zeier, 1973). Plafcan et al (1997) developed an instrument called the *Perry tool,* which was used to quantify posterior scapular displacement in normal subjects in both weighted and unweighted upper extremity conditions.

The tool, which consists of a T-shaped frame and measurement scales, was placed on the subject's back over the "most distal aspect palpable on the medial border," often near the inferior angle of the scapula (Plafcan et al, 1997). This allowed the examiner to quantify the amount of posterior scapular displacement near the inferior angle of the scapula. ICCs ranged between 0.97 and 0.98 for intrarater reliability and between 0.92 and 0.97 for interrater reliability. The test provides reliable measurements but requires a specialized measurement device.

Warner et al (1992) described another method to quantify scapular position—specifically the amount of posterior scapular displacement. Moire topographic analysis, which relies on stroboscopic evaluation of the exact contours of the scapula and spine, was used to measure the scapular contours in normal subjects, subjects diagnosed with unilateral glenohumeral joint impingement, and subjects with unilateral glenohumeral joint instability. Significant bilateral differences in scapular positioning were noted in the subjects with both glenohumeral impingement and instability. The technique of measurement used by the authors, however, is not available in most clinical centers. No other methods for clinically applicable measurement of scapular tipping or posterior scapular displacement have been reported.

Kibler Scapular Assistance Test

Indication

The Kibler scapular assistance test is used to determine the effects of scapular dysfunction on active shoulder range of motion and glenohumeral joint impingement.

About the Test

This test assesses the effect of superimposing increased scapular upward rotation during arm elevation on both active range of motion and pain diminution. As the name implies, during this test the examiner assists the scapula in the movement pattern of upward rotation during arm elevation. This test simulates the function of the serratus anterior and lower trapezius force couple during elevation (Kibler, 1998a, 1998b).

Start Position

The examiner stands behind the patient. The patient starts from a resting posture, with arms comfortably at the side.

Action

The patient is asked to actively elevate the involved shoulder and is instructed to inform the examiner at what point in the range of motion pain occurs. The examiner closely monitors both the quality of the active range of motion and the actual amount of excursion of active elevation. The examiner should note at what point in the range of motion pain occurs. The patient then is asked to lower the involved extremity to the resting position.

The examiner then places the left hand (if examining a right scapula/shoulder) along the superior border of the scapula while placing the thumb of the examiner's right hand (if examining a right scapula/shoulder) along the medial border of the patient's scapula, near the inferior third of the scapula (Figure 4-11). The patient is again asked to elevate the involved shoulder (Figure 4-12). While the patient elevates the involved shoulder, the examiner assists the scapula by upwardly rotating it as the patient continues toward the end range of elevation. The patient then lowers the involved extremity to the resting position at the side.

What Constitutes a Positive Test?

Two clinical findings indicate a positive Kibler scapular assistance test. This first is with respect to pain diminution or alleviation of pain. If the patient reported pain

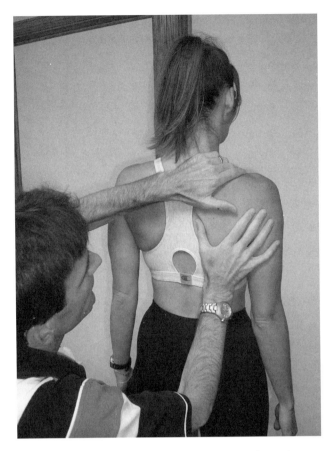

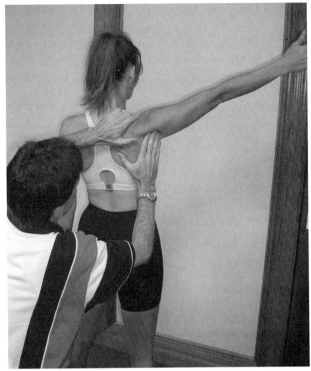

Figure **4-12** Wide-angle photo of the Kibler scapular assistance test.

Figure **4-11** Close-up photo of the Kibler scapular assistance test.

during the initial independent arm elevation, the superimposed upward rotation performed by the examiner during the scapular assistance test often alleviates the pain because of a more optimal scapular component to arm elevation. Increased active range of motion with scapular upward rotation is the second component that renders the scapular assistance maneuver positive. Patients often have greater active range of motion and greater ease of elevation when scapular upward rotation is superimposed by the examiner. "Impingement symptoms are diminished or abolished in cases of muscle inhibition" (Kibler, 1998a, 1998b).

Ramification of a Positive Test

One advantage of a clinical test like the scapular assistance test is that it directs the examiner to a treatment plan or intervention. With a positive Kibler scapular assistance test, the implied ramification is the important component scapular upward rotation plays in the improvement of either active range of motion, or diminution of pain with

active elevation. Superimposing scapular upward rotation raises the overlying acromion from the path of the elevating humerus (Kibler, 1991, 1998a, 1998b). This superimposition by the examiner removes the acromion and may be the mechanism by which pain is diminished.

Upward rotation of the scapula also improves the length-tension relationship of the muscular force couples that control glenohumeral and scapulothoracic movement, and may consequently improve the arc and quality of the active range of motion against gravity (Kibler, 1998). Patients presenting with a positive Kibler scapular assistance test are candidates for scapular strengthening and stabilization programs in rehabilitation (Kibler, 1998a).

Kibler Scapular Retraction Test

Indication

The Kibler scapular retraction test is used to determine the effect of a more retracted scapula on rotator cuff strength indirectly assessed through changes in shoulder elevation and reduction of symptoms with arm movement.

About the Test

This test involves the use of manually imposed scapular retraction by the examiner. This position "confers a stable base of origin for the rotator cuff" and often improves clinical signs and symptoms. The manual support provided by the examiner mimics the function of the stabilizing perimusculature and can help determine the effect of improved scapular positioning on shoulder range of motion and patient self-reported pain levels.

Start Position

The patient is typically examined in a standing position, with the examiner positioned directly behind the patient. The patient is asked to actively elevate the arm in the scapular plane against gravity or externally rotate the shoulder from the neutral position with 90 degrees of glenohumeral abduction in either the scapular or coronal plane (Kibler & McMullen, 2003). The examiner notes the amount and quality of the self-directed shoulder motion, specifically where pain is encountered in the range of motion.

Action

The examiner then stabilizes the medial border of the scapula (Figure 4-13) using both hands along the medial border to maintain a greater amount of scapular retraction during arm movement. The patient is again asked to elevate the shoulder in the scapular plane or externally rotate the shoulder from neutral with 90 degrees of abduction. The examiner notes the amount and quality of motion and asks the patient whether pain is present.

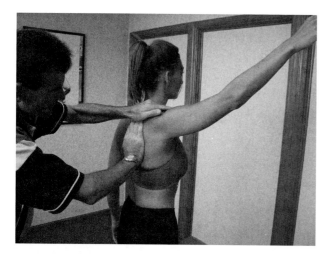

Figure 4-13 Kibler scapular retraction test.

What Constitutes a Positive Test?

A positive scapular retraction test occurs when either an increase in active range of motion in the patient's involved shoulder occurs during manually imposed scapular retraction or pain is abated or disappears. Use of the pretest active motion serves as a benchmark or baseline to which range of motion and pain levels are compared against during manual stabilization.

Ramifications of a Positive Test

Similar to the ramifications of a positive scapular assistance test, a positive scapular retraction test implies that inadequate scapular stabilization, in this case scapular retraction, is present, so that abnormal scapulohumeral biomechanics produce an effect on the patient's shoulder movement and pain presentation. A positive finding directs the clinician to perform interventions to enhance scapular stabilization and to focus particularly on scapular retraction, the major superimposed manual correction applied during this testing maneuver. Kibler reported improvement in symptoms and arm movement in patients with internal impingement as the manually applied retraction removes the posterior glenoid impingement from the excessively protracted impingement position during testing (Kibler & McMahon, 2003).

Scapulothoracic "Conductor's" Test

Indication

The scapulothoracic "conductor's" test is a simple maneuver to monitor the relative movement of bilateral upper extremities to movement of the scapulothoracic articulation.

About the Test

Based on the scapulohumeral rhythm and, most specifically, research by Bagg and Forrest (1988) and Doody et al (1970), who have reported movement ratios just under 1:1 in the movement arc between 80 and 120 degrees, this test merely compares upward rotation movement of both scapulae during elevation of the glenohumeral joint in the scapular plane.

Start Position

The examiner stands directly in front of the patient, who is examined in a standing position. The patient actively elevates the arms in the scapular plane to approximately 70 to 80 degrees. The examiner reaches under the arms of the patient to palpate the lateral border of the scapula near the lower third of the scapulae bilaterally.

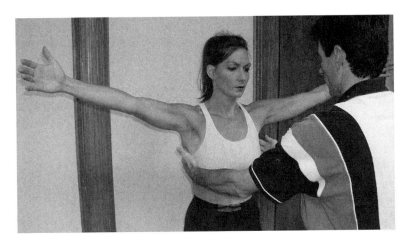

Figure **4-14** Scapular conductor's test.

Action

The patient is instructed to actively elevate both extremities between approximately 80 and 150 degrees in the scapular plane repeatedly while the examiner palpates the motion of the scapula, making a visual note of the movement of the extremities (Figure 4-14). The repeated waving of the arms is similar to that of a conductor of an orchestra, for which this maneuver is named.

What Constitutes a Positive Test?

There is technically no positive or negative aspect to this maneuver; it simply provides the clinician with an estimate of how well the patient's scapulothoracic joints are moving relative to humeral elevation. According to research outlined earlier, the arc of 80 to 120 degrees of scapular plane elevation should produce close to a 1:1 pattern of scapulothoracic and glenohumeral joint motion. This is easily palpated and assessed using this maneuver.

Patients with capsular hypomobility, such as those diagnosed with adhesive capsulitis, demonstrate early and excessive scapular motion relative to the movement of the humerus, whereas other patients may exhibit unilateral humeral motion without concomitant upward rotation of the scapula. Patients with glenohumeral joint instability and impingement often have abnormal scapular upward rotation because of abnormal muscular recruitment patterns (McMahon et al, 1996).

Ramifications of a Positive Test

Unilateral abnormalities in this maneuver direct the clinician to focus on treatment strategies that promote more optimal dynamic stabilization and movement of the scapulothoracic joint. In the case of the patient with exaggerated scapular motion resulting from restricted glenohumeral joint motion, this test directs the clinician to strategies to enhance capsular mobility and improve glenohumeral joint motion.

Flip Sign

Indication

The flip sign is a test or sign noted during manual muscle testing of the glenohumeral joint to indicate scapulothoracic stabilization.

About the Test

This test or sign identifies the position of the scapula during routine manual muscle testing of the infraspinatus (external rotation), which is performed during clinical evaluation of the patient with shoulder dysfunction.

Starting Position

The position of manual muscle testing, as recommended by Kelly et al (1996) for the infraspinatus, is used. This test position is described on page 133 and consists of testing the patient with the arm at the side and in a position of 45 degrees of internal rotation.

Action

During traditional manual muscle testing, the examiner is positioned so that the medial border of the scapula is visible during testing. Standard manual muscle testing overpressure is exerted on the distal aspect of the forearm while the scapula is observed and the performance of the infraspinatus muscle is graded.

What Constitutes a Positive Test?

A positive flip sign occurs when the medial border of the scapula protrudes away from the thoracic spine during the overpressure phase of the manual muscle test (Figure 4-15). The extent of the movement away from the thorax is noted and compared with the condition of the scapula on the contralateral side.

Ramifications of a Positive Test

A positive flip sign indicates that the patient is unable to stabilize the scapula during a resisted movement requiring rotator cuff activation. This sign alerts the clinician to a deficiency in the stabilization of the scapula and directs him or her to further test the scapulothoracic joint, as well as integrate treatment strategies to improve the strength and muscular endurance of the scapular musculature.

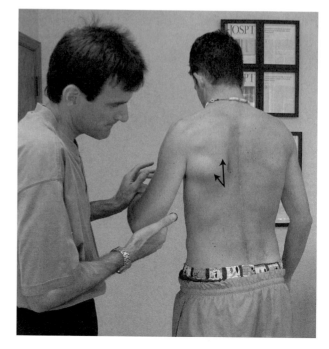

Figure **4-15** Scapular flip sign.

Related Referral Joint Testing

INTRODUCTION

Before the clinician can ultimately focus on a particular joint or complex, the joints and adjoining segments, both proximal and distal to the area being examined, must be cleared to rule out the referral of symptoms from those joints. This chapter describes the important steps that should be taken before evaluating the shoulder joint to ensure that adjoining segments are not involved in the patient's symptom presentation and to rule out pathology in the adjoining structures.

GENERAL SCREENING

In addition to the musculoskeletal screening process, which includes testing the joint or joints below the injured area and the joint or joints proximal to the injured area, general screening to rule out or screen the patient for nonmusculoskeletal causes of shoulder-specific pain syndromes is a crucial part of the comprehensive examination process. This process, termed *differential diagnosis,* can be difficult in the patient with shoulder pain, because pain that is felt in the shoulder often affects the joint as though the pain were originating in the joint (Mennell, 1964).

Figure 5-1 outlines the musculoskeletal and systemic structures that can refer pain to the shoulder. A brief overview of some specific referral patterns for the shoulder and scapula is provided in this chapter; for a more complete overview, the reader is referred to Boissonnault (1995) and Goodman and Snyder (2000).

The use of an extensive medical history and screening process is important for all patients. The patient presenting with shoulder pain is no exception. Many visceral diseases are known to appear as unilateral shoulder pain. Esophageal, pericardial, or myocardial diseases, as well as diaphragmatic irritation from thoracic or abdominal disease, can all appear as unilateral shoulder pain (Goodman & Snyder, 2000).

Another common referral of shoulder pain occurs after acute injury to the spleen. The typical history and symptoms inherent in a splenic rupture include a history of abdominal trauma, abdominal rigidity, nausea and

vomiting, and reflex pain called *Kehr's sign,* which radiates to the left shoulder and approximately one third of the arm (Klafs & Arnheim, 1981). This pattern of pain radiation is particularly applicable during the evaluation of an athlete involved in a contact sport who presents with left shoulder pain after a traumatic event or contact with either the ground or another player/participant.

Careful questioning regarding the aggravation of symptoms can help to differentiate the common clusters typical in musculoskeletal shoulder pain from visceral causes. One example is shoulder pain caused by pleural irritation. Pleural irritation and other pulmonary diseases create sharp localized pain in the shoulder. Aggravating factors of pleural irritation include respiratory movements that typically do not affect most musculoskeletal shoulder conditions, as well as alleviation of symptoms by lying on the involved shoulder (Goodman & Snyder, 2000). Most musculoskeletal shoulder conditions are aggravated by lying on the involved shoulder. This occurrence is normally attributed to compression, and placement of the scapula in a protracted position, which narrows the subacromial space, can exacerbate many shoulder conditions (Solem-Bertoft et al, 1993). Box 5-1 and Table 5-1 outline the additional systemic causes of shoulder pain. Table 5-2 lists the systemic origin of thoracic and scapular pain based on the specific location of symptoms.

Specific screening for rheumatic disease is also important when performing a comprehensive examination of the patient with shoulder pain. The most fundamental aid to recognizing rheumatic disease in people presenting with shoulder pain is a search for systemic components (Caldron, 1995). Systemic components include new-onset fatigue, fever, weight change, and mucocutaneous signs such as rash, mouth sores, hair loss, skin thickening or tightening, or nodules (Caldron, 1995). Although many systemic symptoms occur with rheumatic diseases, the clustering of these symptoms along with joint pain should lead the clinician to suspect rheumatic disorders, and referral should be made to the appropriate source for further testing. The distinction between inflammatory

Box 5-1   Systemic Causes of Shoulder Pain

Shoulder pain may be referred from the neck, chest (thorax or thoracic spine), and abdomen and from systemic disease. The following have been diagnosed as having the onset or origin of presenting symptoms in the shoulder.

Neck
- Bone tumors
- Metastases
- Tuberculosis
- Nodes in the neck (from metastases, leukemia, and Hodgkin's disease)
- Cervical cord tumors

Chest
- Angina/myocardial infarct
- Postcoronary artery bypass graft
- Bacterial endocarditis
- Pericarditis
- Aortic aneurysm
- Empyema and lung abscess
- Pulmonary tuberculosis
- Pancoast's tumor
- Lung cancer (bronchogenic carcinoma)
- Spontaneous pneumothorax
- Nodes in mediastinum/axilla
- Metastases in thoracic spine
- Breast disease:
  - Primary or secondary cancer
  - Mastodynia
- Hiatal hernia

Abdomen
- Liver disease
- Ruptured spleen
- Spinal metastases
- Dissecting aortic aneurysm
- Diaphragmatic irritation:
  - Peptic ulcer
  - Gallbladder disease
  - Subphrenic abscess
  - Hiatal hernia
  - Pyelonephritis
  - Diaphragmatic hernia
  - Ectopic pregnancy (rupture)
- Upper urinary tract infection

Systemic Disease
- Collagen vascular disease
- Gout
- Syphilis/gonorrhea
- Sickle cell anemia
- Hemophilia
- Rheumatic disease
- Metastatic cancer:
  - Breast
  - Prostate
  - Kidney
  - Lung
  - Thyroid
  - Testicle
- Diabetes mellitus (adhesive capsulitis)

Modified from Zohn DA: *Musculoskeletal pain: diagnosis and physical treatment*, ed 2, Boston, 1998, Little Brown.

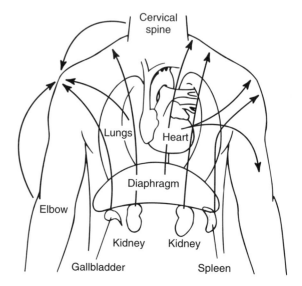

Figure 5-1 Musculoskeletal and systemic structures referring pain to the shoulder. (Adapted from Goodman CC, Snyder TE: *Differential diagnosis in physical therapy*, ed 3, Philadelphia, 2000, WB Saunders, p. 485.)

and degenerative arthritic conditions is rarely difficult to make if the examiner focuses on the historical information listed previously and notes the typical distribution of involved joints (Caldron, 1995).

Finally, one additional area to be discussed in this section is the presence and screening for nonorganic signs. Waddell et al (1980) described five nonorganic signs, each identifiable with one or two simple testing maneuvers that assess a patient's pain behavior. A patient with three or more of the five nonorganic signs is believed to have a clinical pattern of nonmechanical, pain-focused behavior (Waddell et al, 1980; Goodman & Snyder, 2000). Examples of Waddell's signs include deep tenderness felt over a wide nonspecific pattern rather than isolated to a particular region or structure, and diminished sensation following a "stocking-type" pattern rather than dermatomal patterns. Overreaction or disproportionate verbalization, facial expression, or muscle tension during examination maneuvers should also alert the examiner to the presence of nonorganic sources of the patient's pain.

CERVICAL SPINE CLEARING TESTS

The cervical spine can be the source of pain in patients presenting with primary complaints of shoulder and arm pain and disability. Use of the overpressure and Spurling's tests provide valuable insight into the condition of the cervical spine and its related structures (Grimsby & Gray, 1997). Cervical spine overpressure tests are completed

TABLE 5-1   Shoulder Pain

RIGHT SHOULDER		LEFT SHOULDER	
SYSTEMIC ORIGIN	LOCATION	SYSTEMIC ORIGIN	LOCATION
Peptic ulcer	Lateral border, right scapula	Ruptured spleen	Left shoulder (Kehr's sign)
Myocardial ischemia	Right shoulder, down arm	Myocardial ischemia	Left pectoral/left shoulder
Hepatic/biliary:		Pancreas	Left shoulder
Acute cholecystitis	Right shoulder; between scapulae; right subscapular area	Ectopic pregnancy (rupture)	Left shoulder (Kehr's sign)
Liver abscess	Right shoulder		
Gallbladder	Right upper trapezius		
Liver disease (hepatitis, cirrhosis, metastatic tumors)	Right shoulder, right subscapula		
Pulmonary:	Ipsilateral shoulder; upper trapezius	Pulmonary:	Ipsilateral shoulder; upper trapezius
Pleurisy		Pleurisy	
Pneumothorax		Pneumothorax	
Pancoast's tumor		Pancoast's tumor	
Kidney	Ipsilateral shoulder	Kidney	Ipsilateral shoulder
		Postoperative laparoscopy	Left shoulder (Kehr's sign)

From Goodman C, Snyder T: *Differential diagnosis in physical therapy*, ed 3, Philadelphia, 2000, WB Saunders.

after the patient has moved the cervical spine via the cardinal movements of flexion, extension, lateral flexion, and rotation. In the event that active range of motion of the aforementioned movements is within normal limits and does not elicit or reproduce symptoms, passive overpressure is applied at the end of each range of motion. Although the presence of any symptom with these movements and overpressures is important, the reproduction of the patient's symptoms in the shoulder or scapular region is of particular concern because this will ultimately lead the clinician to suspect that the patient's symptoms arise from the cervical spine. Isometrically applied resistance in mid-ranges of cervical spine motion can be applied to stress the contractile elements, with end-range overpressure exerted to stress the noncontractile elements (Davies et al, 1981).

SPURLING'S MANEUVER

Another test recommended for cervical spine clearing is Spurling's test, which is comprised of cervical spine extension with ipsilateral lateral flexion and rotation (Grimsby & Gray, 1997). The position (Figure 5-2) stresses the intervertebral foramen and applies a compressive stress and strain to the facet joints of the cervical spine (Grimsby & Gray, 1997). The patient's shoulder or arm pain may be reproduced from the intervertebral disk via posterolateral compression and an inflamed nerve root, or facet joint. A slight overpressure can be applied as shown in the figure, with stabilization of the contralateral shoul-der to prevent compensatory shoulder girdle elevation. I perform the Spurling's maneuver to both sides to thoroughly stress the cervical structures. Local cervical spine discomfort is often noted, particularly in older patients with glenohumeral joint dysfunction; however, the most significant indication of this test occurs when a patient's shoulder or arm symptoms are reproduced. Ramifications of a positive cervical spine clearing test are for the completion of a more detailed and directed cervical spine examination, because these tests may indicate that the source of the patient's shoulder complaint is centrally derived.

STERNOCLAVICULAR JOINT

Evaluation of the sternoclavicular (SC) joint is an important part of the clearing process in the comprehensive examination of the patient with shoulder dysfunction. This joint undergoes 30 degrees of axial rotation during humeral elevation and receives stabilization from the bony configuration of the joint, as well as both intrinsic and extrinsic ligamentous structures (Kapandji, 1985). Davies et al (1981) recommended clearing the SC joint via active and passive movements of the shoulder girdle. Bilateral comparison of the movement of the SC joint during shoulder girdle elevation/depression, protraction/retraction, and circumduction is recommended. Palpation of the SC joint during these motions can reveal crepitace and grating, as well as either hypermobility or restricted motion. Anterior or posterior subluxation is often noted

TABLE 5-2   Location of Systemic Thoracic/Scapular Pain

SYSTEMIC ORIGIN	LOCATION
CARDIAC	
Myocardial infarct	Midthoracic spine
PULMONARY	
Basilar pneumonia	Right upper back
Empyema	Scapula
Pleurisy	Scapula
Pneumothorax	Ipsilateral scapula
RENAL	
Acute pyelonephritis	Costovertebral angle (posteriorly)
GASTROINTESTINAL	
Esophagitis	Mid-back between scapulae
Peptic ulcer: stomach/ duodenal	Sixth through tenth thoracic vertebrae
Gallbladder disease	Mid-back between scapulae; right upper scapula or subscapular area
Biliary colic	Right upper back; mid-back between scapulae; right interscapular or subscapular areas
Pancreatic carcinoma	Midthoracic or lumbar spine
OTHER	
Acromegaly	Midthoracic or lumbar spine

Adapted from Goodman CC, Snyder TE: *Differential diagnosis in physical therapy*, ed 3, Philadelphia, 2000, WB Saunders, p. 487.

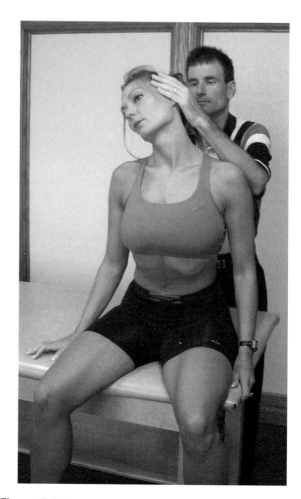

Figure 5-2 Spurling's maneuver, consisting of passive extension, ipsilateral lateral flexion, and rotation of the cervical spine.

via either a prominent proximal clavicle or a sulcus, respectively, as compared with the contralateral uninvolved side. Passive mobility testing of the SC can be difficult and uncomfortable for the patient because of the difficulty in grasping the clavicle itself. Bilateral comparison of anterior posterior glide and superior inferior glide can also assist the clinician in identifying either hypermobility or hypomobility of this joint. Research on the reliability of accessory mobility assessment of this joint is not available. Davies et al (1981) reported that, in cases of anterior SC joint subluxation, a posterior relocation force can be maintained during reexamination of active or passive movements. An assessment of that relocation force's effect on the patient's symptoms has diagnostic implications.

ACROMIOCLAVICULAR JOINT

The joint immediately proximal to the glenohumeral joint is the acromioclavicular (AC) joint. This joint can be a source of shoulder pain secondary to injury or separation, which jeopardizes the intrinsic or extrinsic ligamentous structures that stabilize the joint. Hypermobility of the AC joint can lead to osteophyte production and hypertrophic bone formation, which can encroach on the rotator cuff during arm elevation, leading to primary glenohumeral joint impingement (Neer, 1983). Evaluation of the AC joint consists of initially evaluating the external appearance of the joint and comparing it with the contralateral uninjured side. The external appearance of a unilateral step-down or piano-key sign, where the distal clavicle is higher than the acromion, can indicate a past history of injury to the AC joint (Figure 5-3). In addition to visual inspection and palpation of the AC joint itself, three special examination maneuvers can be used to clear the AC joint. One of these maneuvers is recommended as a clearing test (AC joint passive mobility test, also called the *AC joint shear test*), and the other two (cross-arm adduction impingement test and O'Brien's test) are

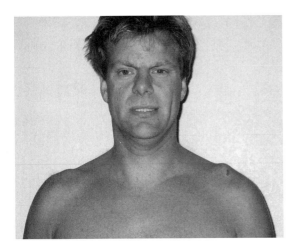

Figure **5-3** Patient with typical step-down sign on the left shoulder from complete acromioclavicular joint separation.

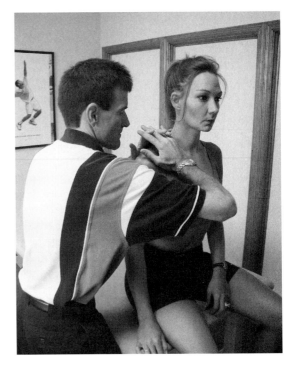

Figure **5-4** Acromioclavicular joint shearing test; lateral view.

component parts of the examination of other structures of the glenohumeral joint complex.

ACROMIOCLAVICULAR JOINT PASSIVE MOBILITY TEST (AC JOINT SHEAR TEST)

The AC joint passive mobility or shear test can be used to provoke the AC joint by producing a shear force across the joint. The AC joint passive mobility test can also be used to compare the actual motion of the AC joint with the contralateral extremity to determine whether movement of that joint reproduces the patient's pain. One significant advantage to this test maneuver is that actual hand contacts are not placed close to the AC joint itself. Unlike other AC joint direct examination techniques, this technique produces movement of the clavicle and scapula using proximal hand placements, thereby reducing the chance of producing pain simply by palpating and attempting to grasp the clavicle and acromion near the AC joint.

This test is performed with the patient in either the seated or standing position. The patient's arm is positioned at the side or in the lap if seated. The examiner stands on the same side of the patient's shoulder being examined. Using clasped hands (Figure 5-4), the heels of the hands are located near the midpoint of the clavicle anteriorly and on the spine of the scapula posteriorly. With a compressing-type action, the anterior hand presses posteriorly on the clavicle, while the posteriorly placed hand presses anteriorly on the spine of the scapula in an oscillating-type pattern. Several oscillations of movement are performed, with particular attention paid to both the amount and quality of the motion with bilateral comparison carried out. Reproduction of pain is also an important factor in this test. The

test is considered positive when the patient's superiorly directed pain is reproduced unilaterally with the shearing movement. Normal responses to this test are for bilaterally symmetric anterior posterior shear motions of the AC joint without symptoms.

CROSS-ARM ADDUCTION IMPINGEMENT TEST

This examination maneuver is discussed in detail with the other impingement tests (see page 92). The reproduction of superior shoulder discomfort over the AC joint with the cross-arm adduction test is thought to indicate AC joint pathology as a result of compression of the distal clavicle toward the acromion.

O'BRIEN'S TEST (ACTIVE COMPRESSION TEST)

This test is described in detail in the labral testing section of this text. The O'Brien's test can be used to identify both AC joint pathology and superior labral pathology. A positive O'Brien's test, with specific pain being reproduced and identified, indicates AC joint pathology.

ELBOW JOINT

Additional clearing of the extremity is indicated for the patient with shoulder dysfunction, including the joint distal to the shoulder complex. Radiation of symptoms distally often produces complex pain patterning in the region of the elbow joint. Examination maneuvers to screen the ulnohumeral and radiohumeral joints are part of the patient's comprehensive evaluation. Tests listed in this section can be used to screen the structures that can produce medial, lateral, and posterior elbow joint pain.

VALGUS STRESS TEST

The valgus stress test is used to evaluate the integrity of the ulnar collateral ligament. The position used for testing the anterior band of the ulnar collateral ligament is characterized by 15 to 25 degrees of elbow flexion and forearm supination. The elbow flexion position is used to unlock the olecranon from the olecranon fossa and decreases the stability provided by the osseous congruity of the joint. This places a greater relative stress on the medial ulnar collateral ligament (Morrey & An, 1983). Reproduction of medial elbow pain, in addition to unilateral increases in ulnohumeral joint laxity, indicates a positive test. Grading the test is typically performed using the American Academy of Orthopaedic Surgeons (AAOS) guidelines of 0 to 5 mm grade I, 5 to 10 mm grade II, and greater than 10 mm grade III (Ellenbecker et al, 1998).

Use of greater than 25 degrees of elbow flexion increases the amount of humeral rotation during performance of the valgus stress test and provides misleading information to the clinician's hands. Lateral movement by the clinician's distal hand grasping the patient's distal forearm is countered by the blocking of the clinician's proximal hand on the lateral aspect of the joint. This produces a levering effect, with opening of the medial aspect of the joint to stress the medial ulnar collateral ligament. The test is typically performed with the shoulder in the scapular plane, but it can also be performed with the shoulder in the coronal plane to minimize compensatory movements at the shoulder during testing (Figure 5-5).

VARUS STRESS TEST

The varus stress test is performed using similar degrees of elbow flexion and shoulder and forearm positioning. This test assesses the integrity of the lateral ulnar collateral ligament and should be performed along with the valgus stress test to completely evaluate the medial/lateral stability of the ulnohumeral joint. Hand placements are reversed, such that the proximal blocking by the clinician's hand is now situated on the medial side of the elbow, while the clinician's distal hand makes a medially directed motion of the distal forearm (Figure 5-6). The varus test is positive if lateral elbow pain is reproduced with unilateral increases in joint laxity. This test is graded using the same criteria as those for the valgus stress test.

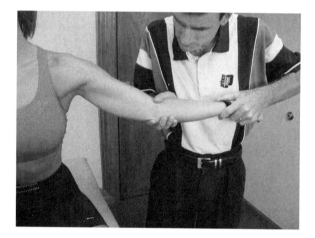

Figure 5-5 Valgus stress test performed with 15 to 25 degrees of elbow flexion, with the shoulder placed in the coronal plane to minimize compensatory humeral rotation during testing.

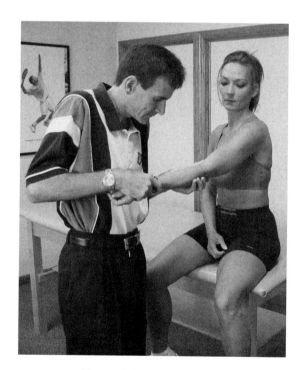

Figure 5-6 Varus stress test.

VALGUS EXTENSION OVERPRESSURE TEST

The valgus extension overpressure test has been reported by Andrews et al (1993) to determine whether posterior elbow pain is caused by a posteromedial osteophyte abutment with the medial margin of the trochlea and the olecranon fossa. This test is performed by passively extending the elbow while maintaining a valgus stress to the elbow

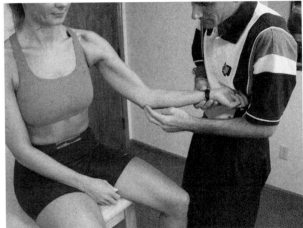

Figure 5-8 Tinel's test demonstrating percussion over the cubital tunnel retinaculum.

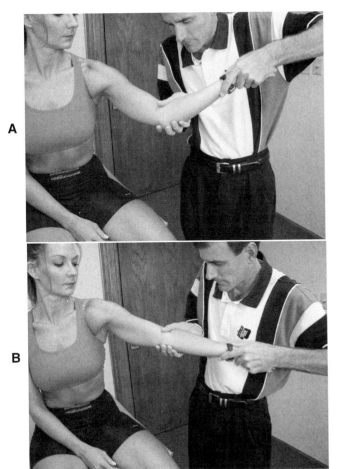

Figure 5-7 Valgus extension overpressure test. **A,** Valgus stress exerted with elbow in flexion, **B,** with maintained valgus stress as elbow is extended.

(Figure 5-7). The valgus test is meant to simulate the stresses imparted to the posterior medial part of the elbow during the acceleration phase of the throwing or serving motion. Reproduction of pain in the posteromedial aspect of the elbow indicates a positive test. The examiner's finger can be placed across the posterior part of the olecranon tip to palpate during the valgus extension overpressure force to feel for grating and crepitace.

PROVOCATION TESTS

Provocation tests can be used when screening the muscle tendon units of the elbow. These tests consist of manual muscle tests to determine pain reproduction. Specific tests used to screen the elbow joint of a patient with suspected shoulder pathology include wrist and finger flexion and extension, as well as forearm pronation and supination

(Ellenbecker, 1995). These tests can be used to provoke the muscle tendon unit at the lateral or medial epicondyle. Testing of the elbow at or near full extension can often re-create localized lateral or medial elbow pain secondary to tendon degeneration (Kraushaar & Nirschl, 1999). Reproduction of lateral or medial elbow pain with resistive muscle testing (provocation testing) may indicate concomitant tendon injury at the elbow and directs the clinician to perform a more complete elbow examination. The presence of overuse injuries in the elbow occurring with proximal injury to the shoulder complex or with scapulothoracic dysfunction has been widely reported (Ellenbecker & Mattalino, 1996; Ellenbecker, 1995; Morrey, 1993; Nirschl, 1988a, 1988b).

TINEL'S TEST

This test involves tapping the ulnar nerve in the medial region of the elbow over the cubital tunnel retinaculum (Figure 5-8). Reproduction of paresthesias or tingling along the distal course of the ulnar nerve indicates irritability of the ulnar nerve (Morrey, 1993) and can help explain the distal radiation of symptoms in a patient with upper extremity pathology.

LOWER EXTREMITY SCREENING

One test that has been advocated by Kibler (1998b) as a screening test for patients with glenohumeral and scapulothoracic dysfunction is the one-leg stability test. This test assesses the ability of the patient to perform a unilateral squat while maintaining proper alignment of the spine and lower extremities. The test is initiated with the subject in a standing position on one leg, with the

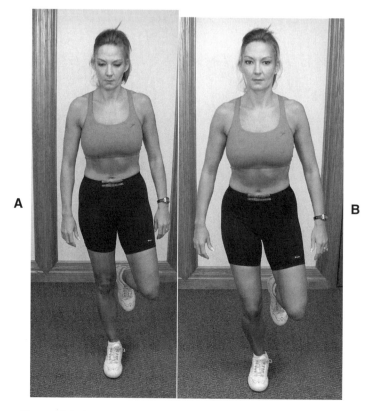

Figure **5-9** One leg stability test. **A,** Start position. **B,** End position.

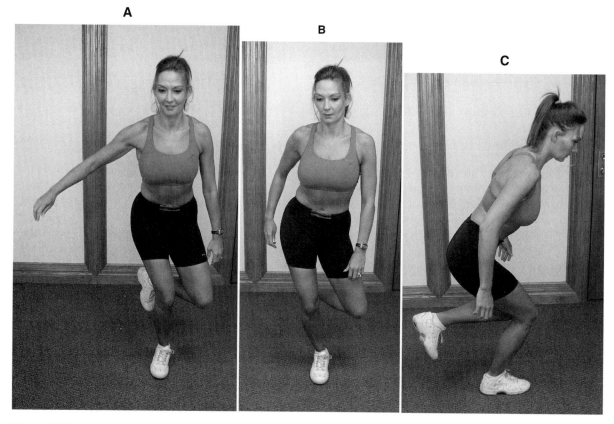

Figure **5-10** Common compensations during the one-leg stability test. **A,** Increased valgus angulation at the knee. **B,** Trendelenburg sign. **C,** Increased trunk flexion.

contralateral limb flexed to 90 degrees (Figure 5-9, *A*). The arms are resting at the patient's sides. The examiner asks the patient to perform a squat on the weightbearing limb, bending that limb's knee to 30 to 45 degrees (Figure 5-9, *B*). During the performance of the squat, the patient's overall alignment is noted. Presence of a Trendelenburg pattern (dropping of the contralateral hip and pelvis), corkscrew (twisting accompanying the squat maneuver), or excessive trunk flexion all indicate weakness of the hip and pelvic musculature and would lead the clinician to include a broader exercise base in the patient's rehabilitation program, including stabilization training of the trunk and lower extremities (Figure 5-10). The important role of the lower extremity and trunk in the overall function of the shoulder is best illustrated by the discussion of the kinetic link principle in Chapter 17.

SUMMARY

Although many tests can ultimately be used to clear the segments and joints both proximal and distal to the injured shoulder, the combination of these specific related referral tests with a detailed subjective evaluation can ensure that the clinician has adequately screened for pathology in the adjoining segments and joints, thereby enabling identification of a specific shoulder pathology.

Neurovascular Testing

INTRODUCTION

Complete patient evaluation must include specific techniques to establish the neurovascular integrity of the extremity being examined. These techniques are most often used when the initial patient evaluation does not produce typical musculoskeletal pain patterns.

SENSATION

In most musculoskeletal evaluations, light touch sensation can be examined in a cursory fashion following the dermatomal patterns (Figure 6-1). Figure 6-1 also shows the cutaneous sensory distribution of the upper extremity. Specific notation of locations of sensory loss or deprivation should be followed. Focused areas of sensory loss may be present during the postoperative evaluation of a patient after open surgical exposure of the shoulder. The use of a Semmes Weinstein Monofilament Test Kit is recommended to better quantify the sensory pattern in the patient with identified sensory involvement. This test kit consists of a series of monofilaments with different diameters that can be used to test the patient's sensation, thereby providing an objective method to evaluate patient sensation. Bilateral comparison forms the basis for most sensory measurement during musculoskeletal shoulder evaluations.

REFLEXES

The biceps (C5, C6), brachioradialis (C5, C6), and triceps (C7, C8) reflexes should be checked, not only for their presence but also for hyperactivity or bilateral differences. If these reflexes are difficult to obtain, Davies et al (1981) recommended having the patient clench the jaw and look to the side opposite that being tested; this is termed the *Jendrassik's maneuver* and facilitates the reflex response.

STRENGTH

Specific manual muscle tests have been covered elsewhere in this text; Chapter 14 contains detailed descriptions of isokinetic testing and interpretation. From a neurologic standpoint, however, using simple but sequenced manual muscle tests helps the clinician to establish distal motor function in the upper extremity before proceeding with specific special tests and strength tests for the proximal muscle groups.

One example of a sequence for manual muscle testing that encompasses the cervical and upper thoracic nerve roots is listed in Table 6-1. Although many sequences can be used, following a standardized sequence that includes each level is recommended.

THORACIC OUTLET TESTING

Although it is beyond the scope of this text to completely review the complex pathophysiology and diagnostic testing of thoracic outlet syndrome (TOS), its common symptoms and clinical tests must be described. The use of clinical screening tests to rule out TOS is a crucial part of the complete evaluation of the patient who presents with atypical musculoskeletal pain patterning in the upper extremity. These patients are often referred with the diagnosis of shoulder pain or arm pain, and a systematic and detailed examination by the clinician is required to identify and/or rule out TOS.

TOS is a controversial topic in clinical medicine, and skeptics doubt its existence (Rayan, 1998). TOS can be defined as neurovascular compression of the thoracic inlet. The thoracic inlet, also called the *superior outlet,* is a pyramidal-shaped space containing the subclavian artery and vein, and the lower trunk of the brachial plexus. Numerous muscular structures insert onto the first rib, including the scalenus anticus, scalenus medius, scalenus minimus, intercostals, serratus anterior, and subclavius. In addition to the structures originating and inserting in this area, the space between the first rib and clavicle narrows with arm elevation (Telford & Mottershead, 1948).

TOS is typically classified into three categories: proximal, middle, and distal. Proximal TOS results from neurovascular entrapment at the interscalene triangle between the anterior and middle scalene muscles (Rayan, 1998). Middle TOS occurs at the interval between the first rib and the clavicle, and the less common distal TOS occurs

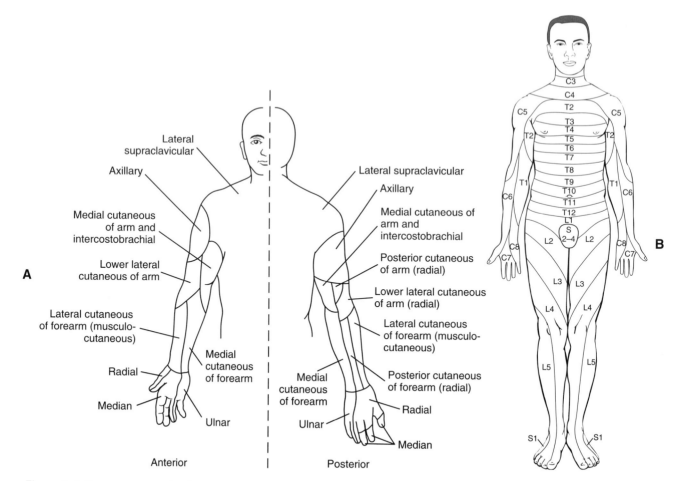

Figure 6-1 Cutaneous sensation distribution of the **A,** upper extremity, and **B,** dermatomes of the upper extremity. (*A* from Ellenbecker TS, Mattalino AJ: Anatomy and biomechanics of the elbow. In *The elbow in sport: injury treatment and rehabilitation*, Champaign, IL, 1996, Human Kinetics Publishers. *B* from Jenkins DB: *Hollinshead's Functional anatomy of the limbs and back*, ed 8, Philadelphia, 2002, WB Saunders.)

TABLE 6-1   Upper Extremity Motor Screening Manual Muscle Test Sequence

MUSCLE	TEST ACTION	NERVE/LEVEL
Deltoid	Resisted abduction (coronal plane)	Axillary nerve (C5, 6)
Biceps	Resisted elbow flexion (supinated forearm position)	Musculocutaneous nerve (C5, 6)
Triceps	Resisted elbow extension	Radial nerve (C7, 8)
	Extensor carpi radialis	
	Extensor carpi ulnaris	
	Resisted wrist extension	Radial and deep radial nerve (C6, 7, 8)
Interossei dorsales	Resisted finger abduction	Ulnar nerve (C8, T1)

Adapted from Hislop HJ, Montgomery J: *Daniels and Worthingham's Muscle testing: techniques of manual examination*, ed 7, Philadelphia, 2002, WB Saunders.

at the level of the coracoid process and pectoralis minor muscle. The age of onset of TOS, although variable, occurs most frequently between 20 and 40 years (Rayan, 1998).

TOS can be further classified into neurologic TOS and the much less common vascular TOS. Neurologic TOS is characterized by symptoms that are purely neurologic without vascular symptoms, whereas vascular TOS has arterial and venous symptoms without neurologic symptoms. Neurologic symptoms can be either motor or sensory (Rayan, 1998).

PROVOCATION TESTS FOR THORACIC OUTLET SYNDROME

Clinically, physical therapists use provocation tests to screen for TOS. These tests have serious limitations, but no other clinical testing methods are currently recommended to more effectively screen or examine the patient with suspected TOS. Most of the provocation tests use certain positional maneuvers, with the clinician closely monitoring the patient's neurologic and vascular responses to these positions. Although there are many variations of these tests to screen for TOS, four of the most commonly used provocation tests—Adson's, Allen's, costoclavicular, and hyperabduction maneuvers—are covered in more detail here.

In 1927, Adson and Coffey reported that cervical rib symptoms could be provoked by head position. This led to the development of Adson's maneuver, which is performed with the patient in a seated position, with the arm held by the examiner in approximately 15 degrees of abduction in the coronal plane. The patient is then asked to inhale deeply and hold the breath, with the head tilted backward and the head and neck rotated to the ipsilateral side, so that the chin is elevated and pointing toward the examiner, who should be immediately beside and slightly behind the patient being examined (Figure 6-2). The examiner palpates the radial pulse volume at the patient's wrist. The radial pulse (vascular response) is recorded as *no change, diminished,* or *occluded.* The patient is then allowed to breathe normally, keeping the head in the testing position for approximately 1 minute. If present, paresthesias (neurologic response) are recorded as mild, moderate, or severe, and their distribution is noted (Rayan, 1998).

Allen's test, another provocation maneuver, is performed exactly as described by Adson; however, the patient looks to the contralateral side (away from the examiner) during testing. Similar recording and procedures are used in this examination maneuver.

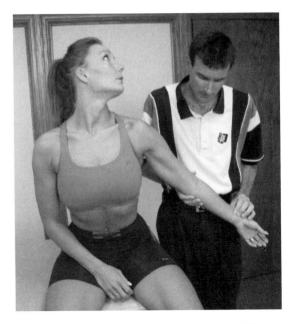

Figure 6-2 Adson's test for screening for TOS.

The costoclavicular maneuver is performed by simulating an exaggerated military-type posture (Rayan, 1998). The patient is in a seated position, with the arms toward the side in the coronal plane (Figure 6-3). The patient is asked to retract and depress the scapulae, protrude the chest outward, and tuck the chin, holding this position for 1 minute. Changes in radial pulse are noted and the presence of paresthesias is recorded.

Finally, the hyperabduction or Wright's maneuver is performed by palpating the radial pulse, initially with the arms at the side and repeated with the arms in a hyperabduction position. Hyperabduction is typically performed with external rotation of the shoulder and elbow extension without head movement. Changes in radial pulse and/or the presence of paresthesias are recorded, with sampling for 1 minute. Several modifications of this maneuver are recommended. The first is to verify that the elbow is extended beyond 45 degrees to ensure that compression of the ulnar nerve does not unfairly bias or influence the result of the distal paresthesias (Rayan, 1998). Also, the effects of gravity may influence the radial pulse diminution; therefore performing the test with the patient in the supine position neutralizes the effects of gravity in the overhead position. The use of this test is specific with regard to position for many industrial and athletic patients who report symptoms only with overhead positions.

Rayan and Jensen (1995) tested the prevalence of positive responses with TOS provocation tests in a normal population to determine the incidence of false-positive

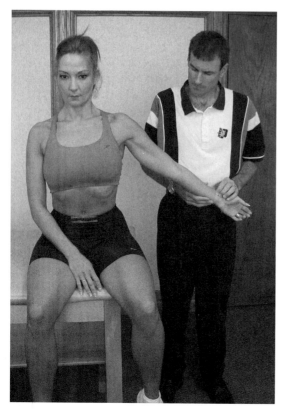

Figure 6-3 Costoclavicular test used for screening for TOS.

results. Provocation examination maneuvers were performed in 200 upper extremities of 100 volunteers. Provocation tests were assessed for both the vascular response (diminution of the radial pulse) or neurologic response (paresthesias). The vascular response was present in 13.5% of the normal volunteer extremities for the Adson's maneuver, 47% of the extremities for the costoclavicular maneuver, and 57% of the extremities for the hyperabduction maneuver. The neurologic response was present in 2% of extremities for the Adson's maneuver, 10% of the extremities for the costoclavicular maneuver, and 16.5% of the extremities for the hyperabduction maneuver. The authors concluded that the vascular response was far more common than the neurologic response in the normal population. Caution must be taken when interpreting the results of the vascular portion of these clinical TOS maneuvers as a result of the high incidence of positive findings in a normal population. The neurologic response, consisting of replication of paresthesias in the distal upper extremity with positional provocation, is far more discriminating and less commonly occurs in the normal population. Further research is needed to better define the validity and reliability of these clinical TOS tests.

One final test has been reported in the literature for TOS. As reported by Roos (1966), in this test the patient opens and closes the hands quite rapidly for 3 minutes, with the arms in an overhead position. A positive response to this test consists of a neurologic response such as paresthesias, fatigue, heaviness, and a sudden drop of the limb. This test can also be performed with the patient in the "surrender" position, which places the elbows in 90 degrees of flexion. No reliability and typical response pattern or incidence have been reported in the normal population with this test.

SUMMARY

These neurovascular clinical evaluation tests are essential to determine the integrity of the neurovascular structures before specific musculoskeletal tests for the shoulder complex are performed. Ruling out involvement of the neurovascular structures that supply the upper extremity is essential for performing both an efficient and accurate musculoskeletal examination of the shoulder.

CHAPTER

7

Palpation

INTRODUCTION

Palpation is a widely used technique among physical therapists to identify structures and determine the presence and location of patient-described pain patterns. Various positions have been advocated to place the shoulder in an advantageous position to optimally palpate the tendons of the rotator cuff and surrounding structures (Mattingly & Mackarey, 1996). The optimal shoulder position for palpation and the typical location of specific structures in that position are reviewed to assist the clinician in obtaining the most accurate information during this portion of the clinical examination.

ROTATOR CUFF TENDONS

The four rotator cuff tendons are not directly palpable because of the overlying deltoid and acromion. The recommended shoulder position to best palpate the supraspinatus tendon was originally described by Cyriax and Cyriax (1993) and included shoulder adduction, full internal rotation, and slight extension, such that the patient's forearm and hand are placed behind the body in the lower back region. In this position, the supraspinatus is palpable just off the anterior medial aspect of the acromion and "passes near vertical, lateral and parallel to the bicipital groove" (Cyriax & Cyriax, 1993; Mattingly & Mackarey, 1996). One limitation of this position for many patients with shoulder pain is the lack of the available range of internal rotation to achieve the position behind the back, similar to the Gerber lift-off test position (pages 99–100). For these patients, Hawkins and Bokor (1990) recommended a modified position that includes shoulder adduction, medial rotation, and less extension, such that the patient's forearm is placed against the stomach. This position places the supraspinatus tendon just off the anterolateral aspect of the acromion and allows the patient's extremity to be examined in a position of greater comfort that nearly all patients can achieve, even after a surgical procedure (Figure 7-1) (Hawkins & Bokor, 1990).

The infraspinatus and teres minor tendons insert on the lower facets of the greater tuberosity of the humerus,

and several positions have been recommended for palpation. Cyriax and Cyriax (1993) and Magee (1997) both recommended using a position where the patient is prone on elbows, with the affected shoulder in slight flexion, adduction, and lateral rotation. In this position, the infraspinatus is located just off the posterolateral corner of the acromion, with the teres minor immediately below the infraspinatus (Tomberlin, 2001). A limiting characteristic of this position is that it requires both a prone position by the patient and slight weightbearing through the humerus. Mattingly and Mackarey (1996) recommended maximal exposure for the infraspinatus and teres minor tendons, which is similar to the position of the statue "The Thinker" by Rodin. The shoulder is placed in 90 degrees of flexion, 10 degrees of shoulder adduction, and 20 degrees of lateral rotation (Figure 7-2). The patient can place the ulnar side of the hand against the side of the face to achieve this position. The infraspinatus and teres minor can be palpated just inferior to the posterolateral corner of the acromion (Mattingly & Mackarey, 1996).

The subscapularis tendon does not require extensive positioning for palpation. Mattingly and Mackarey (1996) found the optimal position of the shoulder to be in adduction against the side of the body, with neutral flexion/extension and internal/external rotation. In this position, the subscapularis can be palpated in the middle of the deltopectoral triangle. Landmarks for the subscapularis tendon are inferior to the clavicle, lateral to the coracoid and bicep short-head tendon, and medial to the bicep long-head tendon in the intertubercular groove of the humerus. Use of this shoulder position and palpation location allow the examiner to palpate the subscapularis with the intervening presence of the deltoid (Mattingly & Mackarey, 1996).

ADDITIONAL PALPATION CONCEPT FOR THE ROTATOR CUFF

Codman (1934) described palpation of full-thickness tears of the supraspinatus. This transdeltoid palpation has become known as the *rent test*. This defect or "sulcus" produced a rent in the supraspinatus tendon, which was

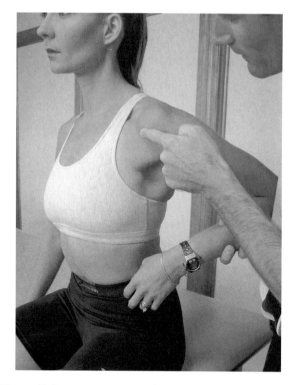

Figure 7-1 Position for palpation of the supraspinatus tendon.

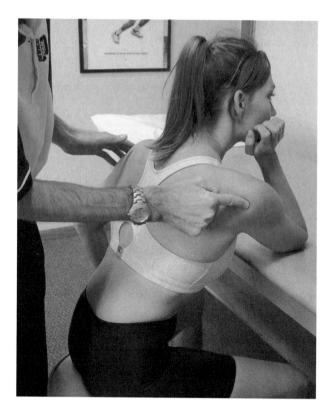

Figure 7-2 Position for tendon palpation for the infraspinatus tendon (thinker's position).

palpable through the deltoid (Wolf & Agrawal, 2001). The technique of transdeltoid palpation requires a relaxed patient, with palpation performed just anterior to the anterior margin of the acromion through the deltoid. The patient is evaluated in the seated position, with the arm dangling next to the side to promote relaxation. With one hand, the examiner grasps the forearm, with the patient's elbow in 90 degrees of flexion. The examiner's grasp on the forearm is meant to allow for rotational control of the extremity while the examiner's other hand performs the palpation. The arm is brought into extension while the patient's extremity is rotated internally and externally. According to Wolf and Agrawal (2001), both an eminence and a rent are palpated as the arm is brought from extension to slight flexion and internally and externally rotated. The eminence represents the greater tuberosity that is more prominent because of a full-thickness tear of the rotator cuff tendon. The rent is a soft tissue defect (Figure 7-3) created by the rotator cuff that avulsed from the tuberosity. The examination should be performed bilaterally to appreciate the anatomy of the uninvolved shoulder and compare it with the symptomatic side (Wolf & Agrawal, 2001).

Lyons and Tomlinson (1993) correlated clinical palpation using the rent test with the size of the tear at time of surgery. They reported sensitivity of 91% and a specificity of 75% in a population of 42 patients. Wolf and Agrawal (2001) prospectively studied 109 consecutive patients using the rent test. Results of the transdeltoid palpation were compared with arthroscopic findings at the time of surgery. A sensitivity of 95.7% and specificity of 96.8% for the diagnosis of a full-thickness tear of the supraspinatus tendon were reported. The authors concluded that in the trained examiner, transdeltoid palpation is highly accurate. Although the ability of each clinician to palpate the torn rotator cuff via the deltoid and determine the presence of a full-thickness rotator cuff tear remain in question, this information is relevant based on the specific description of both the technique used and the exact location of palpation and positioning of the patient. Determining specific diagnostic conclusions from the palpation of the rotator cuff may not be indicated in the physical therapy evaluation of the patient with shoulder pathology; however, use of this technique can be recommended based on its success in the literature.

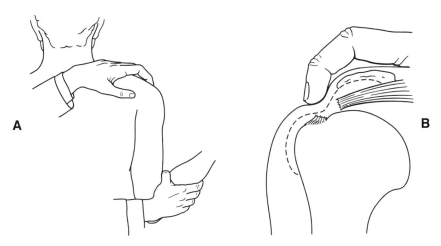

Figure **7-3 A,** Position of the hands for the rent test with **B,** demonstration of the tip of the finger palpating the eminence and rent. (From Codman EA: *The shoulder: rupture of the supraspinatus tendon and other lesions in or about the subacromial bursa,* Boston, 1934, Thomas Todd; Reprint edition. Melbourne, FL, 1984, Krieger.)

BICEPS LONG-HEAD TENDON

Mattingly and Mackarey (1996) also reported maximal exposure of the biceps long-head tendon. This tendon was most exposed with the glenohumeral joint in adduction and 20 degrees of internal rotation, placing the biceps long-head tendon in the deltopectoral triangle (Figure 7-4). The tendon is less accessible with either neutral rotation or lateral rotation because it is under the deltoid muscle. To assist with palpation of the long head of the biceps, the examiner can rotate the humerus back and forth while gently palpating for the biceps long-head tendon as it slides back and forth with humeral rotation.

ADDITIONAL CONCEPTS FOR SHOULDER PALPATION

Davies and DeCarlo (1995) reported that palpation used during the examination of the shoulder provides information regarding changes in skin temperature that might suggest an inflammatory process, locate areas of sensation loss or deficiency, identify specific sites of swelling, check circulatory status via distal pulses, and identify point tenderness. Davies teaches palpation using similar sequences on each patient to ensure that related areas are checked consistently during the comprehensive evaluation process. The following sequence has been recommended: Starting at the sternoclavicular joint anteriorly, the examiner pro-

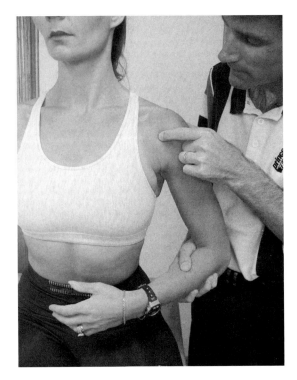

Figure **7-4** Position for tendon palpation of the biceps long-head tendon in the deltopectoral triangle with 20 degrees of internal rotation.

gresses laterally along the margin of the clavicle to the acromioclavicular joint. After palpating the acromioclavicular joint, the examiner drops inferiorly to palpate the coracoid process, lesser tubercle, and subscapularis insertion. By taking hold of the arm at the patient's elbow, the examiner palpates the biceps tendon in the intertubercular groove and, with internal rotation of the humerus, palpates the greater tuberosity and the supraspinatus insertion while the arm is being slightly extended, as mentioned earlier in this chapter. Rotation of the humerus from internal to external rotation allows the examiner to move from the lesser tuberosity to the intertubercular groove, and finally to the greater tuberosity while palpating. The lateral aspect of the acromion is then palpated and, after slight flexion and lateral rotation, the infraspinatus and teres minor are encountered just inferior to the posterolateral corner of the acromion with posterior palpation. Continuation of the palpation sequence involves the margins of the scapula posteriorly. Systematically following this sequence allows the examiner to palpate nearly all of the palpable structures around the shoulder girdle. This systematic approach helps to avoid skipping or forgetting less common areas of involvement that can occur when the areas that are most obvious or subjectively directed by the patient are palpated first. Box 7-1 lists commonly associated pathology with the compartment of palpation from Davies and DeCarlo (1995). This list is not meant to imply a direct relationship between the location of tenderness or pain reproduction with palpation, but it is included here as a guide for the examining clinician.

Box 7-1   Shoulder Complex Compartments for Palpation

1. Anterior Compartment
   Bicipital tendinitis
   Subscapularis tendinitis
   Coracoacromial ligament pain secondary to rotator cuff impingement
   Anterior capsule pain secondary to chronic subluxations, status post macrotraumatic dislocation
   Sternoclavicular joint sprain
   Clavicular fracture
2. Superior Compartment
   Acromioclavicular joint sprain
   Supraspinatus tendinitis
   Subacromial/subdeltoid bursitis
   Upper trapezius strain
   Levator scapula strain/spasm
3. Lateral Compartment
   Supraspinatus tendinitis
   Subacromial/subdeltoid bursitis
   Sulcus sign indicating a multidirectional instability
4. Posterior Compartment
   Infraspinatus tendonitis/strain
   Teres minor tendonitis/strain
   Posterior capsule pain secondary to chronic subluxation
   Posterior impingement

Modified from Davies GJ, DeCarlo MS: *Examination of the shoulder complex: current concepts in rehabilitation of the shoulder,* LaCrosse, WI, 1995, Sports Physical Therapy Association Home Study Course.

Range of Motion Testing

INTRODUCTION

One of the unique characteristics of the evaluation process used by physical therapists and other medical professionals in physical rehabilitative medicine is the careful assessment of range of motion. Historically, joint motion during clinical examination was evaluation via visual observation (Berryman-Reese & Bandy, 2002). Early editions of the *Joint Range of Motion Guide* published by the American Academy of Orthopaedic Surgeons suggested that visual observation of joint range of motion was equal or superior to goniometric evaluation. As early as 1949, Moore supported the use of the universal goniometer but outlined its inherent errors, including lack of standardized technique, patient positioning, and numerical expression. Later research has shown both the effectiveness and reliability of goniometric assessment of joint range of motion in human subjects, and the universal goniometer initially described by Clark in 1920 is used worldwide to objectively document joint range of motion during clinical examination (Berryman-Reese & Bandy, 2002).

This chapter highlights important concepts needed to objectively measure active and passive range of motion during clinical evaluation of a patient with shoulder pathology. The reader is referred to three sources that provide detailed descriptions and copious references on joint range of motion assessment and normal values (Berryman-Reese & Bandy, 2002; American Academy of Orthopaedic Surgeons, 1994; Norkin & White, 1985).

RANGE OF MOTION ASSESSMENT

Measurement of both active and passive range of motion is indicated during the complete evaluation of the patient with shoulder pathology. It is important to understand the relationship between scapulothoracic and glenohumeral motion when evaluating shoulder joint range of motion. The reader is referred to pages 17–18 for a discussion of scapulohumeral rhythm. It is imperative that the clinician observe and document the patient's ability to elevate the shoulder in flexion, abduction, and scapular plane elevation, with particular emphasis to not only the actual movement performed with documented endpoint, but also the quality of the motion and rhythm between the glenohumeral and scapulothoracic joints.

Measurement of isolated glenohumeral joint elevation in the sagittal, frontal, or scapular planes is not clinically applicable above the first 30 degrees of glenohumeral joint elevation (Inman et al, 1944), and it is recommended that measurement be performed to assess the combined movement of these articulations when assessing humeral elevation in those three planes (Berryman-Reese & Bandy, 2002). Measurement of the patient in a supine position can assist with scapular stabilization to some degree during humeral elevation measurements; however, complete isolation of humeral motion is unlikely except in controlled laboratory conditions. Typical range of motion measures can be classified as *combined* or *isolated*.

COMBINED SHOULDER ACTIVE RANGE OF MOTION TESTS

The most popular combined motion tests used in clinical examination are the Apley's scratch tests (Hoppenfeld, 1976; Magee, 1997). These tests combine the motions of abduction with external rotation (top arm [dominant left arm], Figure 8-1) and adduction and internal rotation with slight extension (bottom arm [nondominant right arm], see Figure 8-1). Additional positions include the movement of cross-arm adduction and internal rotation where the patient should reach across to touch the outer aspect of the acromion of the contralateral shoulder. Hoppenfeld (1976) suggested that these movements be observed for symmetry and for any break in normal rhythm. As a quick assessment, these movements can provide a visual marker for combined range of motion restrictions that can assist the clinician in coupling these range of motion restrictions with the patient's subjectively reported functional limitations in activities of daily living. Another use of the combined movement tests lies in the visual demonstration of bilateral range of motion differences in overhead athletes. Loss of internal rotation range of motion in the dominant shoulder of elite tennis

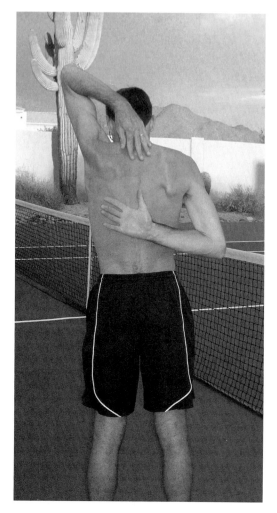

Figure 8-1 Posterior view of Apley's scratch test with combined glenohumeral joint abduction/external rotation in the left dominant arm, and adduction/internal rotation with the right nondominant arm in a senior tennis player.

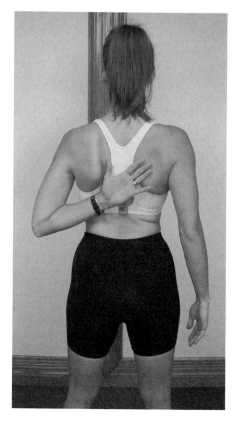

Figure 8-2 Combined glenohumeral joint measurement technique using hand placement behind the back to assess highest maximal vertebral level contact.

and baseball players has been widely documented (Ellenbecker, 1992; Ellenbecker et al, 2002b). The vast difference between the top and bottom arm (see Figure 8-1) observed when the dominant arm is performing the lower movement (adduction, internal rotation, and extension) can clearly identify to the patient and coaches the degree of range of motion adaptation or loss (Roetert & Ellenbecker, 1998).

In addition to the observation of the combined movements suggested by Hoppenfeld (1976), many clinicians document which spinous process the patient can touch during each of the combined motions bilaterally. Documentation using the combined movement of adduction and internal rotation (hand behind the back) movement

(Figure 8-2) is particularly popular among clinicians for assessing glenohumeral joint internal rotation. Edwards et al (2002) evaluated the intraobserver and interobserver reliability of this measurement technique using three male subjects, with 11 orthopaedic surgeons and 2 physical therapists as examiners. All examiners measured internal rotation based on maximal vertebral level achieved between T4 and L5 with an extended thumb. Radiographs were used to establish the true level the thumb was placed over. Results showed poor interobserver reliability (intraclass correlation coefficients [ICC] 0.12 to 0.27), with an average error of 1 vertebral level. Intraobserver reliability ranged between ICC 0.18 and 0.82, with a mean of 0.44; the average error was 1 level. Even within a single examiner, repeated bouts of testing using this combined method to document internal rotation via an extended thumb are prone to error on an average of 1 vertebral level.

Additional research testing the validity of the combined method to assess maximal internal rotation active range of motion via vertebral level was performed by Mallon et al (1996) during radiographic analysis. Posteroanterior radiographs were used to determine actual movement of the scapulothoracic and glenohumeral joints. The movement of maximal internal rotation behind the back occurs at a ratio of 2:1, with 2 degrees of glenohumeral joint motion occurring with 1 degree of scapulothoracic motion. The scapulothoracic motion was more important in actually placing the hand behind the back, with essentially all internal rotation range of motion occurring with the hand in front of the body (Mallon et al, 1996). The actual act of reaching toward the maximal vertebral level is achieved by elbow flexion and thumb hyperextension, not continued internal rotation. Mallon et al (1996) concluded "that measuring shoulder internal rotation by the maximal vertebral level reached by the patient's thumb greatly oversimplifies the concept of internal rotation and that limitations in this motion may not be strictly due to a loss of internal rotation at the glenohumeral joint." Use of this combined pattern may give the clinician an indication of the combined movement of the glenohumeral and scapulothoracic joints, but should not be substituted for measurement of isolated internal rotation of the glenohumeral joint.

ISOLATED GLENOHUMERAL JOINT RANGE OF MOTION TECHNIQUES

As mentioned earlier, it is beyond the scope of this chapter to provide the detailed review of every isolated measurement technique for the shoulder girdle. However, several important concepts, particularly regarding measurement of rotational range of motion, are pertinent. Table 8-1 provides descriptive data on normal range of motion for the human shoulder. Riddle et al (1987) examined intratester and intertester reliability of measuring the shoulder with a universal goniometer in 50 subjects with shoulder pathology. Passive range of motion measurements for flexion, abduction, and external rotation ranged from 0.87 to 0.99 for intertester reliability, with values of 0.26 to 0.55 for horizontal abduction/ adduction and internal rotation. They concluded that the reliability of shoulder range of motion measurement using a goniometer was motion specific. Norkin and White (1995) summarized the intrarater reliability for goniometric assessment of shoulder range of motion using a large universal goniometer. They reported ICCs ranging from 0.84 to 0.98 for shoulder flexion, extension, and abduction, and ICCs ranging between 0.87 and 0.99 for internal and external rotation. By comparison, Norkin and White (1995) reported ICCs for elbow extension/flexion range of motion at greater than 0.90.

Analysis of Table 8-1 shows relatively consistent readings for some motions, such as flexion and abduction, and a wide variation of normal responses in others. One area with a particularly wide variation is glenohumeral joint internal and external rotation. This range of motion is often measured in 0 or 45 degrees of abduction in the initial evaluation after surgery or injury, and more frequently measured in 90 degrees of abduction as patients progress in rehabilitation (Ellenbecker & Mattalino, 1999b). Also, the contribution of the scapulothoracic joint to glenohumeral motion has been widely documented (Inman et al, 1944; Mallon et al, 1996) and is one of the variables that can lead to extensive variation of rotational measurement in the human shoulder.

Active rotational range of motion measures were taken bilaterally in 399 elite junior tennis players using two differing measurement techniques and a universal goniometer (Ellenbecker et al, 1993). A total of 252 subjects were measured in the supine position for internal and external rotation with 90 degrees of glenohumeral joint abduction, with no attempt to stabilize the scapula (Figure 8-3); 147 elite junior tennis players were measured for internal and external rotation active range of motion in 90 degrees of glenohumeral joint abduction using scapular stabilization. Stabilization was provided by a posteriorly directed force applied by the examiner's hand placed on the anterior aspect of the shoulder over the anterior acromion and coracoid process (Figure 8-4). Results of the two groups showed significantly less internal rotation range of motion when using the measurement technique with scapular stabilization (18% to 28% reduction in range of motion). Changes in external rotation range of motion were

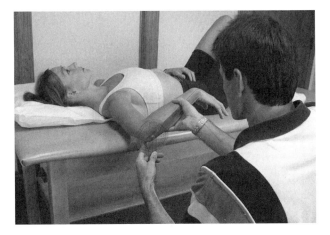

Figure **8-3** Glenohumeral joint internal rotation range of motion measurement technique without scapular stabilization in 90 degrees of abduction.

TABLE 8-1   Normal Range of Motion Values for the Shoulder*

Joint	AAOS	Boone & Azen	Clark	CMA	Daniels & Worthingham	Dorinson & Wagner	Ewsch & Lepley	Gerhardt & Russe	Hoppenfeld	JAMA	Kapandji	Kendall & McCreary	Weichec & Krusen
Flexion	180	167	130	170	—	180	170	170	—	150	180	180	180
Extension	60	62	80	30	50	45	60	50	45	40	50	45	45
Abduction	180	184	180	170	—	180	170	170	180	150	180	180	180
Internal rotation	70	69	90*	60*	90	90	80	80	55	40	95	70	90
External rotation	90	104	40*	80*	90	90	90	90	45	90*	80	90	90

Adapted from American Physical Therapy Association promotional material, Fairfax, VA.

*Measurements obtained with the shoulder in 0 degrees of abduction. Normal range of motion (in degrees) according to various authors.

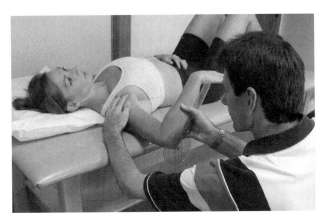

Figure 8-4 Glenohumeral joint internal rotation range of motion measurement technique with scapular stabilization provided by a posteriorly directed force on the anterior aspect of the shoulder.

TABLE 8-2   Glenohumeral Joint Internal Rotation Values from 138 Patients with Glenohumeral Joint Instability and Impingement

Internal rotation with scapular stabilization	38.8 degrees
Internal rotation without scapular stabilization	67.4 degrees
Maximal vertebral level	T7

From Ellenbecker & Davies, 1997.

smaller between groups, with 2% to 6% reduction in active range of motion.

One common finding confirmed by this research is significantly less (approximately 10 to 15 degrees) dominant arm glenohumeral joint internal rotation in elite junior tennis players (Ellenbecker, 1992; Ellenbecker et al, 1996). In this study, however, this difference between extremities in internal rotation range of motion was identified only when the scapula was stabilized. Failure to stabilize the scapula did not produce glenohumeral joint internal rotation range of motion measurements that identified a deficit. This study clearly demonstrates the importance of using consistent measurement techniques when documenting range of motion of glenohumeral joint rotation. Based on the results of this study, I highly recommend the use of scapular stabilization during measurement of humeral rotation to obtain more isolated and representative values of shoulder rotation.

Ellenbecker and Davies (1997) studied 138 patients undergoing rehabilitation for rotator cuff impingement and glenohumeral joint instability. Patients were measured for internal glenohumeral joint rotation using three methods: isolated supine glenohumeral joint internal rotation in 90 degrees of abduction without scapular stabilization, isolated glenohumeral joint internal rotation with 90 degrees of glenohumeral joint abduction with scapular stabilization, and determination of maximal vertebral level reached behind the back. Internal rotation range of motion was almost twice as large without scapular stabilization, as compared with the condition when the scapula was stabilized. The average vertebral level achieved by these patients was T7 (Table 8-2).

TOTAL ROTATION RANGE OF MOTION CONCEPT

The concept of total rotation range of motion combines the glenohumeral joint internal and external rotation range of motion measure by adding the two numbers to obtain a numerical representation of the total rotation range of motion available at the glenohumeral joint (Figure 8-5). Kibler et al (1996) and Roetert et al (2000) found that decreases in the total rotation range of motion arc in the dominant extremity of elite tennis players correlated with increasing age and number of competitive years of play. Ellenbecker et al (2002b) measured bilateral total rotation range of motion in professional baseball pitchers and elite junior tennis players. The professional baseball pitchers had greater dominant arm external rotation and significantly less dominant arm internal rotation compared with the contralateral nondominant side. The total rotation range of motion, however, did not differ significantly between extremities (145 degrees dominant arm, 146 degrees nondominant arm) (Figure 8-6). This research shows that, despite bilateral differences in the actual internal and/or external rotation range of motion in the glenohumeral joints of baseball pitchers, the total arc of rotational motion should remain the same.

In contrast, Ellenbecker et al (2002b) tested 117 elite male junior tennis players and found significantly less internal rotation range of motion on the dominant arm (45 degrees versus 56 degrees), as well as significantly less total rotation range of motion on the dominant arm (149 degrees versus 158 degrees). The total rotation range of motion did differ between extremities (Table 8-3, see Figure 8-6); approximately 10 degrees less total rotation range of motion can be expected in the dominant arm compared with the nondominant arm of the uninjured elite junior tennis player.

Use of normative data from population-specific research can assist clinicians in interpreting normal range of motion patterns and identify when sport-specific adaptations or clinically significant maladaptions are present (see Table 8-3) (Ellenbecker et al, 2002b). Further research on additional subject populations is needed to outline the total rotation range of motion concept.

Clinical application of the total rotation range of motion concept is best demonstrated by a case presentation of a unilaterally dominant upper extremity athlete. During initial evaluation of a high level baseball pitcher, if the clinician finds a range of motion pattern of 120

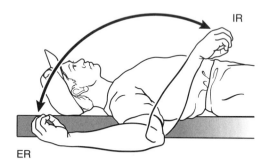

Figure 8-5 Total rotation range of motion concept.

degrees of external rotation and only 30 degrees of internal rotation, there may be some uncertainty as to whether that represents a range of motion deficit in internal rotation that requires rehabilitative intervention via stretching and specific mobilization. If measurement of that patient's nondominant extremity rotation reveals 90 degrees of external rotation and 60 degrees of internal rotation, however, the current recommendation is to avoid extensive mobilization and passive stretching of the dominant extremity, because the total rotation range of motion in both extremities is 150 degrees (120 ER + 30 IR = 150 dominant arm/90 ER and 60 IR = 150 total rotation nondominant arm). In elite level tennis players, total active rotation range of motion can be expected to be up to 10 degrees less on the dominant arm before a clinical treatment to address internal rotation range of motion restriction would be implemented. This total rotation range of motion concept can be used to guide the clinician during rehabilitation, specifically in the application of stretching and mobilization. Careful measurement of range of motion can best determine what glenohumeral joint requires additional mobility and which extremity should

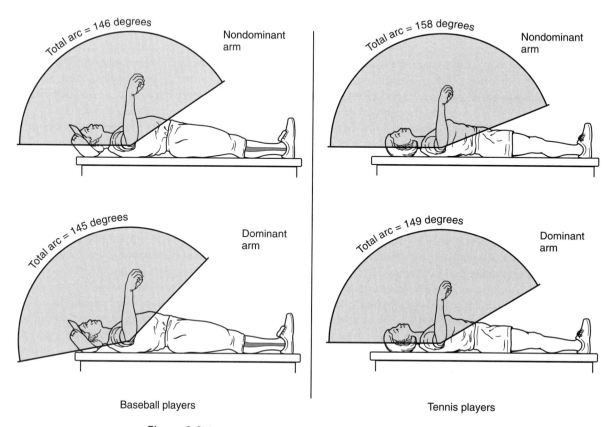

Figure 8-6 Summary of total rotation range of motion research.

TABLE 8-3   **Bilateral Comparison of Isolated and Total Rotation Range of Motion from Professional Baseball Pitchers and Elite Junior Tennis Players**

SUBJECTS	DOMINANT ARM	NONDOMINANT ARM
BASEBALL PITCHERS		
External rotation	103.2 ± 9.1 (1.34)	94.5 ± 8.1 (1.19)
Internal rotation	42.4 ± 15.8 (2.33)	52.4 ± 16.4 (2.42)
Total rotation	145.7 ± 18.0 (2.66)	146.9 ± 17.5 (2.59)
ELITE JUNIOR TENNIS PLAYERS		
External rotation	103.7 ± 10.9 (1.02)	101.8 ± 10.8 (1.01)
Internal rotation	45.4 ± 13.6 (1.28)	56.3 ± 11.5 (1.08)
Total rotation	149.1 ± 18.4 (1.73)	158.2 ± 15.9 (1.50)

All measurements are expressed in degrees. Standard error of the mean in parentheses.
From Ellenbecker TS, Roetert EP, Bailie DS, et al: Glenohumeral joint total rotation range of motion in elite tennis players and baseball pitchers, *Med Sci Sports Exerc* 34(12):2052-2056, 2002b.

not have additional mobility because of the obvious harm induced by increases in capsular mobility, which can lead to an increase in humeral head translation during aggressive upper extremity exertion.

Loss of internal rotation range of motion is significant for several reasons. The relationship between internal rotation range of motion loss (tightness in the posterior capsule of the shoulder) and increased anterior humeral head translation has been scientifically identified (Tyler et al, 1999; Gerber et al, 2003). The increase in anterior humeral shear force reported by Harryman et al (1990) was manifested by a horizontal adduction cross-body maneuver, similar to that incurred during the follow-through of the throwing motion or tennis serve. Tightness of the posterior capsule has also been linked to increased superior migration of the humeral head during shoulder elevation (Matsen and Artnz, 1990).

Koffler et al (2001) studied the effects of posterior capsular tightness in a functional position of 90 degrees of abduction and 90 degrees or more of external rotation in cadaveric specimens. Imbrication of either the inferior aspect of the posterior capsule or the entire posterior capsule altered the humeral head kinematics. In the presence of posterior capsular tightness, the humeral head shifts in an anterosuperior direction, compared with a normal shoulder with normal capsular relationships. With more extensive amounts of posterior capsular tightness, the humeral head shifted in a posterosuperior fashion. These effects of altered posterior capsular tensions experimentally representing in vivo posterior glenohumeral joint capsular tightness highlight the clinical importance of using a reliable and effective measurement methodology to assess internal rotation range of motion during examination of the shoulder. Burkhart et al (2003) clinically demonstrated the concept of posterior superior humeral

head shear in the abducted externally rotated position with tightness of the posterior band of the inferior glenohumeral ligament (See Chapter 17 for a more complete description relative to the throwing athlete.)

The Tyler posterior shoulder tightness test is another test that can be used to measure cross-arm adduction range of motion to assess posterior shoulder tightness (Tyler et al, 1999). This test assesses the limitation in shoulder cross-arm adduction and is thought to measure tightness in the posterior capsule and the muscle tendon units of the posterior shoulder muscles. The patient is placed in a side-lying position on a plinth, approximately half the length of the humerus away from the edge of the plinth. The hips are flexed to approximately 45 degrees, with 90 degrees of knee flexion to stabilize the patient. Males are measured with no shirt and females in a sports bra or gown to expose the scapular area. The acromion is aligned perpendicular to the plinth, with the nontested extremity placed under the patient's head. The tester stands facing the patient (Figure 8-7) and grasps the extremity to be measured at the elbow near both epicondyles, and passively moves the patient's shoulder to 90 degrees abduction in neutral rotation. The scapula is then stabilized in a position of retraction by using the examiner's other hand along the lateral border of the scapula (see Figure 8-7). With the position of the scapula maintained, the patient's shoulder is lowered passively and gently into horizontal adduction in neutral rotation. The humerus is lowered with the patient relaxed, until motion has ceased or rotation of the humerus occurs, indicating end range of motion. At the end of the achieved range of motion, the examiner takes a carpenter square (60 cm) and measures the distance from the top of the plinth to the patient's medial epicondyle and records that value. Testing is repeated for the contralateral shoulder. A greater distance

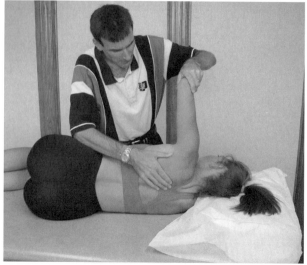
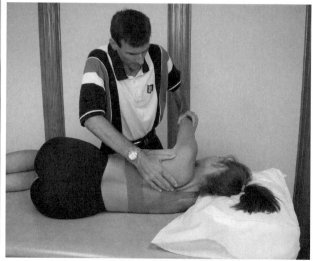

Figure 8-7 Tyler posterior shoulder tightness test demonstrating starting position with **A,** scapular stabilization, and **B,** end position.

represents decreased posterior shoulder flexibility, and a smaller distance between the top of the plinth and the medial epicondyle indicates greater flexibility of the posterior shoulder structures (Tyler et al, 1999).

Tyler et al (1999) reported intratester reliability using ICCs ranging between 0.92 and 0.95 and intertester reliability of 0.80. They also reported a significant correlation between the Tyler posterior shoulder tightness test and isolated glenohumeral joint internal rotation range of motion, with 90 degrees of abduction and scapula stabilized ($r = 0.61$), as well as significant differences ($P < 0.001$) between the dominant and nondominant extremities in posterior shoulder tightness in NCAA division I college baseball pitchers. Greater posterior shoulder tightness was identified in the dominant arm. In addition to testing on nonimpaired subjects and athletes, Tyler et al (2000) tested shoulders in patients diagnosed with shoulder impingement. The Tyler posterior shoulder tightness test was positive in the involved shoulder in patients with subacromial impingement when the impairment was in the dominant or nondominant extremity. The authors recommended this test for measuring posterior shoulder tightness in clinical applications.

END FEEL CLASSIFICATION

An additional concept important in the determination and measurement of both physiologic and accessory range of motion testing is end feel. Cyriax and Cyriax (1983) described end feel as the feeling transmitted to the examiner's hands at the extreme range of passive motion (Table 8-4). Normal end feels are considered as bony, capsular,

and soft tissue approximation. Abnormal end feels are spasm, springy block, and empty end feels (Cyriax & Cyriax, 1983). End feels for human joint movements have been established, with normal expected end feels for glenohumeral joint motions being listed as capsular. One exception is the movement of cross-arm adduction. On some individuals with substantial muscular development of the pectorals and biceps, the end feel for cross-arm adduction can be interpreted as soft tissue approximation as the muscles become superimposed against one another at or before end range of motion.

An example of a common situation in which abnormal end feels may be present during passive range of motion assessment in the clinical examination of the patient with shoulder dysfunction is the empty end feel felt in patients with an acute onset of shoulder pain, where no measurable resistance is encountered during the patient's range of motion before pain is encountered. The spasm end feel is also often encountered during apprehension testing of the patient with glenohumeral joint instability as the arm is brought toward abduction and external rotation. Finally, a heavy capsular end feel at early ranges of motion is often encountered during passive range of motion assessment of the patient with adhesive capsulitis (Magee, 1997). Interpretation of end feel can provide the clinician with valuable information with which to formulate a treatment program. For example, a patient with an empty, painful end feel is not a candidate for early aggressive strengthening. In general the concept of "pain before resistance" indicates an acute condition whereby the clinician uses caution regarding range of motion and strengthening

TABLE 8-4   **Classification and Description of End Feels**

CLASSIFICATION	DESCRIPTION
Bony	Two hard surfaces meeting, bone to bone (i.e., elbow extension)
Capsular	Leathery feel, further motion available (shoulder external rotation)
Soft tissue approximation	Soft tissue contact limits further motion (elbow flexion, shoulder cross-arm adduction)
Spasm	Muscular spasm limits motion (vibrant twang)
Springy block	Intraarticular block prohibits motion (rebound is felt)
Empty	Movement causes pain, pain limits movement

From Ellenbecker TS, Mattalino AJ: Comparison of open and closed kinetic chain upper extremity tests in patients with rotator cuff pathology and glenohumeral joint instability, *J Orthop Sports Phys Ther* 25:84, 1997.

(Cyriax & Cyriax, 1983). Pain encountered with resistance indicates a subacute condition requiring light and gentle range of motion and strengthening; resistance before pain indicates a more chronic condition where vigorous interventions would be indicated to restore range of motion and strength to the injured segment or segments (Cyriax & Cyriax, 1983).

Hayes and Petersen (2001) studied the reliability of end-feel assessment and the pain-resistance sequence in subjects with painful shoulders and knees. Two physical therapists performed examinations to assess end-feel and pain-resistance sequences in two knee motions and five shoulder motions. Intrarater reliability for end-feel and pain-resistance sequences was "generally good," with kappa coefficients ranging from 0.65 to 1.00 for end-feel and 0.59 to 0.87 for pain-resistance sequence. Interrater reliability coefficients were not acceptable for end-feel classification or pain-resistance sequence. With reference to the shoulder, Hayes and Peterson (2001) found more discrepancy in the end-feel classification of shoulder abduction. They attributed this discrepancy to the lack of standardized stabilization of the scapula, which could lead to confusing interpretations of end feel based on the amount and technique of scapular stabilization used by the examiner. This finding again points to the importance of scapular stabilization and the use of examination methods that are standardized to enhance reliability and effectiveness (Ellenbecker et al, 1996; Hayes & Peterson, 2001).

SUMMARY

This chapter has provided important concepts for assessing the physiologic mobility of the glenohumeral and scapulothoracic joints. The combination of the information obtained during measurement and analysis of this physiologic movement of the shoulder, coupled with the accessory mobility assessment covered in the section on glenohumeral joint instability testing, gives the clinician vital information for formulation of an evidence-based treatment program to address hypermobility or hypomobility of the glenohumeral joint.

SPECIAL
TESTS

Glenohumeral Joint
Instability Testing

INTRODUCTION

Historically, one of the primary methods to test for glenohumeral joint instability was the apprehension test (Hoppenfeld, 1976). Although the apprehension test is still used in today's clinical evaluation of the shoulder, many additional tests are now available to more accurately identify and classify glenohumeral joint instability. The close association between glenohumeral joint instability and rotator cuff pathology requires the use of these tests in virtually all clinical evaluations of the shoulder (Jobe & Bradley, 1989; Ellenbecker, 1995).

In addition to identifying the presence of apprehension with shoulder movement in patients with glenohumeral joint instability, the clinician must be able to assess the amount and degree of humeral head translation in three directions, as well as the effects of humeral head translation on pain reproduction in the individual with suspected instability. This chapter describes tests to diagnose glenohumeral joint instability based on three primary factors—pain provocation, apprehension, and humeral head translation.

CLASSIFICATION OF GLENOHUMERAL JOINT INSTABILITY

Many classification schemes and terms can be used to describe glenohumeral joint instability including acute versus chronic, first-time versus recurrent, traumatic versus atraumatic, voluntary versus involuntary, and subluxation versus dislocation (Hawkins & Mohtadi, 1991). Each of these descriptions can be addressed during both subjective questioning of the patient and objective testing. It is important that instability of the glenohumeral joint be thought of as a spectrum of disease or pathology (Hawkins & Mohtadi, 1991). Table 9-1 presents one way of classifying many of the components of glenohumeral joint instability.

By incorporating many of the components in Table 9-1, Matsen et al (1991) described two acronyms, *TUBS* and *AMBRI,* to classify shoulder instability. These represent both ends of the instability spectrum.

TUBS refers to a patient with *t*raumatic *u*nidirectional instability with a *B*ankart lesion, which usually requires *s*urgery to correct. The classic example of a TUBS patient is a football quarterback who is tackled with the shoulder in a position of abduction and external rotation while preparing to throw. The forceful movements into greater degrees of external rotation, horizontal abduction, and abduction in this example often lead to an anterior unidirectional dislocation of the shoulder that requires surgery to repair the Bankart lesion (detachment of the anterior inferior labrum from the glenoid) in order to restore glenohumeral joint stability. The TUBS patient is also commonly referred to as the "torn loose" patient, based on the traumatic incident that produced the unidirectional dislocation.

The AMBRI type of instability has an *a*traumatic onset and is most often *m*ultidirectional in nature, occurring in patients with *b*ilateral glenohumeral joint laxity and generalized joint laxity. These patients typically respond best to *r*ehabilitation and, if surgery is required, an *i*nferior capsular shift is most often performed. The AMBRI patient is also commonly referred to as the "born loose" patient. A classic example of an AMBRI patient is a young female volleyball player with anterior shoulder pain and inability to perform overhead movements.

DIRECTIONS OF GLENOHUMERAL JOINT INSTABILITY

As a precursor to the discussion of specific tests to identify glenohumeral joint instability, it is imperative to describe the actual directions of glenohumeral joint instability. Three typical directions are discussed in the literature: anterior, posterior, and multidirectional (Hawkins & Mohtadi, 1991; Jobe & Bradley, 1989). They are named according to the direction of movement of the humeral head relative to the glenoid.

Anterior glenohumeral joint instability results when the humeral head traverses excessively in an anterior direction relative to the glenoid, producing symptoms of pain, apprehension, or loss of function. Dislocations of the

TABLE 9-1   Classification of Glenohumeral Joint Instability Using Five Main Components

COMPONENTS	
Timing/frequency	Acute versus chronic
	First time versus recurrent
Direction	Anterior
	Posterior
	Multidirectional (inferior)
Onset	Traumatic
	Atraumatic
	Overuse
Volition	Voluntary
	Involuntary
Degree	Dislocation
	Subluxation

Adapted from Hawkins RJ, Mohtadi NGH: Clinical evaluation of shoulder instability, *Clin J Sports Med* 1:59-64, 1991.

shoulder account for approximately 45% of the dislocations in the human body (Kazar & Relovszky, 1969); of those, 85% are anterior glenohumeral joint dislocations (Cave et al, 1974). Subcoracoid dislocation is the most common type of anterior glenohumeral joint dislocation (Matsen et al, 1998). The usual mechanism of subcoracoid dislocation is a combination of glenohumeral joint abduction, extension, and external rotation forces that produces a challenge to the anterior capsule and capsular ligaments, glenoid rim, and rotator cuff mechanism (Matsen et al, 1998).

Posterior glenohumeral joint instability occurs when there is excessive movement of the humeral head in a posterior direction relative to the glenoid, producing symptoms. The most common posterior glenohumeral joint dislocation is the subacromial dislocation. Posterior dislocations are frequently locked (Hawkins et al, 1987). They are reported to occur only 2% of the time; however, they are also the most frequently missed diagnosis with respect to shoulder instability (Matsen et al, 1998).

Carter Rowe (1962) was the first to report that atraumatic instability could occur in more than one direction. Neer and Foster (1980) called the combined type of instability *multidirectional*. Multidirectional instability consists primarily of an inferior instability with excessive inferior movement of the humeral head relative to the glenoid, with concomitant anterior and/or posterior excessive symptomatic mobility.

ADDITIONAL TERMINOLOGY

It is important to note the difference between instability and laxity. *Laxity* can be defined as translation of the

humeral head relative to the glenoid when stress is applied (Matsen, 1992). When defining laxity, reference should be made to both humeral position and the direction of the force applied (Borsa et al, 1999). A minimal amount of humeral head translation or laxity is required for normal glenohumeral joint rotation to occur (McFarland et al, 1996). Glenohumeral translation associated with humeral rotation has been called *coupled* or *obligate motion* (Harryman et al, 1990; Hawkins et al, 1996).

Instability can be defined as excessive symptomatic translation of the humeral head relative to the glenoid when stress is applied. According to Matsen (1992), this excessive or "unwanted" translation compromises shoulder function and produces clinical symptoms. It is important to use these terms in proper context when evaluating the patient with glenohumeral joint pathology, because individuals possess varying amounts of glenohumeral joint laxity but only those with clinical symptoms and functional limitations can be described as having instability.

TESTS TO EVALUATE FOR GLENOHUMERAL JOINT INSTABILITY

As mentioned previously, glenohumeral joint instability tests rely on three primary factors: apprehension, humeral head translation, and pain provocation/replication.

Apprehension Test

Indication

The apprehension test is a test used to determine glenohumeral joint instability.

About the Test

This test uses the common instability movement pattern of abduction, external rotation, and horizontal abduction/extension to provoke the patient's shoulder.

Start Position

The patient is typically examined in a seated position to minimize compensatory movements during examination, but the patient can be evaluated in the standing, supine, or even prone position (Rowe & Zarins, 1981; Andrews & Wilk, 1994). The examiner should be positioned so that careful monitoring of the intended patient response can occur. Figure 9-1 shows the clinician positioned behind the patient. This clinician-patient alignment is particularly effective when a mirror or reflection allows the clinician to clearly see the patient's facial response. In an alternative position, the clinician stands to the lateral side of the involved extremity or directly in front of the patient.

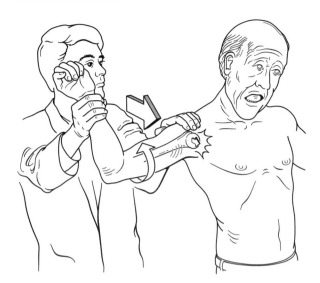

Figure 9-1 Apprehension test. (Modified from Hoppenfeld S, Hutton R: Physical examination of the shoulder. In Hoppenfeld S: *Physical examination of the spine and extremities*, Norwalk, CT, 1976, Appleton-Century-Crofts.)

Action

The clinician passively brings the patient's affected arm into 90 degrees of abduction and full external rotation, while slightly horizontally abducting/extending the extremity just posterior to the coronal plane of the patient's body. One of the examiner's hands is placed just proximal to the wrist on the distal aspect of the patient's involved extremity, and the other hand is placed on the posterior aspect of the humerus (see Figure 9-1). If the patient's initial movement is well tolerated, pressure may then be applied to the posterior aspect of the shoulder, pushing the humeral head in an anterior direction to further provoke the patient's extremity (Davies et al, 1981).

What Constitutes a Positive Test?

The apprehension test does not actually measure the translation of the head of the humerus in any way. It uses solely the position of instability (90 degrees of glenohumeral abduction with external rotation) as a provocation to induce apprehension by the patient. The patient's response is the only criterion evaluated during this maneuver. The test is similar to the patellar apprehension test, which is used to diagnose dislocation of the patella (Hoppenfeld, 1976).

Ramifications of a Positive Test

A positive apprehension test indicates anterior glenohumeral instability and informs the clinician that the patient cannot tolerate this position because of a lack of stability in the glenohumeral articulation. This test can be

used during initial evaluation of a patient with a clinical history consistent with anterior glenohumeral joint instability, as well as a criterion test in returning the athletic or industrial patient back to function after rehabilitation. Unlike other tests that attempt to quantify the amount of humeral head translation, this test indicates the patient's willingness and confidence in the 90/90 position inherent in many functional activities in both sport and industry.

Modifications of the Apprehension Test

Indication

Variations of the classic apprehension test can be used to further provoke the patient with glenohumeral joint instability. These variations use alternative patient positions and forces applied to the proximal humerus.

About the Tests

Magee (1997) described the apprehension crank test for patients with anterior glenohumeral joint instability. The test is performed with the patient in the supine position with 90 degrees of glenohumeral joint abduction. The examiner externally rotates the shoulder slowly, monitoring the patient's expression and muscle guarding. A positive test is indicated by a look or feeling of apprehension on the patient's face. Resistance to further motion and patient reporting that the shoulder feels like it did on prior episodes of instability also characterize a positive test.

The Rowe test (Rowe, 1988) for anterior instability is also performed with the patient in the supine position. The patient places a hand behind the head, such that the glenohumeral joint is placed in abduction and external rotation. The examiner places one hand (clenched fist) under the proximal aspect of the posterior humeral head and pushes gently in an anterior direction, while the examiner's other hand flexes the shoulder via a downward-directed force at the patient's elbow (Figure 9-2). A look of apprehension or reproduction of the patient's pain is considered a positive indicator for anterior glenohumeral joint instability.

Objective Evidence Regarding These Tests

No formal research has been reported on any of the apprehension tests for diagnosing glenohumeral joint instability.

Humeral Head Translation Tests

Introduction

The most important tests that identify shoulder joint instability are humeral head translation tests (McFarland et al, 1996a, 1996b; Gerber & Ganz, 1984). These tests

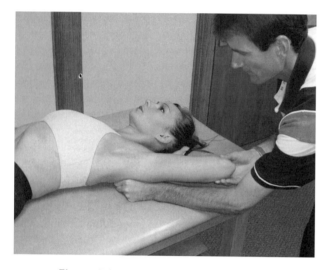

Figure **9-2** Rowe test for anterior instability.

attempt to document the amount of movement of the humeral head relative to the glenoid through the use of carefully applied directional stresses to the proximal humerus.

Harryman et al (1992) measured the amount of humeral head translation in vivo in healthy, uninjured subjects using a three-dimensional spatial tracking system. This device was pinned percutaneously to the humerus and scapula of eight normal subjects. They found a mean of 7.8 mm of anterior translation and 7.9 mm of posterior translation using an anterior and posterior drawer test (see pages 74–78). Translation of the human shoulder in an inferior direction was evaluated using a multidirectional instability (MDI) sulcus test (see pages 68–70 for description of this test). During the in vivo testing of inferior humeral head translation, an average of 10 mm of inferior displacement was measured. Results from this detailed laboratory-based research study indicate that approximately a 1:1 ratio of anterior to posterior humeral head translation can be expected in normal shoulders with manual humeral head translation tests. The research did not provide a definitive interpretation of bilateral symmetry in humeral head translation.

In vivo assessment of human glenohumeral joint translation was also reported by Borsa et al (1999), in normal healthy shoulders using a laboratory-based, instrumented arthrometer. Results of their testing, which examined the shoulder in 20 degrees of scapular plane elevation and neutral rotation (a position similar to that used during clinical testing with the load and shift test [pages 71–74]) showed no significant difference between extremities

(dominant/nondominant). Mean anterior humeral head translation was 8.0 mm, with mean posterior translation of 6.0 mm. Although a wide variation existed in anterior and posterior humeral head translation in this study, most subjects had less than 10 mm of anterior or posterior translation.

Results of these studies (Harryman et al, 1992; Borsa et al, 1996) support the theory reported by Speer (1995), that a wide spectrum of laxity with a normal distribution exists among healthy shoulders.

By using an ultrasonic measurement technique, Krarup et al (1999) documented anterior humeral head translation bilaterally in asymptomatic subjects and patients diagnosed with anterior glenohumeral joint instability. Bilateral differences of only 1.9 mm in healthy shoulders and 4.9 mm in unstable shoulders were reliably documented with patients in a seated position. Ellenbecker et al (2000a) used a stress radiography technique to measure anterior humeral head translation in asymptomatic, healthy professional baseball pitchers (Figure 9-3). The glenohumeral joint was assessed with 90 degrees of glenohumeral joint abduction in both neutral rotation and 60 degrees of external rotation. No significant difference in anterior humeral head translation was reliably measured between extremities in either position of humeral rotation.

These studies have identified relative symmetry between paired extremities (dominant/nondominant) in both normal subjects and overhead athletes. Both Harryman et al (1992) and Borsa et al (1999) reported similar values for average anterior and posterior humeral head translation between 6 and 8 mm. These objective studies can guide the clinician during the use of manual humeral head translation tests.

Grading Anteroposterior Humeral Head Translation During Manual Clinical Tests

Before discussing the specific humeral head translation tests used in the clinical examination, it is imperative to review the grading methods that can be used to interpret the results of these tests. Assessment of glenohumeral joint mobility during the clinical examination includes both physiologic and accessory range of motion. Physiologic mobility assessment is typically performed using both active and passive range of motion measurement, quantified with a goniometer or other clinically applicable recording system (see Active and Passive Range of Motion). Physiologic movements of the glenohumeral joint include those motions that are under the patient's control (Gould, 1985). Examples of these movements include flexion/extension, abduction/adduction, and

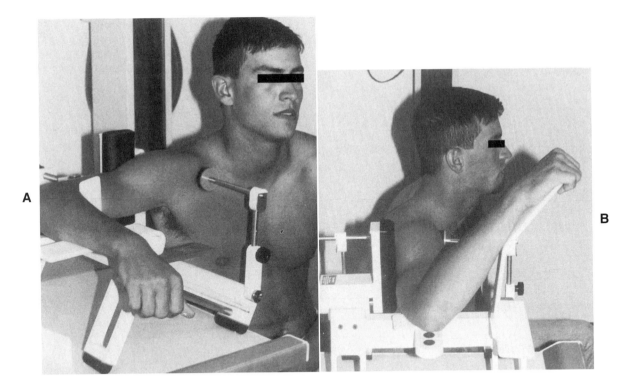

Figure 9-3 Shoulder stress radiography procedure with the shoulder in **A,** neutral rotation, and **B,** 60 degrees of external rotation. (Adapted from Ellenbecker TS, et al: Anterior translation of the humeral head in the throwing shoulder, *Am J Sports Med* 28(2):163, 2000, with permission.)

internal/external rotation. Accessory mobility testing involves measuring the movements that are not under the control of the patient. These motions include anterior, posterior, and inferior gliding, also known as *humeral head translation*. It is these accessory movements of the human shoulder that are tested and graded to facilitate a determination of the underlying accessory mobility status.

Grading humeral head translation has been reported using primarily three systems. These systems use measurement in millimeters of translation (Harryman et al, 1990; Richards et al, 1994), relationship of translation to the glenoid rim (Altchek & Dines, 1993), and percentage of humeral head translated across the glenoid (Hawkins & Mohtadi, 1991).

American Shoulder Elbow Surgeons Grading System

Guidelines established by the American Shoulder Elbow Surgeons (Richards et al, 1994) use techniques to grade or provide an estimation of the amount of humeral head translation. Specific guidelines have been established for anterior/posterior translation testing, as well as inferior humeral head translation testing.

For anterior/posterior tests of humeral head translation, grade 0 translation denotes no translation, grade I translation represents mild translation (0 to 1 cm) up the glenoid face, and grade II represents moderate translation of 1 to 2 cm up to the glenoid rim. Grade III translation is termed *severe translation* and consists of anterior or posterior translation greater than 2 cm and over the glenoid rim.

The American Shoulder Elbow Surgeons guidelines for grading inferior translation include grade 0 (no translation); grade I, mild translation (0 to 1 cm); grade II, moderate translation (1 to 2 cm); and grade III, severe inferior translation (>2 cm).

Some authors believe that estimating humeral head translation in millimeters is inexact and problematic (McFarland et al, 1996a). No study has examined the intraobserver and interobserver error and reliability using this technique. The technique is most applicable when using laboratory-based methods of measuring humeral head excursion such as stress radiography and instrumented arthrometers (Ellenbecker et al, 2000a; Ellenbecker et al, 2002a; Borsa et al, 1999).

TABLE 9-2   **Altchek Humeral Head Translation Grading System**

GRADE	GLENOHUMERAL JOINT TRANSLATION
I	Humeral head rides up the glenoid slope but not over the glenoid rim
II	Humeral head rides up and over the glenoid rim but spontaneously reduces when stress is removed
III	Humeral head rides up and over the glenoid rim and remains dislocated on removal of stress

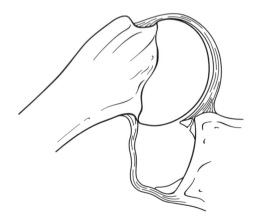

Figure 9-5 Grade II humeral head translation using the Altchek classification. (From Altchek DW, Warren RF, Wickiewicz TL, et al: Arthroscopic labral debridement: a three-year follow-up study, *Am J Sports Med* 20(6):703, 1992.)

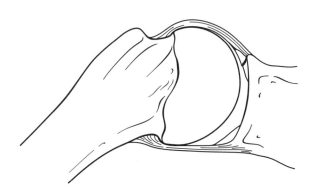

Figure 9-4 Grade I humeral head translation using the Altchek classification. (From Altchek DW, Warren RF, Wickiewicz TL, et al: Arthroscopic labral debridement: a three-year follow-up study, *Am J Sports Med* 20(6):703, 1992.)

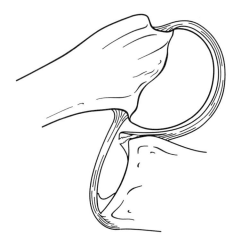

Figure 9-6 Grade III humeral head translation using the Altchek classification. (From Altchek DW, Warren RF, Wickiewicz TL, et al: Arthroscopic labral debridement: a three-year follow-up study, *Am J Sports Med* 20(6):703, 1992.)

Altchek Humeral Head Translation Grading Method (Author's Preferred Method)

Altchek et al (1992) proposed a system for grading anterior and posterior humeral head translation during examination under anesthesia. This system has been widely used and adapted for clinical interpretation of humeral head translation tests (Ellenbecker et al, 2002a) and grades humeral head translation relative to the glenoid. Table 9-2 and Figures 9-4 through 9-6 outline the characteristics of each of the three grades outlined in Altchek's grading system.

In addition to the three grades of humeral head translation listed in Table 9-2, a plus (+) sign can also be used to designate a softer, more compliant end feel during testing and can allow the clinician to further describe humeral head translation (Ellenbecker et al, 2002a). *End feel* has been defined as the feeling transmitted to the examiner's hands at the extreme range of passive motion (Cyriax & Cyriax, 1983) (see End Feels).

Objective Testing of Altchek Grading System

Ellenbecker et al (2002a) studied the intrarater and interrater reliability of the Altchek grading system for anterior humeral head translation in human subjects. Fifteen asymptomatic subjects with varying degrees of anterior glenohumeral joint laxity were clinically tested using anterior humeral head translation tests by two orthopedic surgeons, three physical therapists, and two nonorthopedic physicians. Subjects' identities were shielded from the examiners to prevent bias during testing and retesting the subjects. Examiners were asked to perform the anterior humeral head translation test with 90 degrees of glenohumeral joint abduction and to grade the tests using the Altchek grading system, using the addition of a (+) to designate end feel. Examiners had four possible humeral head translation conditions (I, I+, II, and II+) during bilateral testing and retesting of the 15 subjects. Statistical analysis included the use of a kappa coefficient and coefficient of agreement for the translation conditions, including end feel, and were 0.342 and 54%, respectively, increasing to 0.529 and 81.4%, respectively, when statistical analyses were conducted using only the distinction between grades I and II with no reference to end feel. Results of this study do not support the use of the additional mobility designation for end feel during anterior humeral head translation tests because of the low kappa coefficient and coefficient of agreement.

Interrater reliability with all four possible grades (I, I+, II, II+) resulted in a coefficient of agreement of 37.3% and kappa coefficient of 0.091. When end feel was not considered, the coefficient of agreement increased to 70.4%, with a kappa coefficient of 0.208. Results of this study indicate that both intrarater and interrater reliability of a manual anterior humeral head translation test is improved when only the relationship of the humeral head to the glenoid rim is considered. The addition of an end feel designation to the Altchek grading system results in a decrease in reliability both within and among examiners.

Levy et al (1999) conducted a test-retest reliability study of anterior and posterior humeral head translation tests, as well as the MDI sulcus sign. Asymptomatic NCAA division I athletes served as subjects and were tested initially and again after 3 months. Humeral head translation was graded from 0 to 3+ by four physicians. With the four possible grading conditions (0 [trace], 1+, 2+, and 3+) overall intraobserver reproducibility was 46%, with interobserver reliability of 47%. Improved intraobserver and interobserver reliability was reported when grades 0 and 1+ were combined. These results are similar to the improved reliability coefficients reported by Ellenbecker et al (2002a) with the elimination of the (+) designation for end feel.

Additional Grading Systems to Interpret Anterior and Posterior Humeral Head Translation

Hawkins and Mohtadi (1991) and Hawkins et al (1996) proposed an alternative method to communicate the amount of humeral head translation during manual clinical tests. This method also grades the movement of the humeral head relative to the glenoid but it uses an estimation of the percent width of the humeral head diameter. A mild amount of humeral head translation is considered normal (approximately <25% humeral head diameter). A

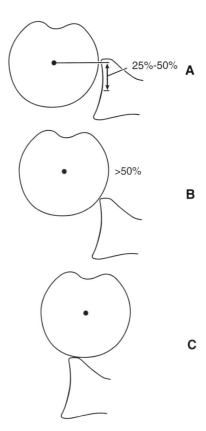

Figure 9-7 Hawkins' humeral head translation grading system. **A,** Grade I. The humeral head is translated in an anterior or posterior position up to 50% of the humeral head diameter. **B,** Grade II. The humeral head is translated greater than 50% of the humeral head diameter. **C,** Grade III. The humeral head is dislocated beyond the confines of the glenoid fossa. (From Hawkins RJ, Mohtadi NG: Clinical evaluation of shoulder instability, *Clin J Sports Med* 1(1):62, 1991.)

feeling of the humeral head riding up the glenoid face to the glenoid rim is designated as grade I translation and is typically estimated from 25% to 50% of the humeral head diameter (Figure 9-7, *A*). A feeling of the humeral head riding over the glenoid rim, but spontaneously reducing with release of the stress, is grade II translation and is estimated as greater than 50% translation (Figure 9-7, *B*). A feeling of the humeral head riding over the glenoid rim, but on release remaining dislocated, is designated grade III translation and is considered a dislocation (Figure 9-7, *C*). This grading system is traditionally applied for anterior and posterior translation only. No study has examined the intraobserver and interobserver error and reliability of this estimation method to describe humeral head translation.

Objective Quantification of Optimal Force Application during Clinical Translation Tests

Borsa et al (2001) measured the loads required to obtain a capsular end point in vivo using an instrumented device. The directions of anterior, posterior, and inferior humeral head translation were studied in asymptomatic subjects in a seated position with the arm in adduction. Loads ranging between 40 and 45 pounds were required to obtain capsular end points, with significantly more force required to obtain the anterior capsular end point as compared with the inferior direction. Borsa et al (2001) found mean translations using the instrumented arthrometer of 14.5, 14, and 13.9 mm for anterior, posterior, and inferior translations, respectively. The objective finding of directional symmetry is in agreement with other authors and supports the circle concept of glenohumeral joint stability (Borsa et al, 2001; Harryman et al, 1992; Sauers et al, 2001a, 2001b).

Application of forces of this magnitude to the shoulder in patients with glenohumeral joint pathology may not be clinically feasible. Further research has involved using smaller amounts of force application during translation testing. McQuade et al (1999) reported that a minimum of 100 newtons (22.4 pounds) was required to reach capsular end points using an electromagnetic tracking system to quantify anterior and posterior translations. Borsa et al (1999, 2000) and Sauers et al (2001a,b) used displacement forces ranging from 0 to 134 newtons (30 pounds) and reported that most nonimpaired shoulders demonstrated force-displacement curves that were still on the rise using the 30-pound force for anterior and posterior humeral head translation.

Comparing results of this research to clinical translation testing in other joints provides perspective when performing glenohumeral translation tests. The KT-1000 (Medmetric Corp., San Diego CA), a clinical device to test knee ligament laxity, uses anterior forces of 10, 20, and 30 pounds. In addition the clinician attempts to translate the tibia anteriorly relative to the femur using their maximal anterior manual force to clinically evaluate and measure knee ligament laxity in vivo. Tohyama et al (2003) reported the magnitude required to measure anterior laxity in the human ankle after injury to the anterior talofibular ligament. In the cadaveric portion of the research, the authors found greater anterior translation after sectioning of the anterior talofibular ligament at 10, 20, 30, and 40 newtons (N) of anterior load. This translation or displacement was significantly greater than the displacement measured with 60 N of anterior force. In vivo examination in the subjects with ankle injury produced greater anterior displacement with 30 N of anterior

load as compared with 60 N. The authors concluded that when evaluating the integrity of the anterior talofibular ligament in cases of acute ankle injury, a low-magnitude load should be used to identify increases in translation.

This research did not provide conclusive guidance with regard to the amount of load to use during examination of the patient with shoulder instability. Further research is needed to better define the exact magnitudes of load needed to identify glenohumeral joint instability without necessarily taking the humeral head to the capsular limit using the high forces reported in the literature. Obtaining the maximum translation with the lowest magnitude of force is desired to attempt to overcome the patient's protective response that is often elicited with larger loads. It is important to follow the specific guidelines contained in this text regarding hand placements and give careful attention to the amount of force and grasp placed on the extremity to accurately assess and interpret glenohumeral joint translation.

MDI Sulcus Sign (Neutral)

The MDI sulcus sign is also known as the *sulcus test* and the *inferior humeral head translation test*.

Indication

This test is used to diagnose multidirectional instability of the glenohumeral joint.

About the Test

This test is the primary method to identify the patient with MDI of the glenohumeral joint. Excessive translation in the inferior direction during this test most often indicates a forthcoming pattern of excessive translation in either the anterior or posterior direction or both. When performed in the neutral adducted position, the test directly assesses the integrity of the superior glenohumeral ligament and the coracohumeral ligament (Pagnani & Warren, 1994). These ligaments are the primary stabilizing structures against inferior humeral head translation in the adducted glenohumeral position (O'Brien et al, 1990).

Start Position

The patient should be examined in the seated position, with the arms in neutral adduction, resting gently in the patient's lap. The elbows are flexed 60 to 90 degrees, with the forearms in a neutral position. This position is used to foster greater muscular relaxation and to place the shoulder in the position of maximal inferior excursion. Helmig et al (1990) reported that maximal inferior excursion of the glenohumeral joint occurs in 20 degrees of abduction and slight internal rotation. The test can be performed with the patient in a standing position; however, control over the exact position of the shoulder is limited, and increased muscle guarding can be encountered with testing in this position (McFarland et al, 1996a). In one modification of this test reported by Rowe (1988), the patient is in a standing position, with 45 degrees of trunk flexion, which places the shoulder in a flexed position. This modified version has been called the *Rowe multidirectional instability test* (Magee, 1997).

Action

The examiner grasps the distal aspect of the humerus using a firm but unassuming grip with one hand, while placing the thumb and index finger on the anterior and posterior lateral corners of the acromion for reference (Figure 9-8). Several brief, relatively rapid downward pulls are exerted to the humerus in an inferior (vertical) direction.

What Constitutes a Positive Test?

A visible *sulcus sign* is usually present in patients with MDI (Hawkins & Mohtadi, 1991). Figure 9-9 shows a patient with a positive sulcus sign as demonstrated by tethering of the skin between the lateral acromion and humerus from the increase in inferior translation of the humeral head and widening subacromial space in patients with MDI.

Mallon & Speer (1995) recommended grading the sulcus sign as grade I, less than 1 cm of inferior translation; grade II, 1.0 to 1.5 cm of inferior translation; and grade III, 1.5 cm of translation. No formal reliability research is available using this grading system for inferior translation.

Ramifications of a Positive Test

A positive test indicates that the patient has increased physiologic laxity of the glenohumeral joint capsule and will possess increased humeral head translation in additional directions during clinical testing and functional use or activities. Increases in inferior humeral head translation in the symptomatic glenohumeral joint have been identified in patients diagnosed with multidirectional glenohumeral joint instability (Hawkins et al, 1996; Warner et al, 1990).

The MDI test should be the initial examination in the clinical evaluation to identify the presence of increased physiologic laxity. If the test is positive, the clinician should expect greater translation of the humeral head during anteroposterior translation tests and other instabil-

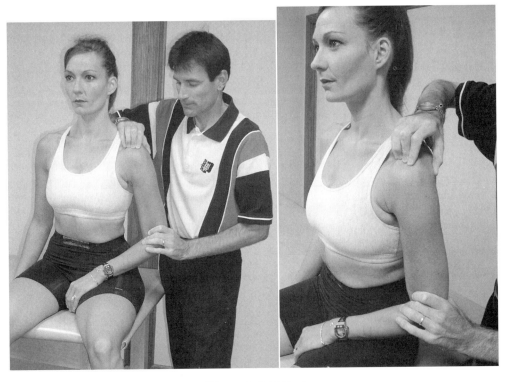

Figure **9-8** MDI sulcus test.

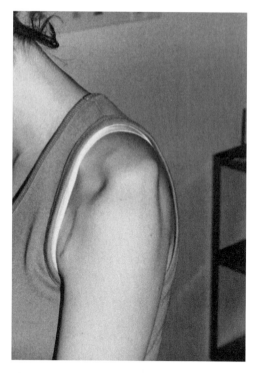

Figure 9-9 Positive MDI sulcus sign in a patient's left shoulder.

found to have grade III translation in any direction, including inferior humeral head translation using an MDI sulcus sign. Also, humeral head translation up to II+ was found in asymptomatic athletes, with as much as 32% of the asymptomatic athletes tested having a bilateral difference in humeral head translation of up to one grade.

Emery and Mullaji (1991) tested 75 British school-children with no history of shoulder pathology; 11% had positive sulcus signs and 26% had asymmetric laxity with respect to bilateral comparison. In another study evaluating 356 high school and college athletes without a history of shoulder symptoms, McFarland et al (1991) reported a grade II sulcus sign in 52%, with 5% of the asymptomatic athletes having a grade III sulcus sign.

Bigliani et al (1997) measured glenohumeral joint range of motion and laxity in 148 asymptomatic professional baseball players; 61% (44 of 72) of the pitchers and 47% (36 of 76) of the position players had a positive sulcus sign on their dominant arm. Of the players with positive sulcus signs, 89% of the pitchers and 100% of the position players had bilateral signs.

These studies provide important descriptive information for the interpretation of manual humeral head translation tests. Unilateral increases in humeral head translation alone, without symptoms, do not necessarily indicate instability. Instability by definition is the excessive symptomatic, unwanted translation of the humeral head that leads to decrements in shoulder function (McFarland et al, 1996a). No additional objective research on the validity of this test has been reported.

MDI Sulcus Sign (90 Degrees Abduction)

This test is also known as the *Feagin test* (Rockwood, 1984).

Indication

The MDI sulcus sign in 90 degrees of abduction is used to identify MDI of the shoulder in the functional position of 90 degrees of glenohumeral joint abduction.

About the Test

This clinical maneuver tests the integrity of the inferior glenohumeral ligament complex and is used in combination with the traditional MDI sulcus sign to provide a complete assessment of inferior stability of the glenohumeral joint.

Start Position

The test is typically performed with the patient in a seated position, but it can also be done with the patient standing, with particular care taken to prevent compensa-

ity tests performed during a thorough evaluation process. Extensive rehabilitation is indicated for patients with positive MDI sulcus signs to improve the dynamic stabilizers of the glenohumeral joint to compensate for the increased capsular mobility identified with this clinical test.

Objective Evidence Regarding the Test

Tzannes and Murrell (2002) found the sulcus sign to have a specificity of 97% for MDI when the sulcus is estimated manually at 2 cm or more. At this level, the sensitivity is relatively poor (28%) (Tzannes & Murrell, 2002). Thus, using the criterion of 2 cm or more of inferior translation during the sulcus test to indicate MDI, 72% of patients would not be diagnosed if only this test were performed. Using a criterion of MDI of a sulcus sign greater than 1 cm, Tzannes and Murrell (2002) reported a sensitivity of 72% and specificity of 85%. A much greater sensitivity using this criterion was reported, but, as often occurs, the specificity decreased from 97% to 85%. Tzannes and Murrell (2002) also reported substantial interobserver error using the sulcus sign with intraclass correlation coefficient values of 0.66 between experienced examiners.

Lintner et al (1996) tested 76 asymptomatic division I athletes using anterior, posterior, and inferior humeral head translation tests. During testing, no athlete was

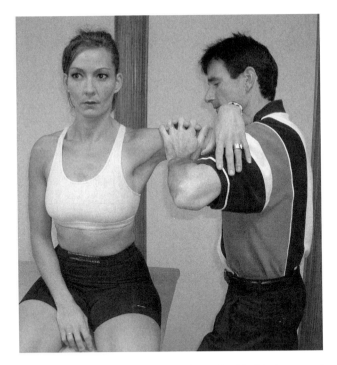

Figure 9-10 MDI sulcus test performed with 90 degrees of glenohumeral joint abduction.

tions from adjoining segments. The examiner sits or stands next to the patient on the involved side of the shoulder to be tested. The glenohumeral joint is abducted 90 degrees in the coronal plane in neutral rotation (Figure 9-10). The patient's elbow can be placed over the examiner's shoulder to provide stability during testing and to allow both hands of the examiner to be free to directly perform the next action.

Action
The examiner's hands are placed such that the fingers are interlocked together, with the ulnar side of the fifth digits placed just lateral to the acromion over the proximal humerus (see Figure 9-10). The examiner then exerts a downward (vertical) force with the glenohumeral joint in 90 degrees of coronal plane abduction. The examiner feels the amount of translation inferiorly and compares that amount with the contralateral extremity.

What Constitutes a Positive Test?
A positive test includes increased inferior humeral head translation in a symptomatic shoulder, a hallmark sign of multidirectional glenohumeral joint instability (Hawkins et al, 1996). The inferior excursion of the humeral head relative to the glenoid is estimated using grading guidelines similar to those proposed for the traditional MDI

sulcus sign in neutral adduction. This recommended grading system, as described by Mallon and Speer (1995), is as follows: grade I, less than 1 cm of inferior translation; grade II, 1.0 to 1.5 cm of inferior translation; and grade III, greater than 1.5 cm of translation. A visible sulcus sign is less prominent and often visible only when substantial inferior translation is present. The MDI test at 90 degrees of abduction requires greater use of estimation and actually feeling the amount of movement by the examiner's hands than the MDI sulcus sign in neutral adduction, which includes the added visual cue of the tethering response in the skin at the lateral border of the acromion.

Ramifications of a Positive Test
A positive MDI sulcus sign indicates increased physiologic laxity of the glenohumeral joint capsule. The specific portion of the capsule being tested is the inferior glenohumeral ligament complex because of its role in providing inferior stability for the humeral head in 90 degrees of glenohumeral joint abduction (O'Brien et al, 1990). Increases in inferior translation identified using the MDI sulcus test at 90 degrees of abduction should also alert the examiner to the likely increase in anterior and posterior translation that will be encountered during anterior and posterior humeral head translation tests. Attenuation of the inferior glenohumeral ligament complex has serious consequences for glenohumeral joint function at 90 degrees of abduction (O'Brien et al, 1990).

Objective Evidence Regarding the Test
No research is available for the MDI sulcus test at 90 degrees of glenohumeral joint abduction.

Load and Shift Test
This test is also known as the *push-pull test*.

Indication
The load and shift test is used to assess anteroposterior humeral head translation.

About the Test
This test measures anterior and posterior humeral head excursion with the glenohumeral joint in a neutral adducted position. In this position the anterior capsule, specifically the superior glenohumeral joint ligament, is stressed with anterior humeral head excursion, and the posterior capsule is stressed with posterior humeral head translation (Pagnani & Warren, 1994). The test is done with the patient in a seated position, which may be advantageous in clinical situations where performing humeral

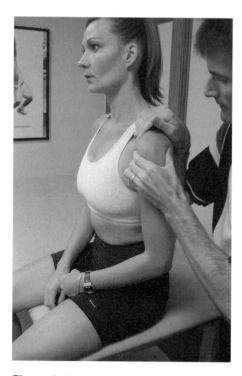 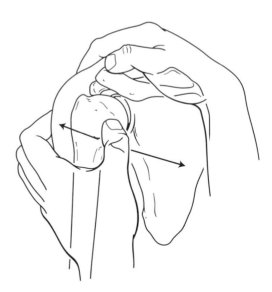

Figure 9-11 Load and shift test. Clinical testing technique depicting underlying shoulder anatomic structures. (From Hawkins RJ, Mohtadi NG: Clinical evaluation of shoulder instability, *Clin J Sports Med* 1(1):63, 1991.)

head translation tests in the supine position is nonoptimal because of transfers or secondary orthopedic and/or general medical complications. Only an adducted glenohumeral joint position can be used because of this seated position.

Starting Position

The patient is examined in a seated position, such that the examiner can either stand or sit directly to the side of the shoulder being examined. Care should be taken to use an upright, erect posture during examination of both extremities, as Kebaetse et al (1999) reported changes in scapular and glenohumeral kinematics with altered thoracic postures. The patient's hands can be placed in the lap to promote muscular relaxation and bilaterally symmetric glenohumeral positions. To test the right shoulder, the examiner's left hand is placed over the patient's shoulder such that the index, second, and third fingers can palpate and rest against the coracoid process and clavicle to stabilize the scapula. The thumb is placed over the posterior lateral aspect of the acromion and oriented nearly horizontally along the spine of the scapula. Flexion of the examiner's wrist is recommended, so that the examiner's

forearm (flexor surface) can provide further stabilization to the scapula. The examiner's right hand grasps the humerus just distal to the humeral head (Figure 9-11). A wide enough grip must be used to contain the humerus and not simply the deltoid and overlying skin, which is a common error when the test is done by inexperienced examiners.

Action

With hands placed on the patient's scapula and humerus, a gentle direct load is placed medially by the hand on the proximal humerus, approximating the humeral head into the glenoid. This maneuver centers the humeral head into the glenoid and provides a neutral, "centered" starting position; this is the "load" portion of the load and shift test. After gently providing the load, the examiner attempts to translate the humeral head in an anteromedial direction, using the thumb posteriorly as the primary point of pressure. It is extremely important to note that the direction of force applied by the examiner to produce translation should be parallel along the line of the glenoid fossa (Figure 9-12). This anteromedial direction of translation displaces the humeral head within the glenoid and

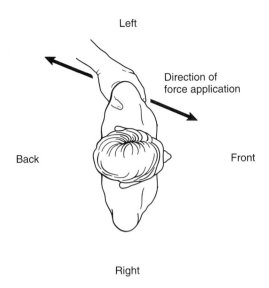

Left

Direction of
force application

Back

Front

Right

Figure 9-12 Load and shift test overhead view with *arrow* showing direction of translation along the lines of the glenohumeral joint for both anterior and posterior humeral head translation.

is oriented at approximately 30 degrees relative to the sagittal plane of the body. Performing translation in the sagittal plane in a straight plane anteriorly and posteriorly results in nonoptimal translation and compression of the humeral head into the posterior glenoid during the posterior part of this test.

The examiner notes the amount of translation, using the criterion reported by Altchek and Dines (1993). Translation within the glenoid without traversing the glenoid rim is considered grade I translation; translation up over the glenoid rim with spontaneous reduction on removal of the anteromedial load is considered grade II.

After the anteromedial translation is assessed, a posterior lateral direction of translation is performed along the line of the joint (Figure 9-11, *posterior arrow*). Similar to the anterior portion of this test, the posterior direction of translation is actually posterolateral, following the line of the glenoid fossa. Careful monitoring of the direction of translation ensures optimal amounts of translation with the applied force. Posterior translation is graded using identical criteria as outlined for anterior translation. Anteromedial and posterolateral translation is typically repeated to optimally assess the amount of humeral head translation. This relatively rapid succession of the anteroposterior translations has led many clinicians to refer to this test as the *push-pull test*.

What Constitutes a Positive Test?

A unilateral increase in humeral head translation in the direction of either anterior or posterior or in both directions in the symptomatic shoulder leads to the diagnosis of either anterior or posterior instability, based on the direction of increased humeral head translation relative to the contralateral, asymptomatic extremity (Hawkins et al, 1996). A unilateral increase in anterior, posterior, or both anterior and posterior, coupled with increased inferior translation during the MDI sulcus test (see pages 68–70) indicates the presence of MDI in the patient's involved glenohumeral joint (Hawkins et al, 1996).

Ramifications of a Positive Test

A positive load and shift test indicates capsular insufficiency of the superior capsular structures because of the adducted position inherent in this test. Unidirectional increases in anterior humeral head translation are indicative of injury to the superior glenohumeral ligament (SGHL) (Pagnani & Warren, 1994) and lead to the diagnosis of unidirectional anterior glenohumeral joint instability. Identification of increased anterior humeral head translation requires the use of rehabilitative exercise to enhance the dynamic stabilization of the posterior rotator cuff in order to attenuate anterior humeral head translation and strain on the anterior capsular structures (Cain et al, 1987). A positive load and shift test in the posterior direction indicates posterior capsular redundancy and leads to the diagnosis of unidirectional posterior instability.

Objective Evidence Regarding the Test

Instrumented laxity testing of the glenohumeral joint, performed by Borsa et al (1999) using the load and shift test, resulted in humeral head translations of 8.0 mm for anterior translation and 6.0 mm for posterior translation. Manual laxity tests are thought to be performed with approximately 67 to 89 N of force. Borsa et al (1999) used similar loads in their instrumented study of normal subjects to produce these translation values. They showed slightly greater anterior humeral head translation with the load and shift test position than posterior humeral head translation. This is in slight contrast to values also measured in vivo by Harryman et al (1990), who found essentially the same amount of anterior humeral head translation as posterior humeral head translation in normal healthy volunteers.

Hawkins et al (1996) tested normal subjects, patients diagnosed with anterior glenohumeral joint instability, and patients with MDI, with all subjects under general anesthesia, using the load and shift tests to measure ante-

TABLE 9-3   Humeral Head Translation of Normal and Unstable Shoulders

SUBJECT TYPE	ANTERIOR	POSTERIOR	INFERIOR
Normal	17%	26%	29%
Anterior instability	29%	21%	40%
Multidirectional instability	28%	52%	46%

Values expressed as percentage of the width of humeral head translated over the glenoid, with 100% being complete dislocation and 0% being no humeral head translation.

From Hawkins RJ, Schulte JP, Janda DH, et al: Translation of the glenohumeral joint with the patient under anesthesia, *J Shoulder Elbow Surg* 5:286-292, 1996.

rior and posterior humeral head translation, as well as the sulcus sign for inferior translation. They used an estimation of the percent width of the humeral head that could be translated out of the glenoid to report humeral head translation. Results of their research are summarized in Table 9-3.

Normal subjects had slightly greater posterior than anterior humeral head translation with the load and shift test. Patients with the diagnosis of anterior glenohumeral joint instability had greater anterior translation than control or normal subjects (almost twice as much), with less posterior translation. Patients diagnosed with MDI had increased anterior, posterior, and inferior translation of the humeral head compared with control subjects, and increased posterior and inferior humeral head translation than the subjects with anterior instability. This study showed how these manual humeral head translation tests can be used to quantify and classify patients into diagnostic categories such as normal, unidirectional, and multidirectional instability.

Lintner et al (1996) used manual anterior, posterior, and inferior humeral head translation tests and found that laxity of up to grade II (Altchek classification) can be expected in any direction in normal healthy shoulders of NCAA division I athletes. The authors reported asymmetric humeral head translation in 32% of the athletes tested, including those from overhead sports. These findings help the examiner interpret clinical findings of anterior and posterior humeral head translation tests. Unilateral increases in translation by one grade (Altchek classification), as well as translations of up to grade II, can be expected in normal healthy subjects. Translation in an extremity without symptoms or functional loss is not considered a positive finding for glenohumeral joint instability.

Tzannes and Murrell (2002) reported the validity of the load and shift test for anterior and posterior directions. They found 50% sensitivity and 100% specificity for the anterior direction, and 14% sensitivity and 100% specificity for the posterior direction. No additional specificity and sensitivity information is available.

Anterior Drawer Test

Indication

The anterior drawer test is a primary test to measure anterior humeral head translation in multiple positions of glenohumeral joint abduction.

About the Test

Gerber and Ganz (1984) and McFarland et al (1996a) believe testing for anterior and posterior shoulder laxity is best performed with the patient in the supine position because of greater inherent relaxation of the patient. This test allows the patient's extremity to be tested in multiple positions of glenohumeral joint abduction, thus selectively stressing specific portions of the glenohumeral joint anterior capsule and capsular ligaments. All three portions of the glenohumeral joint capsular ligament complex (superior, middle, and inferior glenohumeral ligaments) can be assessed using this test.

Start Position

The patient is tested in a supine position. The examiner's left hand is placed on the inside of the patient's left elbow (to assess the left shoulder of a patient), while grasping circumferentially just above the antecubital fossa. The hand grasping the patient's elbow is responsible for maintaining the position of the scapular plane (30 degrees anterior to the coronal or frontal plane) while testing all ranges of abduction. A position of neutral rotation is recommended for all anterior drawer tests to allow the anterior capsule to consistently be measured in a resting position. Examination of the glenohumeral joint in varied positions of humeral rotation can decrease anterior humeral head translation (Ellenbecker et al, 2001).

The examiner's right hand is placed just distal to the patient's left humeral head. The actions listed next should be repeated in three positions of glenohumeral joint abduction to selectively assess the three glenohumeral joint capsular ligaments. Ranges of abduction used in testing as start positions are 0 to 30 degrees, 45 to 60 degrees, and 90 degrees.

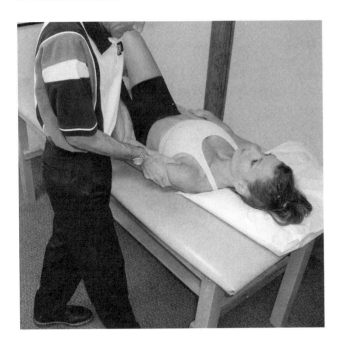

Figure **9-13** Anterior drawer test at 30 degrees of glenohumeral joint abduction.

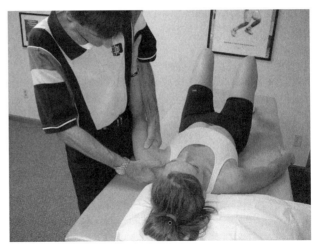

Figure **9-14** Anterior drawer test at 30 degrees of glenohumeral joint abduction using alternative stabilized hand position.

Action

With the glenohumeral joint in the scapular plane, and in the abduction range between 0 and 30 degrees, the examiner's right hand (left shoulder being tested) pushes in an anteromedial direction, translating the humeral head along the face of the glenoid fossa (Figure 9-13). The examiner then removes the stress from the humerus and allows the humeral head to return to the resting position. The translation encountered during testing can be graded using the systems described on pages 66–67. I recommend the use of the Altchek grading system (Altchek et al, 1992), with grade I translation being used to describe translation of the humeral head within the glenoid, and grade II describing translation of the humeral head up over the glenoid rim, with immediate relocation of the head on release of the anteromedial stress.

During the anteromedial loading of the humeral head, some shoulder girdle anterior motion will occur simultaneously. Differentiating shoulder girdle movement from true glenohumeral joint translation can be difficult in inexperienced examiners and requires practice. Use of a fairly rapid and vigorous anteromedial translation force can help minimize movement of the shoulder as a unit and attempts to accelerate the humeral head ahead of the glenoid to produce translation.

An alternative hand placement and translation strategy can be used for clinicians who wish to minimize the movement and contribution of the shoulder girdle during the anterior loading phase of this test. Figure 9-14 shows alternative hand placements that can be used to decrease shoulder girdle movement. This technique requires the examiner to support the patient's extremity under the upper arm and side to allow both hands to be free. To test the left upper extremity of a patient, the patient's arm should be placed under the examiner's left arm. The examiner's left hand grasps just distal to the humeral head from the medial side of the patient arm (axilla), and the examiner's right hand is placed so that the thumb can exert a downward restraining force on the coracoid process of the scapula being tested. The fingers of the supporting hand wrap up over the top of the shoulder to lend greater stabilization. Translation of the proximal humerus is performed in an identical direction and with identical force used during the unstabilized testing method described previously.

Translation is repeated in an anteromedial direction with the glenohumeral joint now placed in 45 to 60 degrees of abduction (Figure 9-15). Finally, a third series of loads in an anteromedial direction is transmitted with the glenohumeral joint abducted 90 degrees (Figure 9-16). The clinician grades the movement of the humeral head in all three positions of abduction and compares the translations with the contralateral extremity.

What Constitutes a Positive Test?

Unilateral increases in anterior humeral head translation in the symptomatic glenohumeral joint indicate anterior glenohumeral joint instability. Movement of the humeral

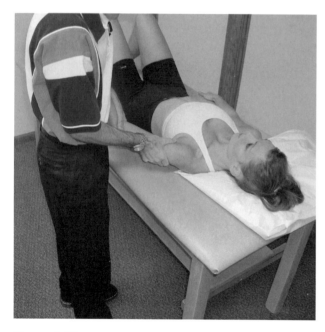

Figure 9-15 Anterior drawer test at 45 to 60 degrees of glenohumeral joint abduction.

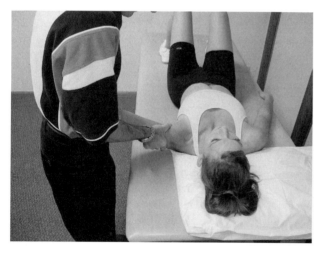

Figure 9-16 Anterior drawer test at 90 degrees of glenohumeral joint abduction.

head may be accompanied by a click, apprehension, or both (Magee, 1997). The click may indicate a labral tear or, most likely, translation of the humeral head over the glenoid rim (Magee, 1997).

Ramifications of a Positive Test

The use of three positions of glenohumeral joint abduction can better isolate specific portions of the glenohumeral capsule. Increased humeral head translation in an

anterior direction with the shoulder between 0 and 30 degrees of abduction indicates laxity or injury to the superior glenohumeral ligament. Increased humeral head translation in an anterior direction, with the shoulder between 45 and 60 degrees of abduction, indicates laxity or injury to the middle glenohumeral ligament. Increased humeral head translation with 90 degrees of glenohumeral joint abduction indicates laxity or pathology to the inferior glenohumeral ligament complex. Labral injury, such as detachment of the anterior inferior portion (Bankart lesion) or superior portion (superior labrum anterior posterior [SLAP] lesion), can also lead to selective increases in anterior humeral head translation with this test (Pagnani & Warren, 1994).

Objective Evidence Regarding the Test

Ellenbecker et al (2002a) studied the intrarater and inter-rater reliability of the anterior drawer test in healthy, uninjured subjects. Using the Altchek system of grading humeral head translation, examiners produced coefficients of agreement of 81.4% when distinguishing between grade I and grade II translation between sessions. This measure of intrarater test-retest reliability decreased to 54% when examiners were asked to further differentiate and identify patients with loose compliant end feels within each of the two Altchek humeral head translation grades (four possible choices: grades I, I+, II, II+). This lower, unacceptable level of reliability among experienced examiners reinforces the recommendation of using the Altchek grading system, recording mainly the relationship of the humeral head to the glenoid rim. Ellenbecker et al (2002a) used the 90-degree abducted position of testing in the scapular plane; however, similar challenges with respect to test-retest accuracy would be expected in the other positions of abduction inherent in the anterior drawer test.

Ellenbecker et al (2000b) tested professional baseball pitchers using a technique of anterior humeral head translation at 90 degrees of abduction with stress radiography. No unilateral difference was noted using radiographs of humeral head translation between the dominant and nondominant extremity. Clinical ramifications of this research lie in the interpretation of clinical humeral head translation tests in athletes from this population. Unilateral increases in anterior humeral head translation in the symptomatic glenohumeral joint are indicative of abnormal static capsular stability and hence lead to the diagnosis of anterior glenohumeral joint instability.

Posterior Drawer Test

Indication

The posterior drawer test is used to assess posterior humeral head translation.

About the Test

This test is similar to the anterior drawer test; the supine position is used to enhance patient relaxation and varied positions of glenohumeral joint abduction are used. This test stresses the posterior capsule and, when applied in 90 degrees of abduction, the posterior band of the inferior glenohumeral ligament complex (Pagnani & Warren, 1994).

Start Position

The patient lies in the supine position. The examiner grasps the patient's elbow circumferentially just proximal to the antecubital fossa with the left hand (for testing the left shoulder of a patient). The humerus is controlled primarily by the distal hand and should be placed in the scapular plane by raising the elbow approximately 30 degrees anterior to the supportive surface on which the patient is lying (30 degrees anterior to the coronal plane) (Saha, 1983). The glenohumeral joint is abducted during the performance of this test, unlike the testing position of glenohumeral joint adduction used during the assessment of posterior humeral head translation in the load and shift test. Some authors recommend testing in 45 degrees of abduction (McFarland et al, 1996a) or in 90 degrees of glenohumeral joint abduction to place selective stress on the posterior band of the inferior glenohumeral ligament complex (Gerber & Ganz, 1984). The examiner's proximal hand (right hand for examination of patient's left shoulder) is placed just distal to the humeral head center, with the thumb placed anteriorly and fingers wrapped posteriorly around the proximal humerus (Figure 9-17). An alternative technique (Figure 9-18) involves a crossed-hand technique that allows the examiner to place the entire heel and palmar surface of the proximal hand over the proximal humerus to increase the surface area of contact with the patient and minimize sensitivity with the posteriorly directed pressure on the anterior structures such as the biceps tendon. Pain elicited during testing will significantly affect the resultant translation during the test.

Action

From the starting position, the examiner presses the humeral head in a posterior and lateral direction along the line of the joint (see Figure 9-17). Several rather rapid,

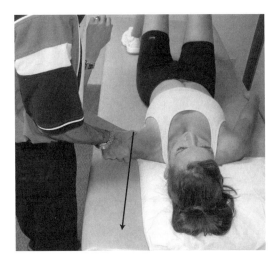

Figure **9-17** Posterior drawer test at 90 degrees of glenohumeral joint abduction. *Arrow* shows posterior lateral direction of translation.

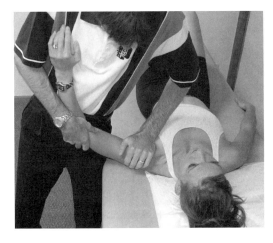

Figure **9-18** Alternative posterior drawer hand placement used to increase surface area of contact on the anterior aspect of the proximal humerus.

firm translations in the posterolateral direction are used. Alternative hand placements to further stabilize the scapula are not necessary with the posterior drawer test because the supporting surface on which the patient is lying provides stabilization against posterior scapular movement with the posterior lateral loading by the examiner.

In some accounts of this test (Magee, 1997), the examiner's distal hand moves in an anterior and medial direction, while the proximal hand pushes the humeral head in the posterior lateral direction. This creates a "pistoning" effect and may further provoke the humeral head in a posterior direction during testing.

What Constitutes a Positive Test?

A positive posterior drawer test identifies unilateral increases in posterior humeral head translation in a symptomatic shoulder. During testing, the examiner carefully perceives the amount of translation of the humeral head in a posterior direction and records the grade of movement accordingly. According to the grading system proposed by Altchek and Dines (1993), posterior translation within the glenoid is graded as grade I. Grade II translation entails movement of the humeral head posteriorly up over the posterior glenoid rim, with spontaneous reduction on removal of the posterior lateral force.

Ramifications of a Positive Test

A positive posterior drawer test indicates increased laxity or pathology in the posterior capsule of the glenohumeral joint. Unlike the specific ligamentous structures found in the anterior capsule of the glenohumeral joint, the posterior capsule is devoid of specific thickenings or ligamentous structures other than the posterior band of the inferior glenohumeral ligament (Pagnani & Warren, 1994). A positive posterior drawer test in isolation indicates unidirectional posterior glenohumeral joint instability. A positive drawer test coupled with a positive MDI sulcus test indicates the presence of MDI (Neer & Foster, 1980).

Objective Evidence Regarding the Test

Levy et al (1999) tested 43 asymptomatic division I collegiate athletes using the posterior drawer test. Intraobserver reproducibility was 52% for the posterior drawer and 73% for the anterior drawer. Significantly greater difficulty was encountered by four experienced surgeons performing and interpreting the translation obtained during the posterior drawer test, as compared with the anterior drawer. Care must be used when performing and interpreting translation during this test. Use of this method with a posterior lateral direction of translation is recommended to ensure that translation follows the angulation of the glenoid so as to prevent compression of the glenohumeral joint surfaces when a force is directed in a straight sagittal posterior plane.

McFarland et al (1991) tested 356 shoulders in high school and college athletes with no history of shoulder pathology; 55% of the athletes had grade II translation using the Hawkins percent humeral head width translation grading system. This finding is consistent with anterior humeral head translation findings reported by Ellenbecker et al (2002a) and Lintner et al (1996), who found that the presence of increased humeral head translation alone, without the presence of symptoms or functional loss, does not constitute glenohumeral joint instability.

Posterior Glide—90 Degrees Flexion Test

Indication

This test assesses the integrity of the posterior capsule with the shoulder in an elevated position and posterior capsule in a more elongated or tensed position.

About the Test

This test is a modification of the test described by Gerber and Ganz (1984) and uses an elevated position of 90 degrees of shoulder flexion. It provides the examiner with an alternative position to examine posterior shoulder stability that approximates the position of many athletic and industrial shoulder stresses such as the posterior pressure imparted to the glenohumeral joint during blocking in football and during an anteriorly directed fall. This test is similar in position and technique to the Norwood stress test for posterior instability (Norwood & Terry, 1984).

Start Position

The patient lies in a supine position and the shoulder is flexed 90 degrees in the sagittal plane. The examiner's left hand (left shoulder examination) is placed at the elbow so that the olecranon process is centered in the palm of the examiner's hand. The examiner's right hand is placed behind the patient's shoulder so that some fingers of the hand are placed on the lateral aspect of the scapula for reference and some fingers are placed on the posterior aspect of the humeral head (Figure 9-19).

Action

The examiner exerts an axial compressive force through the humerus in a posterior and lateral direction using the hand placed at the elbow. The humerus can be brought into slight horizontal adduction beyond neutral, which further tightens the posterior capsule but allows the examiner to place the axially compressed load in a posterior and lateral direction rather than a straight posterior direction (see Figure 9-19). The examiner's other hand palpates and monitors the movement of the humeral head relative to the scapular reference.

What Constitutes a Positive Test?

A positive test occurs when pain, apprehension, and often the feeling of a click occur as the humeral head is pushed over the rim of the posterior glenoid. Replication of the patient's reported episodes of instability or "slipping" also indicates posterior glenohumeral joint instability (Davies & DeCarlo, 1995).

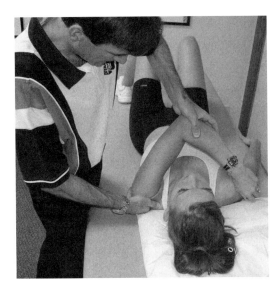

Figure 9-19 Posterior glide with 90 degrees glenohumeral joint flexion and slight horizontal adduction.

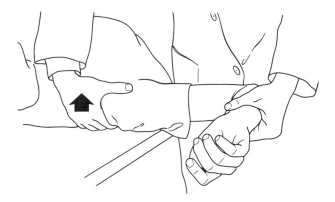

Figure 9-20 Subluxation relocation test (Start). Place the patient supine with the arm off the table at 90 degrees of abduction and external rotation. The examiner gently pushes anteriorly as his fingers grasp the humeral head. No anterior subluxation or apprehension should be evident. Apprehension denotes a previous dislocation. Pain indicates anterior subluxation. (Adapted from Jobe FW, Bradley JP: The diagnosis and nonoperative treatment of shoulder injuries in athletes, *Clin Sports Med* 8(3):427, 1989, with permission.)

Ramifications of a Positive Test

Posterior movement of the humeral head indicates substantial capsular or capsulolabral injury because the posterior capsule in the position of testing (flexion, slight internal rotation, and horizontal adduction) should be tensed or tightened, making it able to resist posterior translation of the humeral head. Excessive posterior movement by the humeral head or reproduction of the patient's apprehension or subluxation in this position also leads the examiner to the diagnosis of posterior instability.

Objective Evidence Regarding the Test

There is no objective evidence with regard to this test.

Pain Provocation Tests

Glenohumeral joint instability tests inherently assess three primary aspects: apprehension, humeral head translation, and provocation or replication of the patient's pain response. This final group of tests uses positions of stress to induce humeral head translation to provoke the pain that patients have primarily with overhead activities such as sport-specific movement patterns or repetitive industrial positions.

Subluxation/Relocation Test

Indication

The subluxation/relocation test is used to identify subtle anterior glenohumeral joint instability and detect posterior impingement.

About the Test

Originally described by Jobe and Bradley (1989), the subluxation/relocation test is designed to identify subtle anterior instability of the glenohumeral joint. Credit for the development and application of this test is also given to Dr. Peter Fowler (Speer et al, 1994a), who described the diagnostic quandary of microinstability (subtle anterior instability) versus rotator cuff injury or both in swimmers. Fowler also advocated the use of this important test to assist in the diagnosis. This test has been advocated to differentiate between occult and subtle anterior instability (Speer et al, 1994a). The subluxation/relocation test uses the position where most patients have symptoms of anterior instability (abduction and external rotation).

Start Position

The patient is positioned supine on a plinth with 90 degrees of abduction of the glenohumeral joint and 90 degrees of external rotation. The examiner stands at the patient's side, facing the patient's head (Figure 9-20). To test the right shoulder, the examiner places the left hand on the patient's right elbow to maintain the position of abduction and external rotation. The examiner's right hand is placed on the proximal aspect of the humerus, near the level of the humeral head. As a landmark, the posterior lateral corner of the acromion can easily be palpated, with hand placement being just distal to the posterior lateral corner of the acromion. Placement of the right hand over the posterior lateral corner of the acromion, or

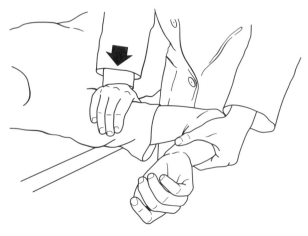

Figure 9-21 Subluxation relocation test (End). After the examiner pushes the humeral head anteriorly and demonstrates anterior pain, the humeral head should be pushed posteriorly. Immediate relief of pain is considered a positive test. (Adapted from Jobe FW, Bradley JP: The diagnosis and nonoperative treatment of shoulder injuries in athletes, *Clin Sports Med* 8(3):427, 1989, with permission.)

proximal to it, results in inappropriate subluxation because the hand is over the scapular portion of the glenohumeral joint, not the humeral head.

Action

With proper right hand placement mentioned previously, the examiner gently subluxes the humeral head anteriorly, while maintaining the position of abduction and 90 degrees of external rotation (see Figure 9-20). During this maneuver, the examiner asks the patient if the mild subluxation movement re-creates the patient's symptoms anteriorly or posteriorly.

If no pain is encountered during this portion of the test, see the Modified Subluxation/Relocation Test (page 82). If pain or symptom replication occurs, the examiner reverses the right hand placement from behind or under the humeral head to a position on top of the humeral head (Figure 9-21). With a soft, cupped hand position to minimize discomfort from the hand interface on the anterior aspect of the shoulder, force is applied in a posterior direction. The posterior force should be directed both posteriorly and slightly laterally, with the examiner realizing that the face of the glenoid is anteverted 30 degrees relative to the frontal or coronal plane (Saha, 1983). The patient is then asked, "Does this decrease the pain in your shoulder?"

What Constitutes a Positive Test?

Reproduction of anterior or posterior shoulder pain with the subluxation portion of this test, with subsequent diminution or disappearance of anterior or posterior shoulder pain with the relocation maneuver, constitutes a positive test.

Ramifications of a Positive Test

A positive subluxation/relocation test detects subtle anterior glenohumeral joint instability. Positive replication of anterior-based symptoms are most likely caused by contact of the rotator cuff superior or bursal surface on the undersurface of the anterior acromion (Figure 9-22). Pressure on the anterior capsule of the glenohumeral joint and bicep long-head tendon could also be a source of pain (Jobe & Bradley, 1989). Morgan et al (1998) reported that a positive subluxation/relocation test can be used to identify a posterior-based type II SLAP lesion.

Development of significant apprehension with this test indicates occult anterior instability and should be differentiated from the pain provoking responses, which indicate milder or more subtle forms of instability.

A positive subluxation relocation test provoking posterior shoulder pain indicates posterior or internal impingement. This relatively new concept involves impingement of the undersurface or articular side of the supraspinatus tendon against the posterosuperior glenoid (Figure 9-23). As the humeral head is translated anteriorly, contact against the posterosuperior glenoid is increased. Halbrecht et al (1999) confirmed via magnetic resonance imaging, performed in the position of 90 degrees of abduction and 90 degrees of external rotation, contact of the undersurface of the supraspinatus tendon against the posterosuperior glenoid in baseball pitchers with arm placed in 90 degrees of external rotation and 90 degrees of abduction (the same initial position used in the subluxation/relocation test). Ten collegiate baseball pitchers were examined and, in all ten, physical contact was encountered in this position.

Effectiveness of the Subluxation/Relocation Test

Speer et al (1994a) tested the diagnostic value of the subluxation/relocation test as it was originally described by Jobe and Bradley (1989) and Fowler (Speer, 1994a). They tested 100 patients undergoing shoulder surgery, using the subluxation relocation test, and assessed patient response to the 90/90 position alone. During testing, specific attention was given to whether the patient reported replication of shoulder pain or a response of apprehension or slipping of the shoulder.

Speer et al (1994a) found that 63 of 100 patients had pain with the 90/90 position alone, with the number reporting pain increasing to 74 of 100 when the anterior subluxation force was applied. Of the patients with pain

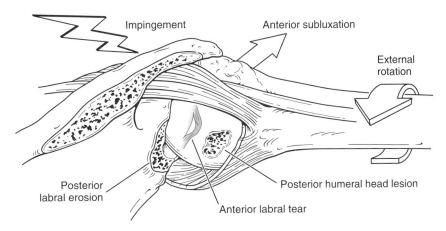

Figure 9-22 Anatomic diagram showing secondary impingement. (Adapted from Jobe FW, Bradley JP: The diagnosis and nonoperative treatment of shoulder injuries in athletes, *Clin Sports Med* 8(3):430, 1989, with permission.)

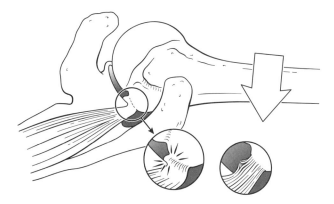

Figure 9-23 Anatomic diagram showing undersurface or internal impingement. (Adapted from Walch G, et al: Impingement of the deep surface of the synospinatus tendon on the posterior superior glenoid rim, *J Shoulder Elbow Surg* 1(5):243, 1992, with permission.)

provocation with the 90/90 position, 59% experienced diminished pain when the relocation force was applied. Patients with pain with anterior loading reported a diminution of pain and symptoms 73% of the time.

Sensitivity of the relocation test reveals the percentage of patients with anterior instability who also had a positive subluxation relocation test. The sensitivity of the test for reproduction of pain with anterior force and diminution of pain with relocation was 54%. Test sensitivity for apprehension was 68%.

Specificity of the relocation test revealed the percentage of patients who had neither anterior instability nor a positive subluxation relocation test. Specificity of the test using pain reproduction as a criterion was 44% for the subluxation relocation test, and specificity using apprehension as the primary criterion was 100%. This test's PPV (percentage of patients who had a positive test and anterior instability) was 45%, increasing to 100% when apprehension was used as the primary criterion. The negative predictive value (NPV) of the test, which indicated the percentage of patients with negative subluxation relocation tests and those who did not have anterior instability, was 53%. This value increased to 78% for apprehension.

Results indicate lower specificity and sensitivity, as well as lower positive and negative predictive values, when pain was used as the diagnostic feature of the test with 90 degrees of glenohumeral joint abduction and 90 degrees of external rotation. Some improvement was noted in the diagnostic value of the test when apprehension was used as the distinguishing diagnostic feature. Also, the anterior subluxation force should be used as a provocation, as both Fowler and Jobe and Bradley (1989) have recommended, as higher specificity, sensitivity, and both PPVs and NPVs are reported when the anterior force is used in the diagnostic sequence. Speer et al (1994a) concluded that the test as originally described by Jobe and Bradley (1989) may have limited effectiveness. Speer et al (1994a) also suggested a modification of the subluxation/relocation test, with increased amounts of external rotation (as much as end range external rotation for each patient) in the 90-degree abducted position. No other research investigations are currently available (see Modified Subluxation/ Relocation Test).

Finally, the Jobe subluxation/relocation test has been used to identify labral pathology. Guanche and Jones (2003) tested 60 shoulders in 59 patients before patients underwent arthroscopic surgery. Sensitivity and specificity values were 44% and 87%, respectively, for the detection of any labral lesion (PPV = 91%, NPV = 34%), and 36% and 63% sensitivity and specificity, respectively, for the identification of SLAP lesions (PPV = 55%, NPV =

45%). Morgan et al (1998) reported the Jobe subluxation relocation test as the primary test used to identify type II posterior SLAP lesions (see pages 115–116). Multiple indications of this test can create confusion regarding the diagnostic interpretation of a positive Jobe subluxation relocation test; however, when this test is used in combination with other instability and labral tests, it can be extremely valuable, particularly in the overhead athlete or individual who functions in the 90/90 position.

Modified Subluxation/Relocation Test

Indication

A modification of the subluxation/relocation test using altered positions of abduction and external rotation to assess subtle anterior glenohumeral joint instability and posterior or internal impingement, particularly in the overhead athlete or industrial patient.

About the Test

Based on the report by Speer et al (1994a), demonstrating limited effectiveness and accuracy of the originally described subluxation relocation test, this modification uses greater amounts of external rotation and abduction to further provoke patients who primarily have pain in this phase of overhead motion (abduction with external rotation).

Start Position

The starting position for this test is nearly identical to the original subluxation/relocation test described previously. Modifications in this test are that testing now occurs in the patient's passive end range of external rotation and at varying positions of glenohumeral joint abduction (Figure 9-24). For many high-level baseball and tennis players (Ellenbecker, 1992; Ellenbecker et al, 2002a), this entails often greater than 100 degrees of external rotation (Figure 9-25).

Action

With the patient's shoulder held and stabilized in the end range of external rotation at 90 degrees of abduction, anterior subluxation is introduced as described for the original subluxation/relocation test (see Figure 9-25). The patient is again asked if this subluxation reproduces the patient's symptoms. Reproduction of patient symptoms of either anterior or posterior shoulder pain with subluxation leads the examiner to reposition a hand on the anterior aspect of the patient's shoulder and perform a posterolateral directed force using a soft, cupped hand to minimize anterior shoulder pain from the hand/shoulder (examiner/patient) interface.

Failure to reproduce the patient's symptoms with end

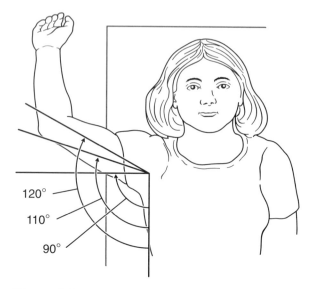

Figure 9-24 Modified subluxation relocation test showing range of glenohumeral joint abduction used during testing. (Adapted from Hamner DL, Pink MM, Jobe FW: A modification of the relocation test: arthroscopic findings associated with a positive test, *J Shoulder Elbow Surg* 9(4):264, 2000, with permission.)

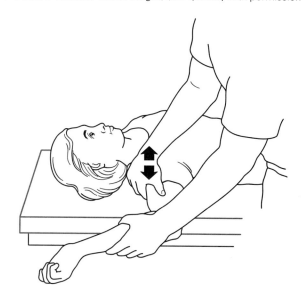

Figure 9-25 Modified subluxation relocation test. Note the use of greater than 90 degrees of external rotation and use of subluxation and relocation forces *(arrows)*. (Adapted from Hamner DL, Pink MM, Jobe FW: A modification of the relocation test: arthroscopic findings associated with a positive test, *J Shoulder Elbow Surg* 9(4):264, 2000, with permission.)

range external rotation and 90 degrees of abduction leads the examiner to reattempt the subluxation maneuver with 110 and 120 degrees of abduction (see Figure 9-24). This modification has been proposed by Hamner et al (2000) to increase the potential for contact between the undersurface of the supraspinatus tendon and the posterior superior glenoid. In each position of abduction (90, 110, and 120 degrees of abduction), the same sequence of initial subluxation and subsequent relocation is performed as previously described.

What Constitutes a Positive Test?

Reproduction of anterior or posterior shoulder pain with the subluxation portion of this test, with subsequent diminution or disappearance of anterior or posterior shoulder pain with the relocation maneuver, constitutes a positive test. Production of apprehension with any position of abduction during the anteriorly directed subluxation force phase of testing indicates occult anterior instability.

Ramifications of a Positive Test

Ramifications of a positive test are the same as described for the traditional subluxation relocation test. The modified test has been advocated as a diagnostic tool in the treatment of shoulder pain in young overhand throwing athletes. In a normal shoulder, the position of arm cocking during throwing occurs in the scapular plane; however, if there has been stretching of the anterior capsular structures, the humerus may be hyperabducted or hyperangulated (Davidson et al, 1995) into the coronal plane (see Chapter 17). As this process of hyperangulation continues and anterior humeral head translation occurs with external rotation of the humerus, the rotator cuff impinges on the posterosuperior labrum. This creates undersurface rotator cuff tears and posterosuperior labral fraying (Hamner et al, 2000).

Objective Evidence Regarding the Test

Hamner et al (2000) performed research using the modified subluxation relocation test in 13 overhand-throwing athletes who failed 3 months of traditional physical therapy and were still unable to perform overhand throwing. The shoulder was evaluated arthroscopically during the subluxation relocation test at 90, 110, and 120 degrees of glenohumeral joint abduction. At 90 degrees of abduction, 8 of 13 patients had physical contact between the undersurface of the rotator cuff and the posterosuperior glenoid; at 110 degrees of abduction, all 13 patients had contact between the undersurface of the rotator cuff and the posterosuperior glenoid; and at 120 degrees of abduction, 12 of 13 patients had similar contact. Six of 13 patients had a positive modified subluxation relocation test in all three positions of glenohumeral joint abduction.

In the study by Hamner et al (2000), posterior impingement of the rotator cuff was associated with a positive modified subluxation relocation test in 63% of patients at 90 degrees of abduction, 69% of patients in 110 degrees of abduction, and 100% of patients with 120 degrees of abduction. No attempt was made to report specificity, sensitivity, or predictive value because no control group was studied. No further research is available using this test.

Paley et al (2000) evaluated the dominant shoulder of 41 professional throwing athletes. With the arthroscope inserted in the glenohumeral joint, all 41 shoulders had posterior undersurface impingement between the rotator cuff and posterior superior glenoid. In these athletes, 93% had undersurface fraying of the rotator cuff tendons and 88% showed fraying of the posterosuperior glenoid. These findings help to explain the type of lesions/pathology found in the dominant glenohumeral joint of overhead athletes and aid in the explanation of the mechanism of pain provocation during specific tests such as the subluxation relocation test described here.

Anterior Release Test

Indication

The anterior release test was developed to physically diagnose occult anterior shoulder instability.

About the Test

This test was originally described by Gross and Distefano (1997) and is a modification of the basic apprehension test. It uses the position of most frequent complaints of glenohumeral joint instability (90 degrees of abduction with external rotation) to provoke/reproduce shoulder pain and apprehension.

Start Position

The patient is examined in a supine position with the involved shoulder hanging just slightly off the edge of the plinth or supporting surface. The patient's arm is abducted 90 degrees. One hand of the examiner holds the patient's involved extremity near the elbow (at the balance point) (see page 6 for description).

Action

The examiner's other hand is placed over the anterior portion of the humeral head, using a soft, cupped hand-patient interface to minimize discomfort from the posterior pressure itself. Keeping the posterior pressure maintained through the humeral head, the examiner externally rotates the shoulder to the extreme end range of external rotation motion (Figure 9-26, *A*). As soon as the end range of external rotation is achieved, the humeral head is released (Figure 9-26, *B*).

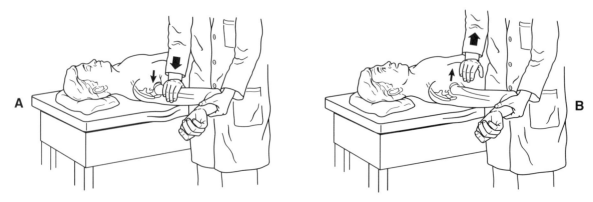

Figure 9-26 Anterior release test. **A,** The humeral head is held in a reduced position while the arm is abducted and brought into maximal external rotation. **B,** Anterior release test drawing showing the release of the humeral head while the external rotation position is maintained. (Adapted from Gross ML, Distefano MC: Anterior release test. A new test for occult shoulder instability, *Clin Orthop* 339:106, 1997, with permission.)

What Constitutes a Positive Test?

The test result is considered positive when the patient experiences a sudden pain on release of the posteriorly directed stress on the humeral head, notes a distinct increase in pain, or states that symptoms have been reproduced.

Ramifications of a Positive Test

Reproduction of pain with the anterior release test identifies instability as playing a role in the patient's pain and functional limitation. Rowe and Zarins (1981) initially described occult anterior instability in patients who had a positive apprehension test that reproduced both pain and apprehension with the 90-degree abducted, externally rotated position. Rowe and Zarins (1981) stated that, in the absence of a positive apprehension test, the examiner should suspect some other cause of shoulder disability. The anterior release test was designed to assist in the evaluation of patients with instability and recognizes that

reproduction of pain often indicates underlying instability of the glenohumeral joint. It also recognizes that patients who do not have apprehension with the 90-degree abducted externally rotated position may indeed have instability as an underlying cause of their shoulder dysfunction (Gross & Distefano, 1997).

Objective Evidence Regarding the Test

Gross and Distefano (1997) performed the anterior release test before induction of anesthesia in 82 patients scheduled to undergo shoulder surgery. The anterior release test was positive in 39 patients and negative in 43. There were five false-positive and three false-negative results, produced a sensitivity of 91.9% and a specificity of 88.9%. The PPV was 87.1% and the NPV was 93%. One of the most significant findings was that in 12 of 14 patients with occult subluxation, the anterior release test correctly identified the instability. No other research has been published using the anterior release test.

Glenohumeral Joint (Rotator Cuff) Impingement

INTRODUCTION

Before an accurate diagnosis of impingement can be made, baseline knowledge of both the types of glenohumeral joint impingement and the underlying mechanism behind impingement must be understood. Significant advancement in the anatomy and biomechanics of the shoulder has led to identification of numerous types of impingement with several underlying pathomechanical causes.

PRIMARY IMPINGEMENT OR COMPRESSIVE DISEASE

Primary impingement, also known as *compressive disease* or *outlet impingement,* is a direct result of compression of the rotator cuff tendons between the humeral head and the overlying anterior third of the acromion, coracoacromial ligament, coracoid, or acromioclavicular joint (Neer, 1972, 1983). The physiologic space between the inferior acromion and superior surface of the rotator cuff tendons is termed the *subacromial space.* It has been measured to be 7 to 13 mm using anteroposterior radiographs in patients with shoulder pain (Golding, 1962) and 6 to 14 mm in normal shoulders (Cotton & Rideout, 1964).

Biomechanical analysis of the shoulder has produced theoretical estimates of the compressive forces against the acromion with elevation of the shoulder. Poppen and Walker (1978) calculated this force at 0.42 times body weight. Lucas (1973) estimated this force at 10.2 times the weight of the arm. Peak forces against the acromion were measured in a range of motion between 85 and 136 degrees of elevation (Wuelker et al, 1994). This position is functionally important for activities of daily living, is inherent in sport-specific movement patterns (Fleisig et al, 1995; Elliott et al, 1986), and is commonly noted in ergonomic activities. The position of the shoulder in forward flexion, horizontal adduction, and internal rotation during the acceleration and follow-through phases of the throwing motion is likely to produce subacromial impingement as a result of abrasion of the supraspinatus, infraspinatus, or biceps tendon against the overlying

structures (Fleisig et al, 1995). These data provide scientific rationale for the concept of primary impingement or compressive disease as an etiology of rotator cuff pathology.

NEER'S STAGES OF IMPINGEMENT

Neer (1972, 1983) outlined three stages of primary impingement as it relates to rotator cuff pathology. Stage I, *edema and hemorrhage,* results from the mechanical irritation of the tendon from the impingement incurred with overhead activity. Stage I is characteristically observed in younger patients who are more athletic and is described as a reversible condition with conservative physical therapy. Primary symptoms and physical signs are similar to the other two stages—a positive impingement sign, painful arc of movement, and varying degrees of muscular weakness (Neer, 1983). The second stage of compressive disease is termed *fibrosis and tendonitis.* This stage occurs from repeated episodes of mechanical inflammation and can include thickening or fibrosis of the subacromial bursae. The typical age range for this stage of injury is 25 to 40 years. Neer's stage III impingement lesion is termed *bone spurs and tendon rupture,* and is the result of continued mechanical compression of the rotator cuff tendons. Full-thickness tears of the rotator cuff, partial-thickness tears of the rotator cuff, biceps tendon lesions, and bony alteration of the acromion and acromioclavicular joint may be associated with this stage (Neer 1972, 1983). In addition to bony alterations that are acquired with repetitive stress to the shoulder, the native shape of the acromion is of relevance.

The specific shape of the overlying acromion process is termed *acromial architecture* and has been studied in relation to full-thickness tears of the rotator cuff (Bigliani et al, 1991; Zuckerman et al, 1992). Bigliani et al (1991) described three types of acromions: type I (flat), type II (curved), and type III (hooked). A type III or hooked acromion was found in 70% of cadaveric shoulders with a full-thickness rotator cuff tear, and type I acromions were associated with only 3% (Bigliani et al, 1991). Also, in a series of 200 clinically evaluated patients, 80% with a positive arthrogram confirming a full-thickness rotator cuff tear had a Type III acromion (Zuckerman et al, 1992).

SECONDARY IMPINGEMENT

Impingement or compressive symptoms may be secondary to underlying instability of the glenohumeral joint (Jobe & Kivitne, 1989; Andrews & Alexander, 1995). Although this concept is relatively common knowledge today, it was not well understood or recognized in the medical community even through the late 1980s. The concept that impingement could occur secondary to instability, rather than as a primary cause, has had significant ramifications, altering evaluation methods and treatment/rehabilitation (Wilk & Arrigo, 1993; Ellenbecker, 1995).

Attenuation of the static stabilizers of the glenohumeral joint, such as the capsular ligaments and labrum from the excessive demands incurred in throwing or overhead activities, can lead to anterior instability of the glenohumeral joint. Because of the increased humeral head translation, the biceps tendon and rotator cuff can become impinged secondary to the ensuing instability (Jobe & Kivitne, 1989; Andrews & Alexander, 1995). A progressive loss of glenohumeral joint stability is created when the dynamic stabilizing functions of the rotator cuff are diminished from fatigue and tendon injury (Andrews & Alexander, 1995; Nirschl, 1988b). The effects of secondary impingement can lead to rotator cuff tears as the instability and impingement continue (Jobe & Kivitne, 1989; Andrews & Alexander, 1995).

POSTERIOR, INTERNAL, OR "UNDERSURFACE" IMPINGEMENT

An additional type of impingement more recently discussed as an etiology for rotator cuff pathology that can often progress to an undersurface tear of the rotator cuff in the young athletic shoulder is termed *posterior, internal* (or *inside*), or *undersurface impingement* (Jobe & Pink, 1994; Walch et al, 1992). This phenomenon was originally identified by Walch during shoulder arthroscopy, with the shoulder placed in the 90/90 position. This shoulder placement causes the supraspinatus and infraspinatus tendons to rotate posteriorly. This more posterior orientation aligns the tendons such that the undersurface of the tendons rub on the posterosuperior glenoid lip and become pinched or compressed between the humeral head and the posterosuperior glenoid rim (Walch et al, 1992). In contrast to the position involved in patients with traditional outlet impingement (either primary or secondary), the area of the rotator cuff tendon that is involved in

posterior or undersurface impingement is the articular side of the rotator cuff tendon. Traditional impingement involves the superior or bursal surface of the rotator cuff tendon or tendons. Individuals presenting with posterior shoulder pain brought on by positioning of the arm in 90 degrees of abduction and 90 degrees or more of external rotation, typically from overhead positions in sport or industrial situations, may be considered as potential candidates for undersurface impingement.

The presence of anterior translation of the humeral head with maximal external rotation and 90 degrees of abduction, which has been confirmed by arthroscopy during the subluxation/relocation test, can produce mechanical rubbing and fraying on the undersurface of the rotator cuff tendons. Additional harm can be caused by the posterior deltoid if the rotator cuff is not functioning properly. The posterior deltoid's angle of pull compresses the humeral head against the glenoid, accentuating the skeletal, tendinous, and labral lesions (Jobe & Pink, 1994). Walch et al (1992) performed arthroscopic evaluation on 17 throwing athletes with shoulder pain during throwing and found undersurface impingement that resulted in 8 partial-thickness rotator cuff tears and 12 lesions in the posterosuperior labrum. Impingement of the undersurface of the rotator cuff on the posterosuperior glenoid labrum may be a cause of painful structural disease in the overhead athlete.

With the use of magnetic resonance imaging, Halbrecht et al (1999) confirmed contact of the undersurface of the supraspinatus tendon against the posterosuperior glenoid in 10 of 10 college baseball pitchers with arms placed in 90 degrees of external rotation and 90 degrees of abduction. Paley et al (2000) found, on arthroscopic evaluation of the glenohumeral joint, that 41 of 41 dominant shoulders of professional throwing athletes had posterior undersurface impingement between the rotator cuff and posterior superior glenoid. In these athletes, 93% had undersurface fraying of the rotator cuff tendons and 88% showed fraying of the posterosuperior glenoid.

ANTERIOR INTERNAL IMPINGEMENT

Anterior internal impingement has recently been described as a source of pain in patients with a stable shoulder and positive traditional impingement signs. Struhl (2002) reported this phenomenon during arthroscopic evaluation of patients who had clinical signs of traditional outlet impingement and anterior pain. Direct visualization during arthroscopy revealed undersurface tears of the rotator cuff resulting from contact between the anterosuperior labrum and undersurface of the rotator cuff, similar to that described by Walch et al (1992) in posterior impingement.

In a series of 10 patients with traditional impingement signs and anterior-based pain presentations, Struhl (2002) reported arthroscopic confirmation of contact between the fragmented undersurface of the rotator cuff tendons and the anterosuperior labrum during the Hawkins impingement test (pages 89–90), viewed from a posterior arthroscopic portal. Understanding this new clinical entity is essential for both diagnosing and treating patients with the clinical appearance of outlet impingement and anterior pain. Jobe hypothesized that shoulder pain seen in swimmers may be the result of anterior internal impingement because pain is frequently reported at hand entry into the water, and, in this position, the humeral position is similar to that of the Neer and Hawkins tests (Struhl, 2002).

NEER IMPINGEMENT TEST

This test is also called the *forward flexion impingement test.*

Indication

The Neer impingement test is used to identify impingement of the rotator cuff against the coracoacromial arch.

About the Test

Originally described by Neer and Welsh (1977), this impingement test places or jams the rotator cuff tendons of the forward flexed shoulder against the undersurface of the anterior acromion. The test is used to identify primary glenohumeral joint impingement.

Start Position

The test is typically described (Neer & Welsh, 1977; Neer, 1972, 1983; Jobe & Kvitne, 1989) with the patient in a standing position. The examiner grasps the patient's elbow near the balance point with one hand (see page 6 for discussion of upper extremity balance point), while the examiner's other hand is stabilizing the mid-thoracic region. This stabilization is important to prevent the patient from arching backward as the arm is elevated toward end range forward flexion. Using a seated position for patient examination during this impingement test is also indicated and helps to minimize the number of possible compensations during arm elevation from the trunk and lower extremity kinetic chain.

Action

The position of the arm to be tested is in slight internal rotation during elevation, so that the hand is placed in a position where the ulnar border of the hand or palm is

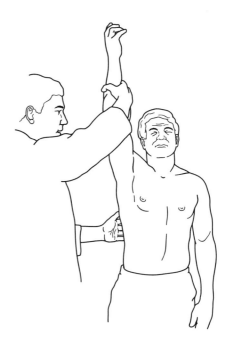

Figure 10-1 Neer impingement test. (From Jobe FW, Bradley JP: The diagnosis and nonoperative treatment of shoulder injuries in athletes, *Clin Sports Med* 8(3):425, 1989.)

facing forward as the arm is elevated (Figure 10-1). Placement of the arm in external rotation would theoretically rotate the greater tuberosity of the humerus away from the overlying acromion and compromise test results because of a lack or decrease in contact of the acromion with the greater tuberosity with external humeral rotation (Inman et al, 1944).

The arm is moved into end range forward flexion in the sagittal plane. At end range, several small movements into and out of terminal end range forward flexion can be performed with careful monitoring of both end feel (see discussion of end feels of the human shoulder, pages 56–57) and patient response.

What Constitutes a Positive Test?

Reproduction of the patient's pain in the subacromial region with the forward flexed position is indicative of a positive test.

Ramifications of a Positive Test

A positive Neer impingement test indicates rotator cuff impingement. Irritability of the rotator cuff tendons, most specifically the supraspinatus tendon, leads to reproduction of pain with compression of the tendon between the greater tuberosity and the undersurface of the coracoacromial arch (Jobe & Bradley, 1989).

Objective Evidence Regarding the Test

Valadie et al (2000) used cadaveric specimens to anatomically study the relationship of the rotator cuff and biceps tendons to the coracoacromial arch during the Neer impingement test. Their results showed contact between the bursal side of the rotator cuff tendons (see discussion of articular versus bursal side rotator cuff tears, page 86) and the lateral aspect of the tendon in 60% of the specimens tested, and contact with the medial aspect of the acromion in 100% (Figure 10-2). Also, the biceps long-head tendon was located beneath the acromion in 60% of the specimens tested. There was no evidence of impingement of the rotator cuff tendons against the coracoid. These findings support the use of the Neer impingement test to produce contact between the undersurface of the acromion and the bursal side of the rotator cuff tendons. Because Valadie et al (2000) reported compression of the biceps long-head tendon below the acromion in many of the samples, caution is warranted regarding interpretation of this test to involve solely the rotator cuff tendons.

Post and Cohen (1986) reported the Neer impingement test to have a sensitivity of 93% in the confirmation of subacromial impingement. Bak and Fauno (1997) tested 36 competitive swimmers and found the Neer impingement test to have no positive results in asymptomatic swimmers. They reported a specificity of 100% and a sensitivity of 39%.

Leroux et al (1995) tested the Neer, Hawkins, and Yocum impingement tests in 55 consecutive patients. Sensitivity was satisfactory for all three impingement tests (78% to 89%); the Neer test's sensitivity was 89%. Despite overall acceptable levels of both sensitivity and specificity in the literature, it is recommended that several impingement tests be used to increase the clinician's ability to identify patients with subacromial impingement.

Calis et al (2000) compared the Neer, Hawkins, and cross-arm impingement tests in patients with and without a positive subacromial injection test. They reported 92% sensitivity and 25% specificity for the Hawkins test, 89% sensitivity and 31% specificity for the Neer impingement test, and 82% sensitivity and 27% specificity for the cross-arm adduction impingement test. These findings are similar to those reported by Leroux et al (1995) and Bak and Fauno (1997).

Finally, MacDonald et al (2000) assessed the diagnostic accuracy of the Neer and Hawkins impingement tests for the diagnosis of subacromial bursitis and rotator cuff pathology. A total of 85 consecutive patients were tested before and after shoulder arthroscopy. The Neer impingement test had a sensitivity of only 75% for the appearance suggestive of subacromial bursitis. The Hawkins test (see later) had a sensitivity of 92%.

For rotator cuff tearing, the Neer test has a sensitivity of 85%, and the Hawkins test had a comparable sensiti-

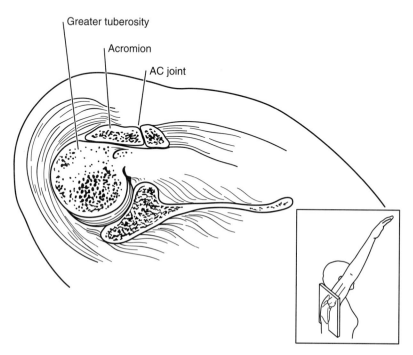

Figure **10-2** MRI showing contact during the Neer impingement test. (From Valadie AL III et al: Anatomy of provocative tests for impingement syndrome of the shoulder, *J Shoulder Elbow Surg* 9(1):40, 2000.)

vity of 88%. The two tests had a high negative predictive value (NPV) (96% for bursitis, and 90% for rotator cuff tearing) when combined. Results of this study indicated that these tests are sensitive for the appearance of subacromial bursitis and both partial and complete rotator cuff tearing. Both the Neer and Hawkins impingement tests are used to formulate a more complete clinical evaluation for the patient with shoulder pathology.

HAWKINS IMPINGEMENT TEST

This test is also known as the *Hawkins-Kennedy impingement test.*

Indication

The Hawkins impingement test is used to test for impingement of the rotator cuff against the coracoacromial arch.

About the Test

Originally described by Hawkins and Kennedy (1980), this test forces the rotator cuff tendons under the coracoacromial arch and against the coracoid process to create mechanical compression or impingement (Leroux et al, 1995).

Start Position

The Hawkins impingement test is typically described with 90 degrees of forward flexion in texts; however, the photos and line art accompanying this clinical test show the arm technically in 90 degrees of elevation in the scapular plane (see scapular plane inset, page 6). The test shows one examiner's hand on the patient's elbow, with the other hand placed at the wrist to provide the internal rotation overpressure (Figure 10-3). My preferred starting technique is shown in Figure 10-4. One of the examiner's hands is placed just distal to the elbow in the extremity balance point position (see page 6) to support the upper extremity with just one hand. The examiner's other hand is placed on top of the shoulder being tested to stabilize the scapular and glenohumeral articulation during the upcoming internal rotation movement. The shoulder being tested is placed near neutral rotation (0 degrees).

Action

Using the hand placements mentioned previously, the patient's shoulder is internally rotated to end range.

What Constitutes a Positive Test?

A positive test is characterized by reproduction of the patient's anterosuperior pain in the subacromial space, either at end range of internal rotation or along the course

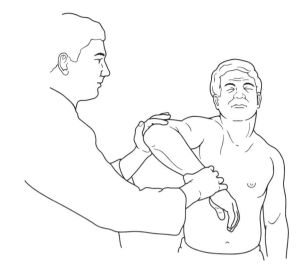

Figure 10-3 Hawkins impingement test. (From Jobe FW, Bradley JP: The diagnosis and nonoperative treatment of shoulder injuries in athletes, *Clin Sports Med* 8(3):426, 1989.)

of movement from the neutral rotation (starting position) to end range (internal rotation).

Ramifications of a Positive Test

A positive Hawkins impingement test indicates irritability of the rotator cuff tendons as they are encroached on the coracoacromial arch.

Objective Evidence Regarding the Test

In a cadaveric study, Valadie et al (2000) found contact between the medial surface of the acromion and the bursal surface of the rotator cuff tendons in 50% of the specimens tested, with contact between the rotator cuff tendons and biceps and the coracoacromial ligament in 100% of the specimens (Figure 10-5). The authors also found contact in all specimens between the articular surface of the rotator cuff tendons and the anterosuperior glenoid rim. In only one specimen tested, the subscapularis tendon was deformed against the coracoid process. Contrary to common belief, the Hawkins test did produce contact between the biceps long-head tendon and the coracoacromial ligament in 50% of the specimens tested. Penny and Welsh (1981) reported that internal rotation of the forward flexed shoulder moved the biceps tendon into a position medial to the coracoacromial arch, making the Hawkins test more specific for rotator cuff impingement. The research by Valadie et al (2000) questions the selective impingement of the rotator cuff by identifying the close association between the biceps tendon to the coracoacromial ligament during the Hawkins impingement maneuver.

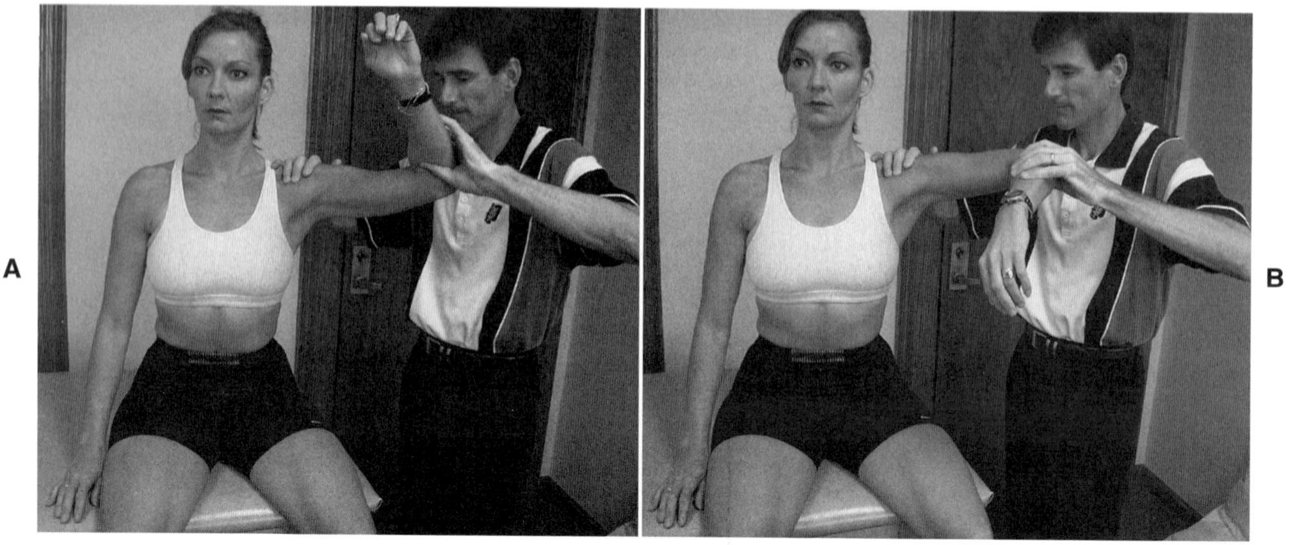

Figure 10-4 Author's preferred technique for the Hawkins impingement test. Note the hand placements, which allow for greater stabilization of the shoulder complex during testing. **A,** Starting position. **B,** Ending position.

Several clinical studies have been performed on the Hawkins impingement test. Bak and Fauno (1997) reported a sensitivity of 80% and specificity of 76% during the examination of 36 elite-level swimmers. Rupp et al (1995) also studied the effectiveness of the Hawkins impingement test in elite-level swimmers. They reported a sensitivity of 44% in a population of 44 shoulders. Leroux et al (1995) reported sensitivity of 87% with the Hawkins impingement test, making it similar to the Neer impingement test, which was 89%. Calis et al (2000) reported 92% sensitivity and 25% specificity, as well as 75.2% positive predictive value (PPV) and 56.2% NPV for the Hawkins test. As mentioned in the previous impingement test discussion, the use of multiple impingement tests is recommended because of the differing locations of contact in the subacromial region and the slightly different levels of both sensitivity and specificity.

CORACOID IMPINGEMENT TEST

This test is a modification of the Hawkins-Kennedy impingement test.

Indication

The coracoid impingement test is used to identify impingement of the rotator cuff against the coracoacromial arch, more specifically the coracoid process.

About the Test

A modification of the original test described by Hawkins and Kennedy (1980), this test also forces the rotator cuff tendons under the coracoacromial arch and against the coracoid process, to create mechanical compression or impingement (Davies & DeCarlo, 1995; Ianotti, 1991).

Start Position

The coracoid impingement test is initiated with 90 degrees of forward flexion in the sagittal plane. The preferred starting technique is shown in Figure 10-6, *A*. One of the examiner's hands is placed just distal to the elbow in the extremity balance point position (see page 6) to support the upper extremity with just one hand. The examiner's other hand is placed on top of the shoulder being tested to stabilize the scapular and glenohumeral articulation during the upcoming internal rotation movement. The shoulder being tested is placed in external rotation.

Action

Using the hand placements mentioned previously, the patient's shoulder is internally rotated to end range as shown (Figure 10-6, *B*), while the shoulder remains in the sagittal plane.

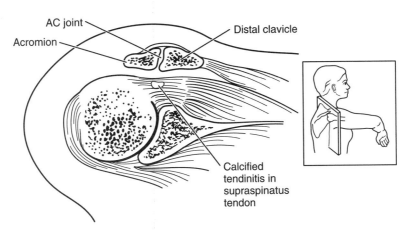

Figure 10-5 MRI showing contact during the Hawkins impingement test. (From Valadie AL III et al: Anatomy of provocative tests for impingement syndrome of the shoulder, *J Shoulder Elbow Surg* 9(1):43, 2000.)

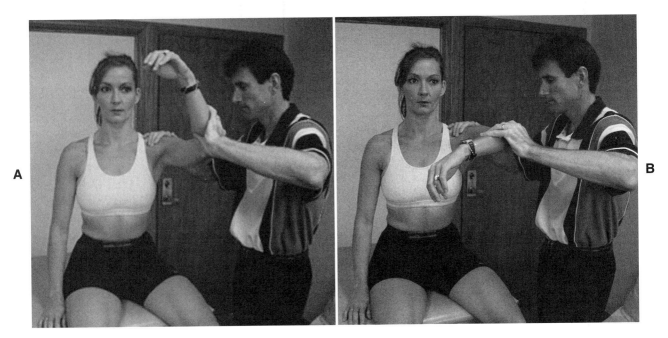

Figure 10-6 Coracoid impingement test. **A,** Starting position. **B,** Ending position.

What Constitutes a Positive Test?

A positive test is characterized by reproduction of the patient's anterior pain in the subacromial space, either at end range of internal rotation or along the course of movement from the neutral rotation (starting position) to end range (internal rotation).

Ramifications of a Positive Test

A positive coracoid impingement test indicates irritability of the rotator cuff tendons as they are encroached on the coracoacromial arch. The more medial position of the humerus during testing (sagittal plane) is theorized to produce greater contact against the coracoid process (hence the test's name), and involves impingement of the subscapularis, supraspinatus, and biceps long-head tendon (Davies & DeCarlo, 1995).

Objective Evidence Regarding the Test

No objective research is available regarding confirmed anatomic contact with this test or either sensitivity or specificity values on human subjects.

CROSS-ARM ADDUCTION TEST

This test is also known as the *crossover impingement test* or *horizontal adduction impingement test.*

Indication

The cross-arm adduction test is used to identify impingement of the rotator cuff against the coracoacromial arch.

About the Test

This test uses the position of cross-arm or horizontal adduction to produce contact between the rotator cuff and biceps long-head tendon and the coracoacromial arch. This test is often used because of the prevalence of this movement pattern in many functional movement patterns, as well as its ability to replicate the position of the glenohumeral joint during the follow-through of the golf swing (right shoulder of a right-handed golfer) and tennis forehand and the preparation position of the tennis backhand (Roetert & Groppel, 2001).

Starting Position

The patient is examined in the seated position (preferred to avoid compensatory movements during testing) or while standing. The examiner grasps the patient's arm with one arm near the balance point near the elbow and places the other hand on the back of the patient's contralateral shoulder to prevent trunk rotation. The hand placed on the posterior aspect of the shoulder and scapula is important for stabilizing the patient during testing.

Action

The patient's extremity to be tested is flexed to 90 degrees with slight internal rotation so that the forearm is pronated and the hand is in the palm-down position. The shoulder is then cross-arm or horizontally adducted to end range across the patient's body (Figure 10-7). Several small oscillations at end range of motion are performed before returning the patient's arm to the resting position at the side.

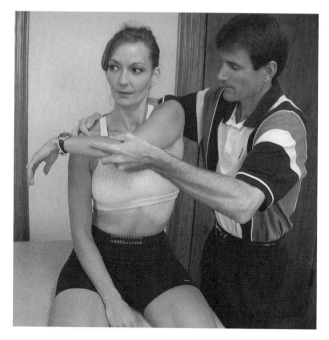

Figure 10-7 Cross-arm adduction impingement test.

What Constitutes a Positive Test?

Reproduction of the patient's anterior shoulder pain at the end range of horizontal adduction or in the process of performing the horizontal adduction movement pattern indicates primary impingement of the rotator cuff against the coracoacromial arch (Davies & DeCarlo, 1995). The test may also produce pain in the superior aspect of the shoulder near the acromioclavicular joint. This is one of the primary tests used to identify acromioclavicular joint pathology because of the compression of the distal aspect of the clavicle against the acromion (Davies & DeCarlo, 1995). Finally, pain produced in the posterior aspect of the shoulder during the cross-arm adduction maneuver may be indicative of posterior capsular tightness (Davies & DeCarlo, 1995).

Ramifications of a Positive Test

A positive cross-arm adduction impingement test indicates irritability of the rotator cuff tendons with compression of the tendons against the coracoacromial arch. A positive test can confirm impingement when it is used with other impingement tests (Neer, Hawkins, coracoid, and Yocum). Results of this test can also be used to guide both resistive exercise programs and the return to functional activity during rehabilitation, as the patient's inability to tolerate this movement pattern suggests that this position should be avoided during exercise and functional activity.

Objective Evidence Regarding the Test

Calis et al (2000) tested the cross-arm impingement test in patients with and without a positive subacromial injection test. The test had a sensitivity of 82% and specificity of 27%, with a PPV of 73% and an NPV of 38%. Despite these values, the authors reported that this test, by compressing forces on the rotator cuff under the acromioclavicular joint, is more likely to be used to investigate acromioclavicular joint osteoarthritis (Calis et al, 2000).

YOCUM TEST

Indication

The Yocum test is used to identify impingement of the rotator cuff against the coracoacromial arch.

About the Test

Initially described by Yocum (1983), the Yocum test is an active impingement test to diagnose subacromial impingement by using the combination of humeral elevation with internal rotation.

Starting Position

The patient places the hand of the involved shoulder on top of the contralateral shoulder (Figure 10-8, *A*). This results in a position of cross-arm (horizontal) adduction and internal rotation. The examiner is not actively involved during administration of this test.

Action

The patient is asked to raise or lift the elbow without raising or elevating the shoulder girdle (Figure 10-8, *B*). The patient's hand is to remain on top of the contralateral shoulder.

What Constitutes a Positive Test?

Reproduction of anterior shoulder pain with elevation of the humerus and compression of the rotator cuff tendons against the coracoacromial arch constitutes a positive test.

Ramifications of a Positive Test

Irritability of the rotator cuff tendons is implied with a positive Yocum test during compression of the tendons against the overlying coracoacromial arch. This test is the only impingement test reported in the literature using an active motion. The others (Neer, Hawkins, coracoid, and cross-arm adduction) use a passive movement provided by the examiner. This test confirms the presence of painful

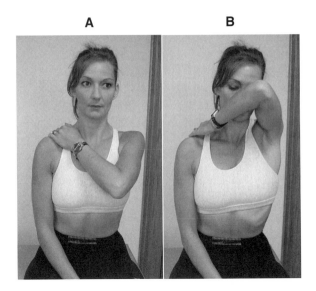

A   **B**

Figure **10-8** Yocum impingement test. **A,** Starting position. **B,** Ending position.

subacromial contact with an active, goal-directed movement by the patient.

Objective Evidence Regarding the Test

Leroux et al (1995) performed preoperative clinical impingement tests on 55 consecutive patients undergoing surgery for Neer's syndrome. Sensitivity of the Yocum test was 78%. This is somewhat comparable to the sensitivities of the Neer and Hawkins impingement tests, which had sensitivities of 89% and 87%, respectively. No formal anatomic study has been performed that outlines the exact region of subacromial contact or any further analysis with the Yocum test.

INTERNAL ROTATION RESISTANCE STRENGTH TEST

Indication

The internal rotation resistance strength test distinguishes between Neer outlet impingement and nonoutlet or intraarticular causes of shoulder pain.

About the Test

This test was first reported by Zaslav (2001) as a test to differentiate between classic Neer-type outlet impingement and other types of intraarticular shoulder pathology. The use of a manual muscle test in a specific position and the subsequent response of the patient to this manual muscle test form the basis for this test.

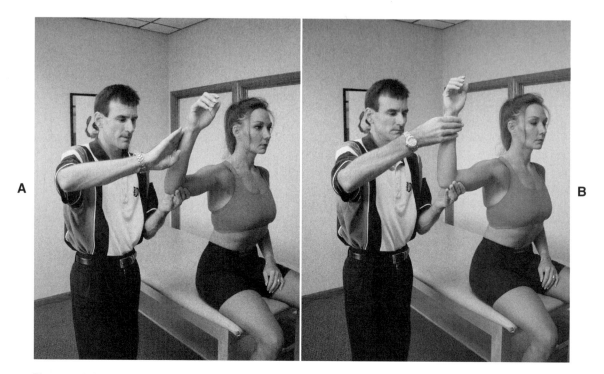

Figure 10-9 Internal rotation resistance strength test. **A,** External rotation resistance. **B,** Internal rotation resistance.

Starting Position

The internal rotation resistance strength test is performed with the patient in a seated position, with the examiner standing directly behind the patient oriented toward the side being tested. The patient's arm is positioned in 90 degrees of abduction in the coronal plane and in approximately 80 degrees of external rotation (Figure 10-9). One of the examiner's hands is placed under the elbow of the patient's extremity to provide support during testing, with the other hand placed at approximately the level of the wrist to perform the manual isometric test.

Action

A manual isometric muscle test is performed for external rotation (examiner's distal hand placed on the extensor or dorsal surface of the patient's wrist) (see Figure 10-9, *A*) followed by a manual muscle test for internal rotation (examiner's distal hand placed on the flexor or palmar surface of the patient's wrist) (see Figure 10-9, *B*).

What Constitutes a Positive Test?

A positive Neer impingement sign and good strength in external rotation and apparent weakness in internal rotation constitute a positive test. Because this is a test of

relative weakness in the pathologic shoulder, strength between the injured and noninjured shoulder is not compared.

Ramifications of a Positive Test

A positive internal rotation resistance strength test (relative weakness in internal rotation) in a patient with a positive Neer impingement sign is predictive of internal (nonoutlet) impingement. A positive Neer impingement sign and greater weakness in external rotation in the 90-degree abducted and 80-degree externally rotated position is suggestive of classic Neer outlet impingement.

Objective Evidence Regarding the Test

Zaslav (2001) examined 115 consecutive patients who had a positive Neer impingement test and were scheduled to undergo arthroscopic evaluation of the injured shoulder. All patients were tested using the internal rotation resistance strength test, and the presence or absence of the index test was compared with intraoperative findings. The sensitivity of the test, defined as the percentage of patients with diagnostic findings of internal impingement and a positive internal rotation resistance strength test, was 88%. Specificity, defined as the percentage of patients with arthroscopic findings of outlet or Neer-type impingement who exhibited a negative internal rotation resistance strength test, was 96%. The PPV (the percentage of patients with a positive internal rotation resistance strength test who actually had internal impingement as the cause of their pain) was 88% and the NPV (patients with a negative test and outlet/Neer impingement as the primary cause of their symptoms) was 96%. Results indicate that this clinical test can be used with confidence by clinicians trying to differentiate between outlet and nonoutlet impingement. Further research, including interrater reliability, will result in further application of this test in the clinical evaluation of patients with shoulder impingement symptoms.

Rotator Cuff Tests

EMPTY CAN TEST

Indication

The empty can test is a manual resistive test to assess the integrity of the supraspinatus muscle-tendon unit.

About the Test

This test position was originally described by Jobe and Moynes (1982) as a position to isolate the supraspinatus muscle-tendon unit for both diagnostic testing and as an exercise position/movement pattern during glenohumeral joint rehabilitation. The test has been called the *supraspinatus test, scaption,* and *empty can position* because of the position's resemblance to a person holding a can and emptying out its contents.

Start Position

The patient can be examined in either the seated or standing position. The examiner is typically in front of the patient in order to observe facial expression or compensation by other parts of the kinetic chain. The patient's extremity is elevated to 90 degrees in the scapular plane (30 degrees anterior to the coronal plane), with full internal rotation of the shoulder so that the patient's thumb is pointing directly toward the ground (Figure 11-1). Care should be taken to ensure that the patient's thoracic posture is erect and consistent with positioning used during testing of the contralateral side. Alterations in muscular strength resulting from the length-tension relationship of the muscle-tendon unit have been reported in the upper extremity (Kebaetse et al, 1999) based on scapulothoracic positioning. Care should be taken to note significant elevation of the shoulder girdle as a compensation by the patient, both during the set-up positioning and resistive portion of the test.

Action

The examiner applies downward pressure to the patient's extremity, with instruction to resist the pressure and maintain the initial starting position. The examiner can apply contact just proximal to the elbow (Jobe & Bradley, 1989) or by using two fingers of pressure just proximal to the ulnar styloid process (see Figure 11-1). It is imperative that consistency be used with regard to the location and intensity of the downward pressure to ensure accurate interpretation of the test.

What Constitutes a Positive Test?

Interpretation of this test is somewhat controversial and deserves further clarification. Several authors consider the test to be positive when there is either muscular weakness or reproduction of pain (Itoi et al, 1999; Jobe & Bradley, 1989; Magee, 1997). Some authors consider the test to be purely a manual muscle test (Kelly et al, 1996). Itoi et al, (1999) published a detailed example of the combined interpretation of this test, noting whether pain was reproduced during the maneuver. They used traditional grading from manual muscle testing (Daniels and Worthingham, 1980) to determine whether there was muscular weakness. Grading of the empty can test was classified from 0 to 5 (Table 11-1).

Using the classification system from Daniels and Worthingham (1980), Itoi et al, (1999) determined that muscle weakness was present when the strength grade was less than 4. Although this classification is somewhat controversial and open to interpretation, I recommend its use, with both pain and muscular weakness being considered positive reactions. Noting whether pain, weakness, or both are present during testing is recommended based on the results of the research discussed in the next section.

Ramifications of a Positive Test

Itoi et al (1999) studied the empty can test and the full can test (scapular plane elevation resistance with the upper extremity in an externally rotated position such that the thumb is pointing upward, similar to the position of someone holding a full can of soda) (Figure 11-2) in patients with suspected rotator cuff pathology. The empty and full can tests were performed in 143 shoulders of 136 consecutive patients, and results of the tests were

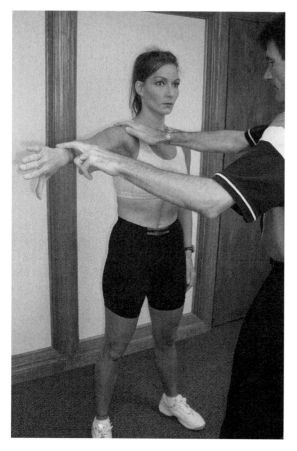

Figure 11-1 Empty can test position.

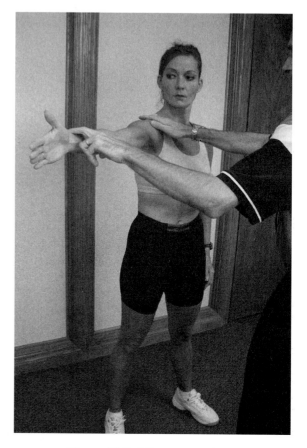

Figure 11-2 Full can test position.

TABLE 11-1   Grading of the Empty Can Test

GRADE	DESCRIPTION
5	Normal amount of resistance to applied force
4	Lesser amount of resistance than grade 5 but greater than grade 3
3	Ability to move the segment through the range of motion against gravity
2	Ability to move the segment through the range of motion with gravity eliminated
1	Presence of a muscular contraction without joint motion
0	No muscular contraction

From Itoi E et al: Which is more useful, the "full can test" or the "empty can test" in detecting the torn supraspinatus tendon? *Am J Sports Med* 27(1):65-68, 1999.

compared with results of high-resolution magnetic resonance imaging (MRI), with 95% proven accuracy for full-thickness rotator cuff tears (Itoi et al, 1999). The empty can and full can tests were considered positive if there was pain, muscular weakness, or both.

The accuracy of the test was greater when muscular weakness rather than pain was the determining feature for both the empty and full can tests. No significant difference existed, however, between the two tests as far as accuracy was concerned in identifying patients with full-thickness rotator cuff tears. There was also no significant difference between the two tests when pain was used as the determining feature. Table 11-2 outlines the specific statistical results of the study by Itoi et al (1999).

Ultimately, both of these tests can be used with varying levels of statistical and clinical confidence when examining the patient with suspected rotator cuff disease. Pain and weakness are important variables when interpreting this test. Table 11-2 shows the difference between these important determinants during the clinical evaluation of the patient with a suspected rotator cuff tear.

Additional Evidence Regarding the Test

Leroux et al (1995) tested 55 consecutive patients using the Jobe empty can test. A positive empty can test producing pain indicated supraspinatus tendonitis, and a

TABLE 11-2   Statistical Results of the Empty Can and Full Can Tests for Supraspinatus Tears

TEST/CONDITION	SENSITIVITY	SPECIFICITY	PPV	NPV	ACCURACY
FULL CAN TEST					
Pain	66%	64%	37%	85%	64%
Weakness	77%	74%	49%	91%	75%
Pain, weakness, or both	86%	57%	39%	93%	64%
EMPTY CAN TEST					
Pain	63%	55%	34%	82%	57%
Weakness	77%	68%	44%	90%	70%
Pain, weakness, or both	89%	50%	36%	93%	59%

PPV, Positive predictive value; *NPV*, negative predictive value.

positive empty can test with muscular weakness indicated tendon rupture (full-thickness tear of the supraspinatus tendon). Sensitivity was 86% and specificity was 50% for the identification of supraspinatus tendonitis; sensitivity was 79% and specificity was 67% for rotator cuff tears. These findings are similar to those reported by Itoi et al (1999) using the empty can test.

GERBER LIFT-OFF TEST

Indication

The Gerber lift-off test, designed by Christian Gerber, an orthopedic surgeon from Switzerland, is used to identify full-thickness tears of the subscapularis tendon.

About the Test

Traumatic rupture of the subscapularis tendon occurs from a forced hyperextension or external rotation of the adducted arm (Gerber & Krushell, 1991). Common clinical symptoms are increased external rotation range of motion and anterior shoulder pain with internal rotation weakness.

Starting Position

The patient is examined in a standing position. The patient is asked to place one hand behind the back such that the dorsal surface of the hand is resting against the patient's lumbar spine (Figure 11-3, *A*). This position places the shoulder in extension and internal rotation.

Action

The patient is asked to lift the dorsum of the hand off the lumbar spine and away from the body (Figure 11-3, *B*).

What Constitutes a Positive Test?

A patient with a full-thickness rupture/tear of the subscapularis tendon will be unable to lift the hand away from the lumbar spine; this is called a *pathologic lift-off test* (Gerber & Krushell, 1991).

Ramifications of a Positive Test

An inability to move the dorsal surface of the hand from the lumbar spine indicates extreme weakness of the subscapularis muscle tendon unit and is thought to represent a full-thickness tear of that tendon. It must be verified, however, that the patient has that range of motion and does not simply lack internal rotation range of motion that, when combined with the shoulder extension and adduction positioning of this test, prevents the patient from any further active motion. Failure to identify this important range of motion restriction before doing this test can lead to inaccurate diagnosis and misinterpretation.

Modifications of the Traditional Gerber Lift-Off Test

Stefko et al (1997) performed an electromyogram (EMG) and nerve block analysis of the Gerber lift-off test. Fifteen subjects were tested in varying positions of shoulder adduction, extension, and internal rotation while indwelling electromyography was performed of several shoulder girdle muscles. Stefko et al (1997) reported that none of the experimental modifications of the Gerber lift-off test isolated either the upper or lower subscapularis from the latissimus dorsi, posterior deltoid, or rhomboid muscles. This finding revealed that this test maneuver did not completely isolate the function of the subscapularis muscle-tendon unit, thus questioning the ability of the test to identify isolated pathology of the subscapularis muscle-tendon unit.

In the second part of this investigation, the subscapular nerve was paralyzed in five human subjects. Patients with a nonfunctional subscapularis were able to perform the lift-off test in its original form as described previously (Gerber & Krushell, 1991), as well as during

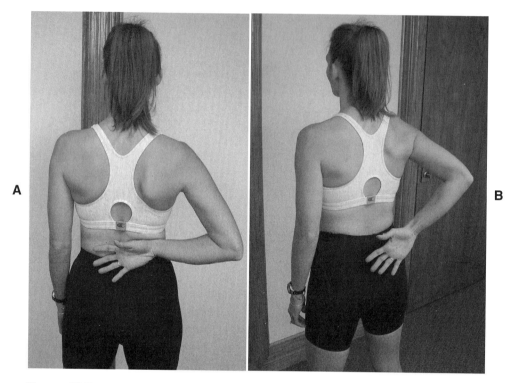

Figure 11-3 Traditional Gerber lift-off test position. **A,** Starting position. **B,** Normal ending position.

several other test modifications. However, one position of testing, the maximal internal rotation lift-off test (Figure 11-4), which consisted of the subject starting from a maximally internally rotated position with the dorsum of the hand near the inferior border of the ipsilateral scapula, was not possible with a nonfunctioning subscapularis. The position was subsequently recommended for better use in isolating subscapularis function or pathology during clinical examination. This maneuver is limited by its need for greater amounts of internal rotation with the shoulder in an extended and adducted position. The range of motion requirement must be checked by the examiner before successful administration of this test.

Objective Evidence Regarding the Test

In their original article, Gerber and Krushell (1991) tested 162 subjects, some with and some without pathology of the rotator cuff. Although they did not report specific statistics on their initial research, 100 subjects with no pathology of the rotator cuff had 100 normal lift-off tests and 27 patients with confirmed rotator cuff tears but with normal subscapularis muscle tendon units had 27 normal lift-off tests. Of nine patients with full-thickness tears

of the subscapularis among those tested, eight had pathologic lift-off tests, and one had a normal test, resulting in a sensitivity of 80% and a specificity of 100%.

Leroux et al (1995) did not find the lift-off test to be as accurate clinically. They found a specificity of 61% and a sensitivity of 0% for the lift-off test in their evaluation of 55 consecutive patients. Kelly et al (1996) reported the lift-off test position (dorsum of hand initially placed against the lumbar spine with extension of the hand away from the lumbar spine) to be the optimal position to test the integrity of the subscapularis muscle-tendon unit.

Greis et al (1996) used EMG to determine muscle activity of the rotator cuff, pectoralis major, teres major, latissimus dorsi, and serratus anterior during performance of the lift-off test. Activity in the upper and lower subscapularis muscle was 70% of maximal voluntary contraction during the lift-off test when the hand was placed in the mid-lumbar region. The level of activity of the subscapularis was statistically higher than for all the other muscles tested during this maneuver. In addition, in agreement with other studies, Greis et al (1996) found approximately 33% more muscle activity when the test was performed with the hand in the mid-lumbar region as

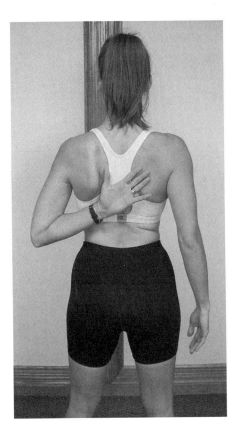

Figure 11-4 Modified Gerber lift-off test position (starting position).

compared with the buttock region. Adding resistance to the lift-off maneuver increased activity in all the muscles except for the pectoralis major. Greater levels of muscular activation are required in the scapular stabilizers during resistance application in this maneuver (Greis et al, 1996). This study further validates the Gerber lift-off test and provides clinically specific information regarding arm/ hand placement during testing.

Gerber and Krushell (1991) concluded that the lift-off test is valid when tested in patients with full passive internal rotation range of motion and when active range of motion is not severely limited by pain. In these conditions, a pathologic lift-off test, coupled with increased external rotation range of motion and decreased internal rotation strength, is indicative of a full-thickness tear of the subscapularis tendon.

NAPOLEON TEST

Indication

The Napoleon test is used to identify a tear of the subscapularis tendon.

About the Test

This test was initially described by Imhoff as a variation of the Gerber belly press test (Burkhart & Tehrany, 2002); it is named for Napoleon's hand position as seen in portraits. The test is an alternative to the Gerber lift-off test when glenohumeral joint internal rotation is too restricted to allow for placement of the hand behind the back in order to detect tears of the subscapularis.

Starting Position

The patient is typically examined in the standing position. The hand is placed directly over the stomach, which places the shoulder in slight forward flexion, abduction, and internal rotation (Figure 11-5, *A*).

Action

The patient is asked to press the hand of the involved extremity against the stomach while the examiner pays particular attention to the position of the patient's involved wrist as the patient presses the hand into the stomach (see later).

What Constitutes a Positive Test?

According to Burkhart and Tehrany (2002), the Napoleon test is graded as negative (normal) when the patient can push the hand against the stomach with the wrist straight. A positive Napoleon sign exists if the wrist must flex 90 degrees while pushing against the stomach (Figure 11-5, *B*). An intermediate grade is given when the wrist flexes 30 to 60 degrees when the patient pushes against the stomach.

Ramifications of a Positive Test

In a patient with a subscapularis tear, the wrist flexes as the patient attempts to press against the stomach because this maneuver allows the patient to harness the power of the posterior deltoid. With a subscapularis-deficient shoulder, the patient cannot rotate the arm internally to full range actively in this position and must flex the wrist to orient the arm so that the posterior deltoid can extend the shoulder back to produce this belly-pressing result. This test can be used in patients with limited function, making the Gerber lift-off test diagnostically inaccurate.

Objective Evidence Regarding the Test

Burkhart and Tehrany (2002) performed the Napoleon test in 25 patients before surgery; 9 had positive tests and 8 of the 9 had tears of the entire subscapularis tendon. The Napoleon test tended to correlate to the size and location of the tear in the subscapularis. Positive Napoleon tests involved full-thickness tears of the

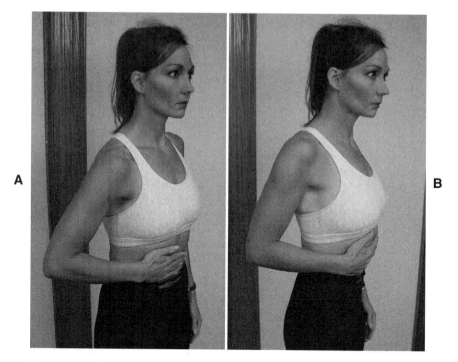

Figure 11-5 Napoleon test. **A,** Positive Napoleon test, characterized by increased shoulder extension and wrist flexion (**B**).

subscapularis in both the upper and lower halves. Negative Napoleon tests were found in patients with only the upper half of the subscapularis torn. Intermediate Napoleon tests were found in patients with more than the upper half of the subscapularis tendon torn, but not a complete tear of both the upper and lower portion. No further objective testing or statistical information is available for the Napoleon test.

DROPPING SIGN TEST

Indication

The dropping sign test is used to assess the integrity of the infraspinatus muscle-tendon unit.

About the Test

This test was designed to evaluate the integrity of the infraspinatus muscle-tendon unit based on its ability to perform and support the distal aspect of the upper extremity against gravity. Neer (1990) described this version of the dropping sign.

Start Position

The patient is typically examined in a seated position. The elbow is flexed to 90 degrees, with the forearm in a neutral position and the arm placed against the side in adduction. The shoulder is externally rotated 45 degrees to the start position by supporting under the patient's elbow and the patient's wrist (Figure 11-6, *A*).

Action

The examiner then performs a manual muscle test by asking the patient to press outward into external rotation. If the patient cannot perform active external rotation and the examiner essentially meets no external resistance, the dropping sign is commenced. The examiner then releases the patient's arm by releasing the patient's wrist (Figure 11-6, *B* and *C*).

What Constitutes a Positive Test?

A positive test occurs when the patient's arm drops into a more neutral rotated position as a result of an inability to support even the weight of the arm in the externally rotated starting position (see Figure 11-6, *C*).

Ramifications of a Positive Test

A positive dropping sign has been correlated with a complete tear of the infraspinatus muscle (Walch et al, 1998).

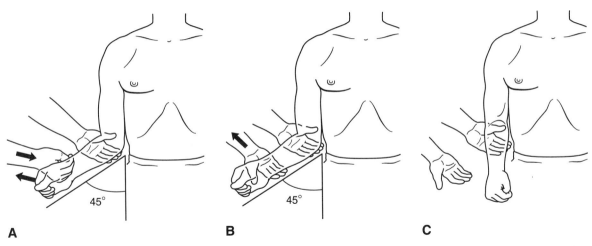

Figure 11-6 Dropping sign. **A,** The examiner places the forearm at 45 degrees of external rotation. The patient then pushes against his hand. **B,** With the patient seated, the shoulder is placed in 0 degrees of abduction and 45 degrees of external rotation with the elbow flexed 90 degrees. The examiner holds the patient's forearm in this position and instructs the patient to maintain it when the examiner releases the forearm. **C,** On releasing the forearm, a positive test is recorded when the patient's forearm drops back to 0 degrees of external rotation, despite efforts to maintain external rotation. (From Walch G et al: The "dropping" and "Hornblower's" sign in evaluation of rotator-cuff tears, *J Bone Joint Surg Br* 80(4):625, 1998.)

Objective Evidence for this Test

Walch et al (1998) tested 54 patients operated on for combined supraspinatus and infraspinatus/teres minor rotator cuff tears. They reported 100% specificity and 100% sensitivity for the dropping sign to identify patients with irreparable degeneration of the infraspinatus muscle-tendon unit. This clinical sign of impaired external rotation (dropping sign) was correlated with fatty degeneration (Goutallier stage 3 or 4) of the infraspinatus. Results indicate severe weakness and impairment of the infraspinatus.

HORNBLOWER'S SIGN

Indication

Hornblower's sign is used to identify severe weakness and degeneration of the teres minor muscle-tendon unit.

About the Test

This test was originally reported in obstetric brachial plexus palsy (Arthuis, 1972). The teres minor is responsible for producing up to 45% of the power in external rotation (Jenp et al, 1996).

Start Position

The patient can be examined in either a standing or seated position, with arms resting against the sides.

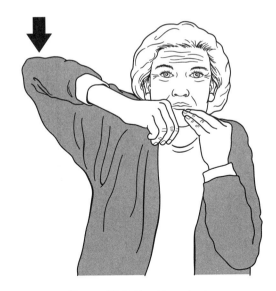

Figure 11-7 Hornblower's sign.

Action

The patient is asked to bring both hands up toward the mouth simultaneously.

What Constitutes a Positive Test?

A positive Hornblower's sign is present when the patient is unable to bring the hand toward the mouth in the same manner as the contralateral side and can only do so in the characteristic compensatory pattern (Figure 11-7), which

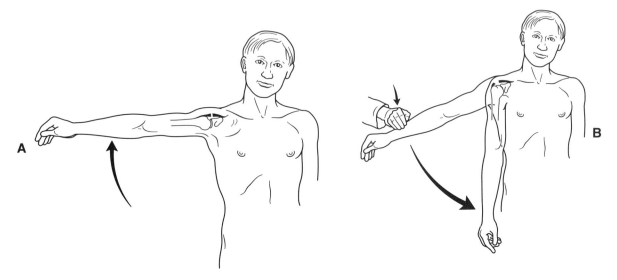

Figure 11-8 Drop-arm test. (Modified from Hoppenfeld S, Hutton R: Physical examination of the shoulder. In *Physical examination of the spine and extremities*, Norwalk, CT, 1976, Appleton-Century-Crofts.)

consists of shoulder abduction in the absence of external rotation.

Ramifications of a Positive Test

A positive Hornblower's sign has been linked to complete full-thickness tears of the teres minor (Walch et al, 1998).

Objective Evidence Regarding the Test

Walch et al (1998) studied 54 patients operated on for rotator cuff pathology. The Hornblower's sign had 100% sensitivity and 93% specificity for irreparable tears of the teres minor. This movement can be used to identify patients with severe teres minor involvement, represented by the characteristic compensatory pattern used with the functional activity of movement of the hands toward the face. No additional research has been conducted on this test.

DROP-ARM TEST

Indication

The drop-arm test is used to detect tears of the rotator cuff.

About the Test

This nonspecific test was originally described by Hoppenfeld (1976) and is based on the important role of the rotator cuff in the deltoid rotator cuff force couple applied in humeral elevation (Inman et al, 1944).

Starting Position

The patient is typically examined in the standing position (Figure 11-8).

Action

The patient is instructed to abduct the shoulder in the coronal plane fully, with the arm placed in slight internal rotation, such that the palm is oriented toward the ground (see Figure 11-8, *A*). The patient is then asked to slowly lower the arm from the abducted position. If there are tears in the supraspinatus muscle-tendon unit, the arm will drop rapidly to the side as the patient lowers the arm from a position of about 90 degrees of abduction. If the arm is able to be held in 90 degrees of abduction, the examiner may gently tap the distal aspect of the patient's arm, which will cause the patient's arm to fall to the side (see Figure 11-8, *B*). It is recommended that the examiner place a hand or hands under the patient's lowering extremity, or one hand under the extremity when tapping, to support and actually catch the weight of the arm after the dropping-type movement begins. This maneuver can help minimize pain.

What Constitutes a Positive Test?

Inability to eccentrically lower the arm in adduction from an abducted position in the coronal plane without dropping as well as dropping of the arm after a light tap on the distal aspect of the extremity are both considered positive drop-arm tests.

Ramifications of a Positive Test

A positive drop-arm test is thought to indicate a full-thickness tear of the supraspinatus muscle-tendon unit. Inability to control the weight of the arm during controlled adduction indicates significant weakness of the rotator cuff secondary to the tear.

Objective Evidence Regarding the Test

Sher et al (1995) conducted MRI evaluations of 96 asymptomatic individuals to determine the presence and prevalence of rotator cuff tears. The overall prevalence of rotator cuff tears was 34%, with 15% being full-thickness tears. The drop-arm test was performed to determine the presence of a substantial rotator cuff tear. All 96 patients had negative drop-arm tests despite a 15% prevalence of full-thickness tears and 20% prevalence of partial-thickness tears.

Calis et al (2000) studied the accuracy of the drop-arm test in a group of patients with and without a positive subacromial injection test. They reported a low sensitivity of 7.8% but a specificity of 97%. The drop-arm test is typically used to clarify whether a complete tear or rupture of the rotator cuff has occurred. The high specificity may have resulted from detection of a rotator cuff tear in patients who tested positive for the subacromial impingement test and perhaps had Neer stage III subacromial impingement (Calis et al, 2000). Further research is necessary, including comparison of the finding to actual surgical findings or MRI reports to better understand the effectiveness of the test. Based on the results of the study by Sher et al, (1995), caution should be used when interpreting results of this test.

Biceps Tests

INTRODUCTION

Injury to the biceps tendon can occur as an isolated entity; however, in most cases problems with this structure occur in conjunction with glenohumeral joint impingement or instability (Eakin et al, 1999). A short discussion of biceps tendon pathology is presented to better understand the role specific tests play in the identification of biceps tendon disorders, as well as to emphasize the role of a comprehensive evaluation to determine the underlying cause of biceps pathology. The close relationship of the biceps long-head tendon to the superior labrum, subscapularis, rotator interval, and coracohumeral ligament has increased interest in its functional anatomy, biomechanics, and evaluation methods (Eakin et al, 1999).

The biceps long-head tendon originates within the glenohumeral joint. After coursing through the bicipital groove between the greater and lesser tuberosities, the tendon joins the short head of the biceps at the level of the deltoid tubercle. Habermeyer et al (1987), in an anatomic study, found that the biceps long head tendon originated from the posterior superior labrum in 48% of specimens examined, from the supraglenoid tubercle in 20%, and from both sites in 28%. Within the glenohumeral joint, the tendon is intraarticular but extrasynovial, ensheathed by a continuation of the synovial lining of the articular capsule (Curtis & Snyder, 1993).

The function of the biceps long-head tendon is controversial. Kumar et al (1989) reported upward migration of the humeral head in 15 cadavers with intraarticular release of the biceps long-head tendon. Dynamic depression of the humeral head was demonstrated by Warner and McMahon (1995) who also showed superior migration of the humeral head relative to the contralateral or control shoulder in seven patients with loss of the biceps long-head tendon. Several studies (Rodosky et al, 1994; Pagnani et al, 1996; Itoi et al, 1993) have identified the function of the biceps long-head tendon as a stabilizer against anterior humeral head translation. The torsional rigidity of the anterior capsule was increased and forces transmitted to the inferior glenohumeral ligament complex were decreased during simulated contraction of the biceps in experimental studies (Rodosky et al, 1994). Detachment of the biceps anchor at the superior labrum increased the strain on the inferior glenohumeral ligament complex up to 120% (Cheng & Karzel, 1997). These studies show the important role the biceps and superior labrum play in the stabilization of the human glenohumeral joint.

Dynamic muscular activity of the biceps has been measured using electromyography (EMG) during both planar motions and functional activities (Glousmann et al, 1988; Yamaguchi et al, 1997). Yamaguchi et al (1997) studied the EMG activity of the biceps in 40 subjects who had their elbow locked in a brace to prohibit elbow movement and isolate shoulder function. Planar shoulder motions were performed, including internal and external rotation and scapular elevation. EMG activity of the biceps ranged from 1.7% to 3.6% of maximal activation levels. No difference was found between subjects with full-thickness rotator cuff tears and normal subjects. The authors concluded that given the EMG results of their investigation, the function of the biceps during isolated glenohumeral motion does not include active contraction of the biceps. Using similar methodology, Levy et al (2001) also found limited EMG activity of the biceps long-head tendon during shoulder motion. They concluded "any hypothesis on biceps function at the shoulder must be a passive role of the tendon or tension in association with elbow and forearm activity."

Glousmann et al (1988) compared the EMG activity in throwing athletes diagnosed with glenohumeral joint instability and in normal throwing athletes. Increases in biceps EMG activity were found during the acceleration phase of the throwing motion in the group of athletes with glenohumeral joint instability. This increased activity in the biceps was thought to improve glenohumeral joint stabilization.

The specific pathomechanics that lead to injury in the biceps long-head tendon typically focuses around impingement or compression of the tendon in the suprahumeral space. According to Neer (1972), in most patients with biceps long-head tendon pathology, the primary source of the pain is glenohumeral impingement, with biceps tendonitis being second. "Both Charles Neer and Charles Rockwood have stressed the fact that 95% to 98% of patients with the diagnosis of biceps tendonitis have in reality a primary diagnosis of impingement syndrome" (Burkhead, 1990).

In addition to impingement as the primary pathomechanical factor in biceps tendonitis, Eakin et al (1999) have described the close association between glenohumeral joint instability and biceps involvement. Forces generated, particularly during overhead shoulder motions in sports on a repetitive basis, eventually exceed the capability of the anterior static restraints of the shoulder. Eventually, progressive attenuation of these restraints can cause a traction injury to both the rotator cuff and biceps tendon. This attenuation can lead to secondary impingement against the coracoacromial arch by the biceps tendon and create further injury (Eakin et al, 1999).

Primary tendinosis has been described as a pathogenesis in biceps long-head tendon injury. Factors leading to the degenerative tendinosis include hypovascularity (Rathburn & MacNab, 1970), fiber failure, and mechanical irritation within the intertubercular groove (Eakin et al, 1999). Kraushaar and Nirschl (1999) described the degenerative response of tendon injury and highlighted the lack of inflammatory cells and high concentration of fibroblasts and vascular hyperplasia in a histologic study of injured tendons. This tendon degeneration can lead to failure and tendon rupture.

Finally, biceps long-head tendon instability has been described as another form of biceps pathology at the glenohumeral joint. Although rare, this condition was thought to be primarily caused by tearing of the transverse ligament, which overlies the bicipital groove of the humerus (Eakin et al, 1999). Cadaveric study, however, has shown that even with transection of the transverse humeral ligament over the groove, the biceps long-head tendon did not subluxate medially (Paavolainen et al,

1983). Walch et al (1994) have highlighted the importance of the rotator interval lesion and the crucial function of the coracohumeral ligament and superior glenohumeral ligament as stabilizers of the biceps long-head tendon.

Table 12-1 lists the classification of biceps tendon pathology at the glenohumeral joint based on the descriptions of Curtis and Snyder (1993). The close association of other glenohumeral joint abnormalities such as rotator cuff impingement and glenohumeral joint instability emphasize the importance of performing a comprehensive examination in the patient with suspected biceps long-head tendon involvement.

SPEED'S TEST

Indication
Speed's test is used primarily to identify biceps tendon pathology.

About the Test
J. Spencer Speed of the Campbell Clinic originally described the Speed's test. The test was invented by Dr. Speed through the frequent use of his own shoulder in an elbow extended, forearm supinated position, elevating the leg of his patients doing a straight leg test for lumbar pathology (Bennett, 1998; Van Moppes et al, 1995). He was subsequently diagnosed with bicipital tendonitis. His test is used to evaluate for biceps tendon pathology as well as SLAP (*s*uperior *l*abrum *a*nterior *p*osterior) lesions (see labral injury section pages 115–117).

Start Position
The patient is preferably in a seated position to minimize compensatory movements; however, the standing position can be used, with feet placed shoulder-width apart. The shoulder is placed in 90 degrees of flexion in the sagittal plane, with the forearm in a supinated position such that the hand is facing directly upward (Figure 12-1). Stabilization by the examiner is recommended by placing a

TABLE 12-1   Classification of Biceps Pathology

PATHOLOGY	DESCRIPTION
Secondary biceps tendonitis	Occurs secondary to either rotator cuff impingement or glenohumeral joint instability
Primary biceps tendonitis	Caused by eccentric overload, hypovascularity, and abnormalities within the bicipital groove, leading to attrition of the tendon
Biceps tendon instability	Occurs infrequently, but may occur with rotator interval lesions or rotator cuff tears
Biceps tendon rupture	Can be acute or chronic; actual tendon rupture can be the end stage of any of the disorders listed in this table

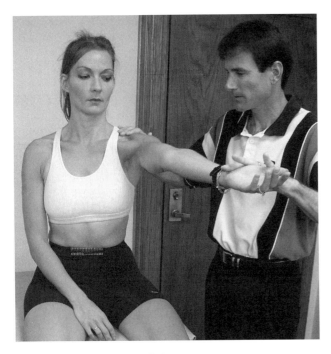

Figure 12-1 Speed's test.

hand on the posterosuperior aspect of the shoulder (Bennett, 1998).

Action

A downward pressure is applied with the shoulder in 90 degrees of shoulder flexion in the sagittal plane. The extremity remains in a position of forearm supination during the test.

What Constitutes a Positive Test?

Reproduction of pain in the anterior aspect of the shoulder over the bicipital groove indicates pathology of the biceps long-head tendon (Bennett, 1998).

Ramifications of a Positive Test

A positive Speed's test indicates primarily bicipital tendon pathology. Because of the intimate blending of the biceps long-head tendon with the superior labrum, reproduction of anterior shoulder pain with this test has been reported to indicate SLAP injury (Bennett, 1998). Detachment of the superior labrum is provoked with the contraction or tensing of the bicipital tendon that occurs with the Speed's test and thus can re-create the patient's anterior shoulder pain during this maneuver.

Objective Evidence Regarding the Test

The specificity of the Speed's test was reported by Bennett et al (1998) by evaluating 46 shoulders in 45 patients with anterior shoulder pain. The clinical evaluation showed that the Speed's test was positive in 40 of 46 shoulders. Arthroscopic evaluation after clinical testing was performed with the use of a neuroprobe that pulled the biceps long-head tendon into the articular portion of the glenohumeral joint. This allowed for direct visualization of the tendon during surgery. Biceps and labral pathology was found only at the time of surgery in 10 of 40 patients with a positive Speed's test. A specificity of 13.8% and a sensitivity of 90% was reported, with a positive predictive value (PPV) of 23% and negative predictive value (NPV) of 83%. This research indicates that the Speed's test is positive for a variety of pathologic shoulder conditions, and the test is nonspecific but sensitive for biceps/labral pathology. Caution should be used when interpreting the results of this lone test for biceps and labral pathology. Clinical reproduction of localized anterior shoulder pain over the bicipital groove has been recognized as the primary positive result with this test; however, objective research findings question the accuracy of this clinical test.

Calis et al (2000) used the Speed's test in patients with and without a positive subacromial injection test. They reported 67% sensitivity and 55% specificity for the Speed's test, with a PPV of 79% and NPV of 41%. The Speed's test was more sensitive but less specific than the Yergason test in patients testing positive for subacromial impingement syndrome via an injection test. Use of this test can play a part in understanding what structure or structures are affected by impingement or compressive disease; however, further research is needed to better outline this test's diagnostic efficiency in identifying bicipital pathology.

YERGASON'S TEST

Indication

Yergason's test is performed to evaluate for biceps long-head tendon pathology. This test uses a more neutral glenohumeral joint position, unlike the 90-degree position of shoulder flexion used during the Speed's test.

About the Test

The test was originally reported by Yergason (1931) as a test to identify biceps pathology.

Starting Position

The patient is seated with the glenohumeral joint in 10 to 20 degrees of passive abduction; the examiner stands directly to the patient's side (same side as shoulder being tested) (Figure 12-2). For examination of the right

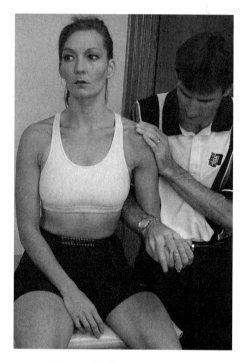

Figure 12-2 Yergason's test.

shoulder, the examiner places his or her left arm under the patient's shoulder, producing 10 to 20 degrees of abduction of the patient's shoulder. The left hand of the examiner grasps the distal aspect of the patient's forearm and wrist (for testing a right shoulder). The right hand of the examiner (again for testing the patient's right shoulder) is placed on the anterosuperior aspect of the right shoulder to stabilize the arm during testing. No significant pressure or compression is performed by the hand stabilizing the proximal aspect of the patient's shoulder.

Action

While keeping the patient's shoulder stationary, the examiner provides resistance on the distal aspect of the patient's forearm and wrist while the patient supinates against that resistance (Davies & DeCarlo, 1995) (see Figure 12-2). Another variation of this test involves simultaneous resistance of external rotation (lateral rotation) during the resistance to forearm supination (Yergason, 1931; Magee, 1997). Additional provocation to the biceps can be obtained by also resisting elbow flexion during the supinatory resistance phase of the Yergason's test (Reider, 1999).

What Constitutes a Positive Test?

Reproduction of the patient's proximal anterior shoulder pain in the bicipital groove indicates a positive test. A painful snap along the bicipital groove may be caused by

subluxation of the long head of the biceps tendon as a result of a second- or third-degree sprain of the transverse humeral ligament (Davies et al, 1981).

Ramifications of a Positive Test

Although objective cadaveric studies that verify the tensile loading of the biceps tendon with the maneuver have not been published, this test is used to assess the irritability of the biceps long-head tendon with the glenohumeral joint placed in a more neutral nonimpingement position. Provocation of anterior pain with biceps contraction in this position would theoretically be less likely to be produced by compression of the rotator cuff or biceps tendon against the coracoacromial arch as a result of the low levels of abduction used during testing. Further research evaluation of this test is needed to determine its efficacy. This test should be used in combination with other biceps and biceps/labral tests.

Objective Evidence Regarding the Test

Calis et al (2000) tested the validity of the Yergason test in a group of patients with and without a positive subacromial injection test, indicating subacromial impingement syndrome. They reported sensitivity values of 37% and specificity of 86%, in addition to a PPV of 86% and an NPV of 36%. By comparison, the Speed and Yergason tests had higher specificity than the traditional impingement tests of Neer, Hawkins, and cross-arm adduction, leading the authors to speculate that bicipital involvement may play a larger part than expected in patients testing positive for subacromial impingement syndrome via the subacromial injection test. Clearly, additional research is needed regarding the effectiveness of this test.

LUDINGTON'S TEST

Indication

Ludington's test was originally used to diagnose rupture of the long head of the biceps; it is also used to test for bicipital tendonitis.

About the Test

Originally described by Ludington (1923) as a test to identify a rupture of the long head of the biceps tendon, this test uses a functional position of abduction with external rotation to test the integrity of the biceps long-head tendon.

Start Position

The patient is preferably in a seated position, although a standing position is equally effective. The examiner asks the patient to interlock the fingers of both hands behind the head, placing the shoulders in approximately 120

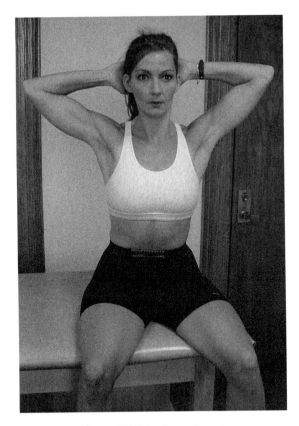

Figure **12-3** Ludington's test.

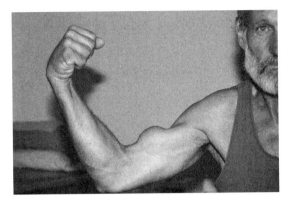

Figure **12-4** Patient with biceps long-head tendon rupture and "Popeye" deformity.

Ramifications of a Positive Test

A positive Ludington's test can be interpreted as indicating pathology of the biceps long-head tendon. Complete rupture of the tendon typically leads to a retraction of the biceps muscle-tendon unit and the appearance of a "Popeye" deformity, resulting in a compacted and enlarged biceps muscle mass (Osbahr et al, 2002) (Figure 12-4). Clinical testing to confirm the ruptured biceps long-head tendon is usually not necessary because of the often obvious muscular adaptation. Reproduction of anterior shoulder pain in the region of the bicipital groove, however, is indicative of biceps long-head tendonitis. The position of the arm in this test (abduction and external rotation) simulates the cocking phase of both the throwing motion (Fleisig et al, 1995) and tennis serve (Elliot et al, 1986) and tests the integrity of the biceps tendon in both a functional position and a position of encroachment by the coracoacromial arch (Valadie et al, 2000).

Objective Evidence Regarding the Test

There is no objective evidence regarding this test in the literature.

GILCHREST'S SIGN

Indication

Gilchrest's sign is a test to determine the presence of biceps long-head tendonitis.

About the Test

This test uses a weight to load the biceps muscle-tendon unit from an overhead position.

Start Position

In a standing position, the patient holds a 2- to 3-kg weight (approximately 5 to 7 pounds) and raises it directly overhead.

degrees of abduction and 90 degrees of external rotation (Figure 12-3). This position creates a relaxation of the biceps muscle-tendon unit by using the interlocking of the hands to support the weight of the extremities (Magee, 1997).

Action

The patient alternately contracts the biceps muscles on each extremity (uninvolved then involved) to produce a forceful contraction of the biceps and tension in the biceps long-head tendon. The biceps long-head tendon can be palpated at the level of the bicipital groove on the proximal humerus to determine whether the tendon has ruptured (Ludington, 1923).

What Constitutes a Positive Test?

As originally described by Ludington (1923), failure to palpate the biceps long-head tendon on the involved extremity indicates a rupture of the long head of the biceps tendon. Davies and DeCarlo (1995) reported reproduction of anterior shoulder pain in the bicipital groove as indicative of biceps tendonitis.

Action

The patient then lowers the arm in the coronal plane from the overhead position in lateral rotation (Figure 12-5).

What Constitutes a Positive Test?

Reproduction of pain in the bicipital groove on lowering the weight in the coronal plane is indicative of biceps tendonitis. An audible click or snapping sensation, most commonly occurring around 90 to 100 degrees of elevation (Magee, 1997), indicates biceps tendon pathology, including instability of the biceps long-head tendon, resulting from interruption of the transverse humeral ligament (Davies et al, 1981).

Ramifications of a Positive Test

Loading of the biceps muscle-tendon unit with the use of an external load indicates pathology of the biceps long-head muscle-tendon unit. This test is most indicated for use in patients who report symptoms only with loads or in overhead reaching applications. Caution is suggested in using this test in patients with easily provoked symptoms or with subjective histories that include microtraumatic mechanisms of overuse because of the presence of the 2- to 3-kg external load.

Objective Evidence Regarding the Test

There is no objective evidence regarding this test in the literature.

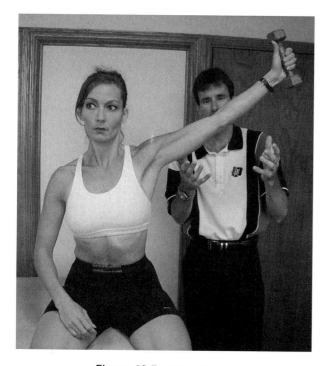

Figure **12-5** Gilchrest's sign.

LIPPMAN'S TEST

Indication

Lippman's test is used to identify biceps tendon pathology.

About the Test

This test was described by Lippman (1943) for the diagnosis of biceps tendonitis.

Starting Position

The patient sits or stands with the involved extremity held in 90 degrees of elbow flexion with one hand by the examiner. The arm is supported by the examiner such that the extremity is relaxed and minimal resting muscle activation is encountered.

Action

The examiner's other hand palpates the biceps tendon in the bicipital groove, moving it from side to side.

What Constitutes a Positive Test?

Lippman's test is considered positive if reproduction of the patient's anterior pain over the biceps tendon at the level of the bicipital groove is produced.

Ramifications of a Positive Test

As with all tests, it is imperative that this test be performed bilaterally. This region (the biceps long-head tendon at the level of the bicipital groove) is often sensitive in patients with rotator cuff and other shoulder pathologies, as well as in the uninvolved extremity. A positive test is often encountered in both extremities.

Objective Evidence Regarding the Test

There is no objective evidence regarding this test in the literature.

TESTS FOR BICEPS TENDON INSTABILITY

Indication

The first reported case of biceps long-head tendon subluxation occurred in 1694 in a woman who was wringing clothes and felt something displace in her shoulder (Burkhead et al, 1998). In patients who have complaints of anteriorly based snapping and popping in addition to symptoms of pain and tenderness, several tests or modifications of tests have been described in the clinical literature as being indicated to test for instability of the biceps long-head tendon.

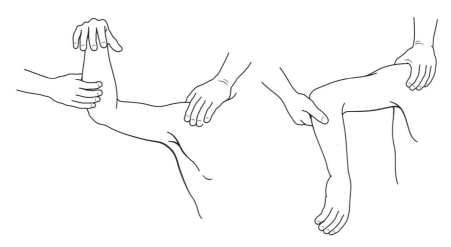

Figure 12-6 Biceps instability test. (From Rockwood CA, Matsen FA III, editors: *The shoulder*, Philadelphia, 1990, WB Saunders.)

About the Tests

These tests use both positional provocation of the tendon and contraction of the tendon in an attempt to dislodge or dislocate the tendon from the intertubercular groove. They are presented in this section as a group because several of the tests also assess the integrity of the tendon itself and are discussed in the previous section.

Tests Used for Biceps Tendon Instability

The primary test used and reported for biceps tendon pathology is the transverse humeral ligament test (Davies & DeCarlo, 1995). This test is performed with the arm at the side in neutral rotation. The patient is asked to actively contract the biceps against the examiner's hand, which is placed on the distal forearm. As the patient is contracting the biceps, the examiner passively rotates the humerus internally and externally in an attempt to sublux the tendon from the groove. A positive test result is present when the tendon subluxates, as well as when the patient's anterior symptoms are reproduced (Davies & DeCarlo, 1995). Reproduction of the patient's perception of subluxation is also considered a positive result.

The second test described in the literature is the biceps instability test. This test was originally described by Abbott and Saunders in 1939. It tests the biceps tendon with the shoulder in abduction. The examiner grasps the arm near 90 degrees of abduction and passively moves the glenohumeral joint from a position of external rotation to a position of internal rotation during palpation of the biceps tendon (Figure 12-6). A positive test occurs when the biceps long-head tendon is forced against the lesser tuberosity with a palpable or audible click.

Additional tests to evaluate the stability of the biceps long-head tendon are described in full detail in the previous section (biceps tests). These tests include Yergason's test and Gilchrist's sign.

Ramifications of a Positive Test

The biceps long-head tendon originates at the supraglenoid tubercle and the glenoid labrum at the most superior aspect of the glenoid. The tendon is 9 mm long on average. The biceps tendon is intraarticular, but extrasynovial. It is stabilized not only by the transverse humeral ligament, but also proximally by the glenohumeral joint capsule. Several capsuloligamentous structures play a key role in stabilizing the biceps long-head tendon in the bicipital groove. The supraspinatus, infraspinatus, subscapularis, and coracohumeral and superior glenohumeral joint capsular ligaments all play a vital role. Paavolainen et al (1983) reported that subluxation of the biceps long-head tendon is nearly impossible, even with complete transection of the transverse humeral ligament. The tendon remained in the intertubercular groove as long as the rotator cuff was intact. These studies inform the examiner of other possible pathology present when biceps long-head tendon instability is encountered during clinical examination. A thorough and complete evaluation of the glenohumeral joint capsular structures is an integral part of the evaluation of biceps instability because of the important role other structures, beyond the transverse humeral ligament, play in stabilizing this important structure.

CHAPTER 13

Labral Testing

INTRODUCTION

The glenoid labrum serves several important functions, including deepening the glenoid fossa to enhance concavity and serving as the attachment for the glenohumeral capsular ligaments. Injury to the labrum can compromise the concavity compression phenomenon by as much as 50% (Matsen et al, 1991). Individuals with increased capsular laxity and generalized joint hypermobility have increased humeral head translation that can subject the labrum to increased shear forces (Kvitne et al, 1995). In the throwing athlete, large anterior translational forces are present at levels up to 50% of body weight during arm acceleration of the throwing motion with the arm in 90 degrees of abduction and external rotation (Fleisig et al, 1995). This repeated translation of the humeral head against and over the glenoid labrum can lead to labral injury. Labral injury can occur either as tearing or as actual detachment from the glenoid.

LABRAL TEARS

Terry et al (1994) reported on arthroscopic evaluation of tears of the glenoid labrum in 83 patients. They classified labral tears into several types, including transverse tears, longitudinal tears, flap tears, horizontal cleavage tears, and fibrillated tears. They also reported the distribution of the location of these tears. Primary tears of the glenoid labrum occurred most commonly in the anterosuperior (60%) or posterosuperior part of the shoulder (18%). Only 1% of tears occurred in the anteroinferior shoulder. Tears were located in more than one location in 22% of cases.

Altchek et al (1992) clinically studied the role of the labrum in the hypermobile shoulder. In a 3-year follow-up evaluation of 40 overhead athletes who underwent arthroscopic labral débridement, 72% initially reported relief of symptoms in the first year after surgery. At the 2-year follow-up evaluation, only 7% of patients reported symptom relief, with a consistent generalized deterioration occurring over time. These authors concluded that arthroscopic labral débridement is not an effective long-term solution for labral tears. They postulated that

the underlying instability of the shoulder that led to labral injury in these overhead athletes must be addressed to effectively return long-term function and symptomatic relief to the patient.

LABRAL DETACHMENT

In addition to the tearing that can occur in the labrum, actual detachment of the labrum from the glenoid rim can occur. The two most common labral detachments encountered clinically are the Bankart and SLAP (*superior labrum anterior posterior*) lesions. Perthes (1906) was the first to describe the presence of a detachment of the anterior labrum in patients with recurrent anterior instability. Bankart (1923, 1938) initially described a method for surgically repairing the lesion that now bears his name.

A Bankart lesion is found in as many as 85% of dislocations (Gill et al, 1997) and is described as a labral detachment occurring between the 2 and 6 o'clock positions on a right shoulder and between the 6 and 10 o'clock positions on a left shoulder (Figure 13-1). This anteroinferior detachment decreases glenohumeral joint stability by interrupting the continuity of the glenoid labrum and compromising the glenohumeral capsular ligaments (Speer et al, 1994b). Detachment of the anterior inferior glenoid labrum creates increases in anterior and inferior humeral head translation.

In addition to labral detachment in the anteroinferior aspect of the glenohumeral joint, similar labral detachment can occur in the superior aspect of the labrum (see Figure 13-1). Snyder et al (1990) classified SLAP into four main types. Type I shows labral degenerative changes and fraying at the edges, but no distinct avulsion. Type II is the most commonly reported superior labral injury (Morgan et al, 1998) and has been described as complete labral detachment from anterosuperior to posterosuperior glenoid rim, with instability of the biceps long-head tendon. The authors further subclassified the type II superior labral lesion into type II anterior, type II posterior, and type II anterior and posterior. Of significance is the increased (threefold) likelihood of type II posterior

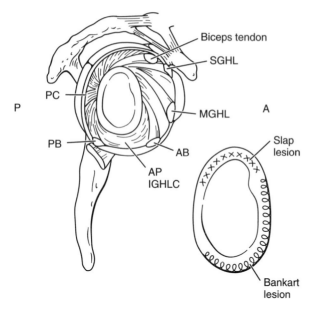

Figure 13-1 Glenoid labrum and depiction of location of Bankart and SLAP lesions. (Adapted from Speer KP et al: Biomechanical evaluation of a simulated Bankart lesion, *J Bone Joint Surg Am* 76(12):1821, 1994.)

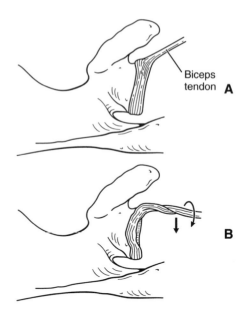

Figure 13-2 A, Superior view of resting position of the biceps-labral complex. **B,** Superior view of the biceps-labral complex in the abducted, externally rotated position, showing peel-back mechanism as the biceps vector rotates posteriorly. (Adapted from Burkhart SS, Morgan CD: The peel-back mechanism: its role in producing and extending posterior type II SLAP lesions and its effect on SLAP repair rehabilitation, *Arthroscopy* 14(6):639, 1998.)

SLAP lesions in throwing athletes, as well as the finding of the Jobe subluxation relocation test as the most accurate and valuable test to identify the type II posterior lesion (Morgan et al, 1998). Type II anterior SLAP lesions are most commonly associated with trauma and are less likely to be found in overhead athletes. A type III labral injury involves the displacement of the free margin of the labrum into the joint in a bucket-handle type fashion with no instability of the biceps long-head tendon noted. A type IV labral lesion is similar to a type III lesion with a bucket handle displacement of the glenoid labrum. In contrast, though, a type IV lesion involves a partial rupture in the direction of its fibers of the biceps long-head tendon (Snyder et al, 1990).

One of the consequences of a superior labral injury is involvement of the biceps long-head tendon and the biceps anchor in the superior aspect of the glenoid. This compromise of both the integrity of the superior labrum and loss of the biceps anchor leads to significant losses in the static stability of the human shoulder. Cheng and Karzel (1997) showed the important role the superior labrum and biceps anchor play in glenohumeral joint stability by experimentally creating a SLAP lesion between the 10 and 2 o'clock positions. They found 11% to 19% decreases in the ability of the glenohumeral joint to withstand rotational force, as well as 100% to 120% increases in strain on the anterior band of the inferior

glenohumeral ligament. This demonstrates a significant increase in the load on the capsular ligaments in the presence of superior labral injury.

Identifying the mechanism of injury for superior labral injury helps the clinician understand the positions used and maneuvers recommended to test for superior labral injury. Andrews and Gillogly (1985) first described labral injuries in throwers and postulated tensile failure at the biceps insertion as the primary mechanism of failure. The Andrews theory was based on the important role the biceps plays in decelerating the extending elbow during the follow-through phase of pitching, coupled with the large distractional forces present during this violent phase of the throwing motion. Recent hypotheses have developed based on the finding by Morgan et al (1998) of a more commonly located posterior type II SLAP lesion in the throwing or overhead athlete. This posterior-based lesion can best be explained by the "peel back mechanism" described by Burkhart and Morgan (1998) (Figure 13-2). The torsional force created when the abducted arm is brought into external rotation is thought to "peel back" the biceps and posterior labrum. Thus several of the tests to identify the patient with a superior labral injury use the position of abduction and external rotation similar to the position Burkhart and Morgan (1998) describe for the "peel back mechanism."

Summary

Understanding the primary types and mechanisms of labral injury when these tests are performed helps the clinician determine whether a labral tear or detachment is present. It is recommended that each clinician have confidence in their ability to perform several of the labral tests outlined in this chapter to optimize the ability to correctly identify injury to this important structure. It is also important to understand the high incidence of additional pathology found at the time of arthroscopic surgery in patients with glenoid labrum injury. Kim et al (2003) evaluated the findings from 544 shoulder arthroscopies. Superior labral lesions were found in 26% of the 544 cases, with 21% being classified as a type II labral lesion. Of clinical importance was the common finding of Bankart lesions in patients less than 40 years old who had a superior labral injury and the high incidence of rotator cuff tears in patients more than 40 years old with a superior labral injury. This study clearly demonstrates the importance of performing a comprehensive examination in any patient with suspected superior labral pathology.

CLUNK TEST

Indication

The clunk test is used to detect the presence of a labral tear or detachment.

About the Test

This test was originally described by Andrews (Andrews and Gillogly, 1985) to detect labral tears in overhead athletes. The test attempts to trap the torn labrum between the humeral head and glenoid by using compression and rotation of the humeral head.

Start Position

The patient is placed in the supine position, with the arm elevated 150 to 160 degrees in the scapular plane. The examiner should face the patient's feet, such that the patient's involved extremity can be placed under the axilla of the examiner to facilitate the use of both hands on the proximal humerus (Figure 13-3). For example, to examine the patient's right shoulder, the patient's right arm is placed under the examiner's left axilla.

The examiner grasps the proximal humerus just distal to the humeral head with both hands. A firm yet relaxed grip must be used to facilitate patient relaxation. Failure to

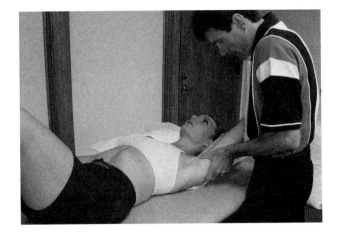

Figure 13-3 Labral clunk test showing set-up and examiner/patient positioning.

grasp the humerus far enough proximally will result in difficulty with the primary action described next.

Action

The examiner compresses the humeral head and initially glides it caudally. A continuation of a circumduction pattern is performed both clockwise and/or anticlockwise while the gentle compression of the humeral head into the glenoid is maintained.

What Constitutes a Positive Test?

A "clunk" that reproduces the patient's symptoms, pain reproduction, and pseudolocking constitute a positive test. Grating and crepitace are often encountered, with no symptom reproduction. This finding of grating and crepitace does not constitute a positive test and is frequently misinterpreted as a labral tear by both informed patients and less experienced examiners. Another common finding in hypermobile shoulders is the movement of the humeral head over the glenoid rim. This finding does not indicate labral dysfunction per se, but should alert the examiner to the hypermobile nature of the patient's shoulder.

Ramifications of a Positive Test

A positive clunk test indicates either labral tearing or labral detachment. Davies and DeCarlo (1995) interpreted the findings of the clunk test. A positive "clunk" or reproduction of symptoms with the humeral head in the position between the 3 and 6 o'clock positions (right shoulder) or the 9 and 6 o'clock positions (left shoulder) implicates a possible Bankart lesion. Positive findings occurring with the humeral head between the 10 and 12 o'clock positions in either the left or right shoulder indicate a SLAP lesion.

Objective Evidence Regarding the Test

In a retrospective review of 100 shoulders in 96 patients, Hurley and Anderson (1990) diagnosed 15 patients with labral pathology using the clunk test before patients underwent shoulder arthroscopy. At the time of surgery, 72 of the 100 shoulders examined had a tear of the glenoid labrum. This finding calls into question the sensitivity (15%) of the clunk test and suggests that the examiner use the test in combination with other evaluative procedures to more accurately identify labral pathology. Other data pertaining to the clunk test have not been published.

CIRCUMDUCTION TEST

Indication

The circumduction test is used to identify labral pathology in multiple glenohumeral joint positions.

About the Test

This test uses principles similar to those previously listed for the clunk test. Compression with rotation of the humeral head is meant to trap the labrum between the humeral head and glenoid. The advantage of this test is that it uses many different positions and can even incorporate humeral rotation in the evaluation process, which is functionally specific for many patients with labral pathology.

Start Position

The patient is in a supine position on a plinth. Initially, the arm is abducted to 90 degrees in the scapular plane. The examiner faces the patient below the patient's abducted humerus. The examiner's right hand (for examining the patient's left shoulder) is positioned at the elbow in the balance point position (see page 6 for description) to allow one-arm support of the patient's extremity by the examiner. The patient's elbow remains flexed approximately 90 degrees during the test. The examiner's hand is placed over the superoanterior aspect of the patient's shoulder to palpate and provide support. No pressure or movement is performed by the examiner's proximal hand (Figure 13-4).

Action

The examiner provides a long axis compression of the humeral head into the glenoid with the shoulder at 90 degrees of abduction in the scapular plane. From that

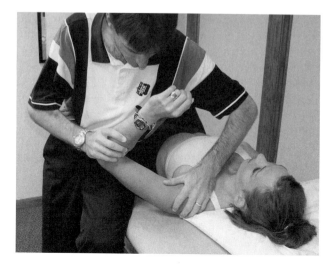

Figure 13-4 Circumduction labral test, set-up position.

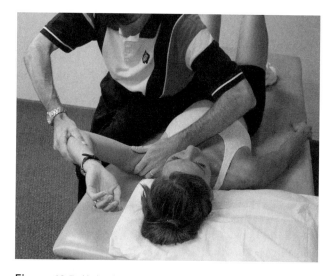

Figure 13-5 Abduction external rotation position of the circumduction test.

starting position (see Figure 13-4), a circumduction or rotating movement is performed by the examiner, so that the patient's glenohumeral joint undergoes a large circumduction pattern (Figure 13-5). In addition to the circumduction pattern, the examiner, via hand placement at the elbow using the balance point position, can provide internal and external rotation as the patient's arm is being moved through the circumduction pattern. This provides a scouring type of motion to entrap the torn labrum and enable manual detection.

One additional cue that can be helpful to a less experienced examiner is to ensure that a large enough circumduction motion is performed during testing. As a guide, the back of the patient's hand and forearm should literally brush the forehead, so that if a baseball cap were being worn by the athlete or patient, it would be knocked off. Coming that far medially with internal rotation of the humerus, followed by a full circle into abduction and external rotation (see Figure 13-5), ensures that the humeral head is traversing the glenoid rim.

What Constitutes a Positive Test?

Reproduction of pain, a "clunk," or pseudocatching may implicate labral pathology.

Ramifications of a Positive Test

A positive circumduction test indicates the presence of labral pathology. This finding can have implications similar to those discussed for the clunk test. Both labral tears and labral detachment may produce pain and catching during the performance of these maneuvers. The use of this test, in combination with other labral tests, can increase the likelihood of making a definitive diagnosis.

Objective Evidence Regarding the Test

There is no evidence regarding this test in the literature.

CRANK TEST

Indication

The crank test is used to identify labral pathology with the arm in an overhead position.

About the Test

This test was originally described by Liu et al (1996b) as a sensitive and specific test for the evaluation of glenoid labrum tears. The test can be performed in both the supine and seated positions, using similar combinations of compression and rotation to determine labral status.

Starting Position

The test can be performed with the patient in either a seated or supine position. In both positions, the glenohumeral joint is elevated 160 degrees in the scapular plane. One of the examiner's hands is placed at the elbow at the balance point position (page 6) to allow the examiner to control the patient's extremity. The examiner's other hand is placed on the superior aspect of the shoulder for support and to palpate (Figure 13-6, *A*).

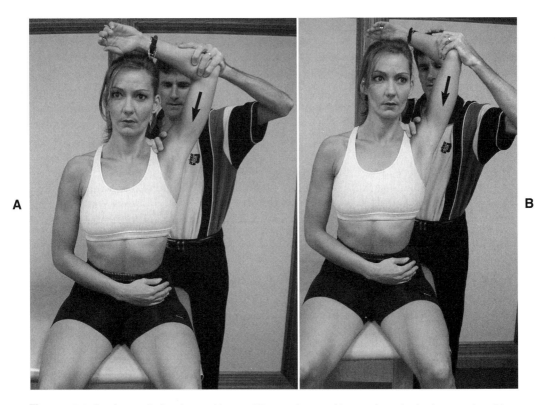

Figure 13-6 Crank test. **A,** Starting position, and **B,** superimposed humeral rotation in the seated position.

Action

The hand placed on the patient's elbow applies a long axis compressive force while the humerus is internally and externally rotated (Figure 13-6, *B*). The combination of compression and rotation is the same whether the patient is seated or supine.

What Constitutes a Positive Test?

A positive test is determined either by pain elicited primarily during external rotation with or without a click or by reproduction of the pain or catching felt by the patient during athletic or work-related activities. According to the originators of the test, the supine position promotes greater patient relaxation, and frequently a positive crank test in the supine position is also positive in the seated position.

Ramifications of a Positive Test

A positive crank test indicates a tear in the labrum. The originators of this examination claim that this test is particularly useful in patients who have stable joints. The presence of labral tears in patients with stable glenohumeral joints include bucket-handle, transverse, flap, longitudinal, horizontal cleavage, fibrillated, and SLAP-type tears (Liu et al, 1996b).

Objective Evidence for This Test

Liu et al (1996b) evaluated 62 patients using the crank test before arthroscopic evaluation of the shoulder; 31 patients (50%) had a positive preoperative crank test. At time of arthroscopy, 32 patients had evidence of labral tears. Two patients who had positive crank tests but no labral tears on arthroscopic examination had partial-thickness undersurface rotator cuff tears. The crank test had a sensitivity of 91% and a specificity of 93%. The positive predictive value (PPV) of the crank test was 94% and the negative predictive value (NPV) was 90%.

In a related work, the same authors (Liu et al, 1996b) compared the accuracy of physical examination in patients with suspected labral injury with the results of magnetic resonance imaging (MRI) (conventional and arthrogram). Results of the physical examination maneuver (crank test) were far superior to the MRI, which had a sensitivity of 59% and a specificity of 85%.

Research by Stetson and Templin (2002) evaluated the effectiveness of the crank test in identifying patients with suspected labral pathology. A complete prospective clinical evaluation was performed by one examiner on 65 patients whose shoulder pain had been present for a mean time of 12 months. The crank test was positive in 29 of 62 patients, 12 of whom (41%) actually had evidence of tears

of the glenoid labrum seen during arthroscopic evaluation. The crank test in this study had a specificity of 56%, sensitivity of 46%, PPV of 41%, and NPV of 61%. These values obtained are significantly lower than reports from the originators of the test.

Guanche and Jones (2003) tested 60 shoulders before undergoing arthroscopy using a series of labral tests. The crank test had a sensitivity of 40%, specificity of 73%, PPV of 82%, and NPV of 29% for the diagnosis of any type of labral lesion. These findings are slightly higher than those reported by Stetson and Templin (2002). When Guanche and Jones (2003) analyzed their results for only diagnosis of SLAP lesions, however, sensitivity and specificity values were 39% and 67%, respectively, with a PPV of 59% and an NPV of 47%, which are much closer to the findings of Stetson and Templin (2002).

Results from these research studies suggest that caution be applied when interpreting a positive crank test. The test should be used in conjunction with other labral tests and a thorough clinical examination to determine the underlying pathology in patients presenting with shoulder pain.

COMPRESSION ROTATION TEST

Indication

The compression rotation test is used to identify the presence of superior labral pathology (SLAP lesions).

About the Test

This test uses a position of 90 degrees of glenohumeral joint abduction to combine the movements of internal and external rotation and compression to determine the status of the superior labrum.

Start Position

The patient is examined in a supine position. The examiner grasps near the elbow of the patient's involved extremity using the balance point (see page 6 for description) with the patient's elbow flexed 90 degrees. The examiner stands below the patient's extremity being evaluated and faces directly toward the patient (Figure 13-7, *A*). To examine the patient's left shoulder, the examiner's right hand is near the elbow and the examiner's left hand is cupped over the superior aspect of the shoulder to palpate and feel for any "clunk" or abnormal catching during the maneuver described next.

Action

The examiner exerts a compressive force via the elbow toward the glenoid to approximate the humeral head into

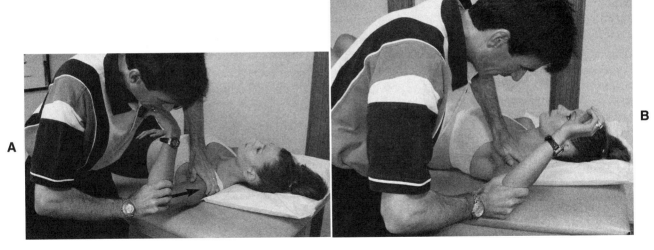

Figure 13-7 Compression rotation test. **A,** Starting position. **B,** Humeral rotation action.

the glenoid while internally and externally rotating the humerus (Davies & DeCarlo, 1995; McFarland et al, 2002) (Figure 13-7, *B*). Magee (1997) described a modification of this test in which the test is performed in only 20 degrees of abduction, rather than 90 degrees as used by Snyder et al (1995), Davies and DeCarlo (1995), and McFarland et al (2002). This lower level of abduction results in a greater superior shear of the humeral head.

What Constitutes a Positive Test?

Reproduction of the patient's pain, a "clunk," or pseudo-catching may implicate a SLAP lesion.

Ramifications of a Positive Test

The use of glenohumeral joint compression with super-imposed rotation is meant to catch the labral fragment, much like the McMurray test of the knee (McFarland et al, 2002). Detachment of the superior labrum from the glenoid may result in instability of the biceps anchor and lead to glenohumeral joint instability (Cheng & Karzel, 1997).

Objective Evidence Regarding the Test

McFarland et al (2002) used the compression rotation test on 426 patients who subsequently underwent shoulder arthroscopy. The compression rotation test was positive in 67 of 274 (25%) control patients (those who did not have a SLAP lesion identified at time of shoulder arthroscopy) and in 7 of 29 patients who did have a type II, III, or IV SLAP lesion at the time of arthroscopy. Of the seven patients who were correctly identified using the compression rotation test, six had pain reproduction and one had pain reproduction and a click.

Based on these finding, the sensitivity of the compression rotation test was 24%, specificity was 76%, and the NPV and PPV were 90% and 9%, respectively. This study clearly showed the difficulty in detecting labral lesions using manual tests in patients who present with shoulder pain. An additional finding that has clinical significance is that most SLAP lesions do not occur in isolation (McFarland et al, 2002); 77% of the patients who had a SLAP lesion at time of arthroscopic examination had an associated intraarticular lesion. This finding is supported by other diagnostic series in the literature, specifically Morgan et al (1998), who found 31% of patients with type II SLAP lesions to have rotator cuff lesions.

In summary, the compression rotation test cannot be used in isolation to accurately identify patients with SLAP lesions. The test is recommended in combination with other manual clinical tests, as well as thorough clinical evaluation and history. Research does not support the need to produce a "clunk" or "click" for the test to be considered positive. Pain reproduction alone, or in addition to a possible clunk or click, is a more appropriate indicator of superior labral pathology.

ANTERIOR SLIDE TEST

Indication

The anterior slide test is used to identify patients with superior labral pathology.

About the Test

This test, initially developed and reported by Kibler (1995), was devised to clinically detect lesions of the superior glenoid labrum with or without a movable free fragment. The test is based on creating an anteriorly and superiorly directed force vector on the humerus relative to the glenoid, which normally is resisted by an intact superior labrum biceps complex (Rodosky et al, 1994).

Start Position

The patient can be examined in either the standing or sitting position. The patient places hands on hips, with the thumbs pointed in a posterior direction. The examiner stands directly behind the patient and places one hand on top of the shoulder from the posterior direction, so that the last segment of the index finger extends over the anterior aspect of the acromion at the glenohumeral joint. Typically this would be the examiner's left hand when examining the patient's right shoulder. The examiner's other hand is placed behind the patient's flexed elbow (Figure 13-8).

Action

Using the hand placed behind the patient's elbow, the examiner exerts a forward and slightly superiorly directed force to the elbow and upper arm. The patient is asked to gently push back against the anterosuperior-directed force.

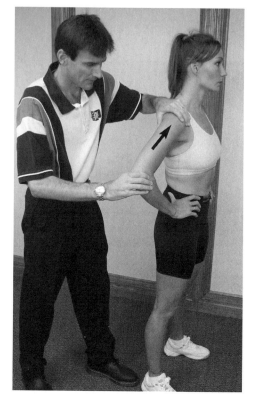

Figure 13-8 Lateral view of the Kibler anterior slide test.

What Constitutes a Positive Test?

Pain localized to the front of the shoulder under the examiner's hand that is placed in an anterosuperior position, and/or a pop or click in the same region, is considered a positive test. Kibler (1995) also interpreted the test as positive if the testing maneuver reproduces the symptoms that occur during overhead throwing or other functional activities.

Ramifications of a Positive Test

A positive Kibler anterior slide test indicates superior labral pathology. The superoanterior-directed force moves the shoulder into internal rotation. Patients who are overhead athletes often have reduced internal rotation active and passive range of motion on their dominant side (Ellenbecker et al, 2002b; Ellenbecker, 1992). Movement produced from internal rotation in the presence of an internal rotation deficit causes increased anterior translation of the humeral head. In the presence of superior labral pathology, the anterior translation of the humeral head can create stress on the superior glenoid labrum and biceps complex, which normally resists this anterior translation.

Objective Evidence Regarding the Test

In his original article, Kibler (1995) used the anterior slide test in 226 patients/subjects to determine the efficacy of the test. Five groups of individuals were tested by Kibler: 46 athletes with arthroscopic confirmation of superior labral tears, 52 patients with arthroscopic confirmation of partial rotator cuff tears (36 of which also had superior labral injury as well), 28 patients undergoing anterior stabilization procedures, 54 asymptomatic overhead throwing athletes, and 46 lower extremity athletes who were also asymptomatic. These groups were chosen to test the anterior slide test in conditions of both isolated and non-isolated superior labral injury, as well as in individuals without superior labral pathology. The anterior slide test was positive 69 times in 88 total superior labral lesions in the testing populations, or a sensitivity rate of 78.4%. The anterior slide test was correct 125 out of 138 times, or a specificity rate of 91.5%. Kibler concluded that the anterior slide test can be added to the evaluation process to aid in diagnosing superior labral lesions because it has a high specificity for superior labral lesions.

McFarland et al (2002) used the anterior slide test to evaluate 426 patients undergoing arthroscopic shoulder surgery. The anterior slide test was positive in 62 of 381 control patients who did not have types II, III, or IV superior labral pathology. The test was also positive in 3 of 38 patients with superior labral pathology. In actual patients with superior labral pathology, the anterior slide test produced pain in only two patients and a click in only one patient. An overall sensitivity was only 8%, specificity was 84%, and PPV and NPV were 5% and 90%, respectively.

ACTIVE COMPRESSION TEST

This test is also known as *O'Brien's test*.

Indication

The active compression test is a clinical test to identify superior labral pathology and acromioclavicular joint involvement.

About the Test

This test, originally developed by Dr. Stephen O'Brien from the Hospital for Special Surgery in New York, uses a combination of glenohumeral joint positioning and active muscle force to provoke the biceps/labral complex and also load the acromioclavicular joint (O'Brien et al, 1998). Both superior labral pathology and acromioclavicular joint degenerative lesions can be identified based on the location of pain produced during the O'Brien provocative maneuver.

Start Position

The test is performed with the examiner standing directly behind the patient. The patient is asked to flex the shoulder forward to 90 degrees in the sagittal plane, with the elbow completely extended. The patient is then asked to adduct the arm horizontally 10 to 15 degrees medial to the sagittal plane of the body, with the arm rotated internally so that the thumb is pointing downward (Figure 13-9, *A*).

Action

The examiner then places a downward force distal to the patient's elbow, with the patient resisting this downward force as in a manual muscle test. The patient is asked whether pain is produced during this maneuver and, if so, to identify its exact location.

The test is repeated using the same position (90 degrees of sagittal plane shoulder flexion, full elbow

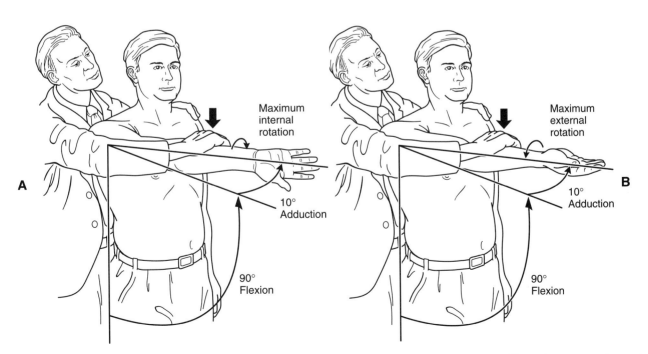

Figure 13-9 O'Brien's test. **A,** Starting position, and **B,** second position. (Adapted from O'Brien SJ et al: The active compression test: a new and effective test for diagnosing labral tears and acromioclavicular joint abnormality, *Am J Sports Med* 26(5):611, 1998.)

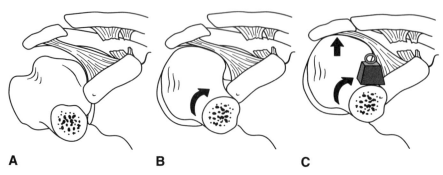

A   **B**   **C**

Figure 13-10 O'Brien's test, anatomic drawing for acromioclavicular (AC) joint. **A,** To demonstrate the anatomic basis of the active compression test, selective cutting was performed to create AC joint instability after testing in the intact situation. **B,** In the unstable AC joint, the highest pressure generated was with the arm forward flexed 90 degrees with approximately 10 to 15 degrees of adduction and maximal internal rotation. **C,** In this position, the greater tuberosity comes over and, by positioning, elevates the relatively depressed acromion and "locks and loads" the AC joint. (Adapted from O'Brien SJ, et al: The active compression test: a new and effective test for diagnosing labral tears and acromioclavicular joint abnormality, *Am J Sports Med* 26(5):611, 1998.)

extension, and 10 to 15 degrees of horizontal adduction medial to the sagittal plane), except that the palm is now placed in the "up" position, with a supinated forearm position and external rotation of the humerus (Figure 13-9, *B*). The uniform downward force is again applied and the patient is asked whether this maneuver produces pain and, if so, its exact location. This test is most effective when the patient is asked to resist the examiner's downward force rather than when the examiner resists the patient's upward force.

What Constitutes a Positive Test?

O'Brien's active compression test is considered positive when the first maneuver (downward pressure with the arm in the internally rotated position) elicits pain and when that pain is eliminated with testing using the second maneuver (downward pressure with the arm in the externally rotated position). Pain indicates a positive test when it occurs in the following locations. For superior labral pathology, the pain must occur deep in the anterior aspect of the shoulder. Pain reproduction with this maneuver or painful clicking is also considered positive for labral pathology. For acromioclavicular joint pathology, the pain must be localized and occur in the superior or top of the shoulder directly over the acromioclavicular joint. Pain in other locations besides the superior aspect (acromioclavicular joint) or deep in the anterior aspect (superior labral pathology) is not considered positive for this test.

Ramifications of a Positive Test

Cadaveric studies were performed with the active compression test to determine the anatomic basis of the test maneuvers. The largest pressure between the acromioclavicular joint surfaces occurred with 90 degrees of shoulder flexion in the sagittal plane, with 10 to 15 degrees of horizontal adduction and internal rotation. Maneuvers that used more than 10 to 15 degrees of horizontal adduction produced a "bayoneting" effect, whereby the unstable acromioclavicular joint was free from pressure as a result of an override effect. This may explain the variable results seen with the cross-arm adduction test for acromioclavicular joint pathology (O'Brien et al, 1998). Abduction of the arm away from the midline of the body produced a relaxation of the acromioclavicular joint. The effect of O'Brien's test for acromioclavicular pathology is further enhanced by the addition of active muscular contraction of the deltoid with anatomic attachment to both the acromion and clavicle, with increased compressive force being measured during simulated contraction (Figure 13-10).

The mechanism for the provocation produced by the active compression test on the superior labrum was identified by arthroscopic evaluation (O'Brien et al, 1998). The position of shoulder flexion and horizontal adduction causes the biceps long-head tendon to displace both medially and inferiorly, tensioning the biceps-labral complex (Figure 13-11). This position may also produce anterosuperior shear forces.

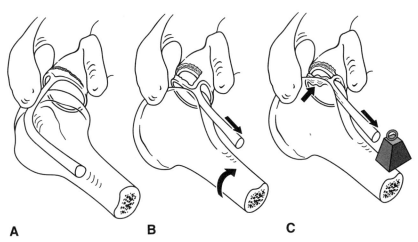

Figure 13-11 O'Brien's test, anatomic drawing for SLAP. **A,** Anatomic drawing of the shoulder in neutral position without force applied. **B,** When the arm is positioned in 90 degrees standard flexion, 10 to 15 degrees of adduction, and maximum internal rotation, the biceps tendon displaces medially and inferiorly, extending the bicipital-labral complex. **C,** Joint load increases because of the wind-up effect of the capsuloligament and musculotendon units. (Adapted from O'Brien SJ, et al: The active compression test: a new and effective test for diagnosing labral tears and acromioclavicular joint abnormality, *Am J Sports Med* 26(5):613, 1998.)

Objective Evidence Regarding the Test

In their original report, O'Brien et al (1998) included a prospective study of 318 patients to measure the effectiveness of their test. In all, 53 of 56 patients whose preoperative examinations indicated a superior labral tear had confirmed labral tears during follow-up arthroscopic surgery; 55 of 62 patients with acromioclavicular joint pain during preoperative testing with O'Brien's test had confirmed pathology and abnormalities at follow-up evaluation.

For labral pathology, the O'Brien active compression test had a sensitivity of 100%, specificity of 98.5%, and PPV and NPV of 94% and 100%, respectively. For acromioclavicular joint pathology or abnormality, the test had a sensitivity of 100%, specificity of 96.6%, and PPV and NPV of 88.7% and 100%, respectively.

McFarland et al (2002) used the active compression test in 426 patients who subsequently underwent diagnostic shoulder arthroscopy. The active compression test was positive in 168 of 371 control patients (those with no arthroscopic evidence of labral pathology). A total of 18 of 38 patients with verified superior labral pathology at time of surgery also had a positive active compression test; none of these 18 patients had a click with the actual test, only pain reproduction. McFarland (2002) reported an overall sensitivity of 47%, a specificity of 55%, a PPV of 10%, and NPV of 91%. These values are far lower than those reported by O'Brien et al (1998). Compared with the anterior slide test and the compression rotation test, which were also used in the population of 426 patients, the active compression test had the highest sensitivity, highest PPV, and lowest overall accuracy. It is important to note that the presence of a click and the location of pain were not particularly reliable diagnostic indicators.

Stetson and Templin (2002) compared the results of the active compression test with the crank test (pages 119–120) and routine MRI in the diagnosis of superior labral pathology. They reported the active compression test to have a sensitivity of 54%, specificity of 31%, PPV of 41%, and NPV of 61%. They concluded that the active compression and crank tests are not sensitive clinical indicators for detecting glenoid labrum pathology, and they found false-positive clinical tests in patients who had rotator cuff tears and impingement. Caution should be used when interpreting the results of these individual clinical tests to detect glenoid labrum pathology.

Finally, Guanche and Jones (2003) used the active compression test during examination of 60 shoulders in 59 patients before shoulder arthroscopy for shoulder pain. Sensitivity values of 63% and specificity of 73% were reported, with PPV of 87% and NPV of 40% for the diagnosis of any labral pathology. Values specifically for SLAP lesions were lower, with sensitivity of 54%, specificity of 47%, PPV of 57%, and NPV of 45%.

BICEPS LOAD TEST

Indication

The biceps load test is used to detect superior labral pathology in individuals who have suffered recurrent anterior glenohumeral dislocations.

About the Test

This test was developed by Kim et al (1999) to test for SLAP lesions in shoulders of patients who have multiple dislocations. The test was called the *biceps load test* to represent the dynamic contribution of the biceps tendon–superior labral complex.

Start Position

The test is performed with the patient in a supine position. The examiner is seated next to the patient on the same side as the extremity being tested. The examiner grasps the patient's elbow and wrist. The shoulder is abducted 90 degrees in neutral rotation, and the forearm is placed in a supinated position (Figure 13-12, *A*). The patient is allowed to relax in this resting position.

Action

An anterior apprehension test is performed with the examiner taking the shoulder back into external rotation while maintaining 90 degrees of abduction. When the patient becomes apprehensive, the external rotation is stopped and the position is maintained. The patient is then asked to flex the elbow while the examiner resists the movement with the hand placed near the patient's wrist (Figure 13-12, *B*). The patient is asked how this affects the feeling of apprehension. To optimize test results, Kim

et al (1999) recommend that the movement be isolated to include only elbow flexion, and that no other direction of resistance be performed simultaneously. Resistance should be strictly in line with the biceps tendon force vector, which is in line with the long axis of the humerus.

What Constitutes a Positive Test?

A positive biceps load test is present when the feeling of apprehension does not change during contraction of the biceps or actually becomes more apprehensive or painful during inducement of the biceps contraction. A negative biceps load test is present when the patient's feeling of apprehension is lessened during contraction of the biceps.

Ramifications of a Positive Test

The biceps load test is positive when the feeling of apprehension is not abated or improved by the contraction of the biceps/labral complex. Normally, the biceps and superior labrum provide extensive stability to the glenohumeral joint (Rodosky et al, 1994), and failure of the biceps contraction to improve the apprehensive feeling in the abducted, externally rotated position indicates that these superior structures are not functioning (Kim et al, 1999).

Objective Evidence Regarding the Test

Kim et al (1999) compared the effectiveness of the biceps load test, including the apprehension test, biceps tension test, and compression rotation test. Tests were performed on 75 consecutive patients with unilateral glenohumeral joint dislocations with a Bankart lesion. The biceps load test was negative in 63 patients and positive in 12. Of the 63 patients with a negative test, 62 showed no evidence of

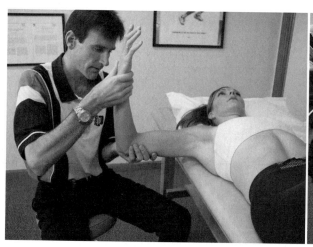
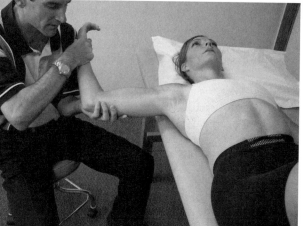

Figure **13-12** Biceps load test. **A,** Starting position. **B,** Ending position.

superior labral injury; one patient had a type II superior labral lesion. Ten of the 12 patients with positive biceps load tests had arthroscopic evidence of superior labral injury. Sensitivity of the biceps load test was 90.9%, specificity was 96.9%, PNV was 83%, and NPV was 98%. The kappa coefficient representing the intraobserver reliability of the test was 0.846. Among the other tests performed by these examiners, the compression rotation test detected only three SLAP lesions.

BICEPS LOAD TEST II

Indication
The biceps load test II is a clinical test to detect isolated superior labral injuries of the shoulder.

About the Test
This test was developed by Kim et al (2001) as a counterpart to the biceps load test (see pages 126–127) to assist in the detection of isolated superior labral lesions. It uses the dynamic contraction of the biceps as an integral part of the test.

Start Position
The test is conducted with the patient in a supine position. The examiner sits directly beside the patient, on the same side as the extremity being tested. The examiner grasps the patient's extremity at the elbow and wrist. The shoulder is abducted 90 degrees in the coronal plane and externally rotated to its maximal point. The elbow remains in 90 degrees of flexion throughout the test, and the forearm is in a supinated position, so that the patient's palm faces directly toward their head.

Action
The patient is asked to flex the elbow while the examiner resists elbow flexion, so that an isometric contraction of the biceps muscle occurs (Figure 13-13). Care must be taken to isolate the resistance to the elbow flexion component to avoid additional loads placed on the shoulder.

What Constitutes a Positive Test?
The test is considered positive if the patient complains of pain during resisted elbow flexion and negative if no pain is elicited, if the pretesting pain level is diminished during the elbow flexion resistance, or if the pain level is unchanged.

Ramifications of a Positive Test
The biceps load test II is a dynamic test to assess the integrity of the superior labrum and is based on three principles, according to Kim et al (2001). First, the

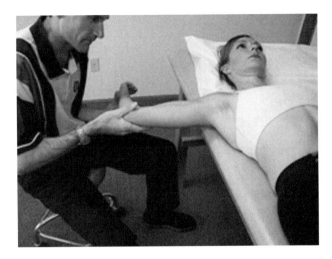

Figure **13-13** Biceps load test II.

contraction of the biceps against the resistance in the abducted and externally rotated position eliminates the standard apprehension of patients with unstable shoulders who have intact biceps-labral complexes as a result of compression of the humeral head into the glenoid and the concavity compression mechanism. Second, active contraction of the biceps against resistance further stresses the attachment of the biceps superior labral complex, by which pain is elicited in the shoulder with a type II SLAP lesion. Finally, based on the results of a cadaveric study by Kuhn et al (1999), the biceps labral complex fails under significantly less force for the cocking position of throwing (60 degrees abduction with maximal 125 degrees of external rotation in the scapular plane) than in a position with less external rotation and abduction. This study suggests the importance of the ultimate position used in testing during the biceps load test II (Figure 13-14). This concept is supported by Burkhart & Morgan (1998), who reported the peel-back mechanism that occurs in the superior labrum with the glenohumeral joint in positions of abduction and external rotation with humeral head translation.

Kim et al (2001), concluded that the reproduction of pain in the abducted externally rotated position used during the biceps load test II is elicited by the forceful traction of the displaced biceps superior labral complex during resistance to the biceps muscle.

Objective Evidence Regarding the Test
Kim et al (2001) reported a prospective biceps load test II in 127 patients undergoing shoulder arthroscopy. A positive biceps load test II was found in 38 patients, which

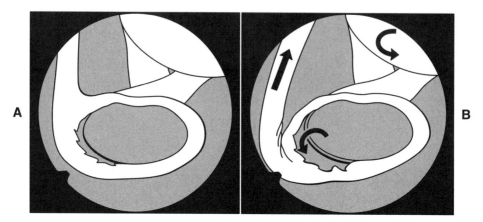

Figure **13-14** Biceps load test II. **A,** In the neutral rotation position of the shoulder, the biceps tendon is parallel to the posterosuperior labrum. **B,** The abduction and external rotation of the shoulder during the biceps load test II changes the relative direction of the biceps fiber in a position that is of an oblique angle to the posterosuperior labrum. This change in the vector of the biceps force increases the pain generated on the superior labrum that is peeled off the glenoid margin during the resisted contraction of the biceps in the abducted and externally rotated position. (From Kim SH, et al: Biceps load test II for SLAP lesions of the shoulder, *Arthroscopy* 17(2):163, 2001.)

correlated positively with 35 superior labral lesions found during subsequent surgical procedures, resulting in a sensitivity of 89.7%, a specificity of 96.9%, a PPV of 92.1% and an NPV of 95.5%. Intraobserver reliability was measured using a kappa coefficient (0.815), which indicates a high level of intraobserver reliability.

No additional research has been reported using the biceps load test II.

MIMORI PAIN PROVOCATION TEST

Indication

The Mimori pain provocation test is used to detect superior labral pathology.

About the Test

This test was developed by Mimori et al (1999) to evaluate the integrity of the superior labrum. This test uses the tension imparted to the biceps long-head tendon to provoke pain and reproduce symptoms in an overhead position inherent in many sport-specific movement patterns and functional activities.

Start Position

The patient is examined in a seated position. The examiner stands behind the patient and grasps the distal aspect of the forearm (examiner's right hand to examine the right extremity of the patient). An abduction angle of 90 to 100 degrees in the coronal plane is used throughout the test. The elbow is placed in 90 degrees of flexion, where it remains during the test. The examiner's other hand is placed over the top of the shoulder to stabilize the arm during the movement described next.

Action

The examiner rotates the shoulder externally, keeping the glenohumeral joint abduction angle in a position of 90 to 100 degrees. This portion of the maneuver is similar to the anterior apprehension test. The Mimori pain provocation test is performed with the forearm in two positions, once in a fully pronated position (Figure 13-15, *A*) and once in a fully supinated position (Figure 13-15, *B*). In each position the shoulder is brought back into end-range external rotation. The patient is asked which of the two forearm positions provoked the most pain.

What Constitutes a Positive Test?

The test is positive for a superior labral tear when pain is provoked only when the forearm is placed in the pronated position, or when pain provoked in the pronated position is greater than pain provoked in the supinated position. The test is negative when there is either no difference in pain between the two forearm conditions, or when the forearm is less painful in the pronated position.

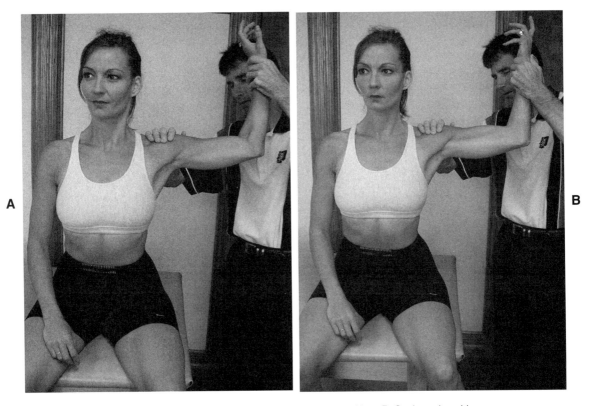

Figure 13-15 Pain provocation test. **A,** Pronated position. **B,** Supinated position.

Ramifications of a Positive Test

Tension in the long head of the biceps is greater when the Mimori pain provocation test is performed with the forearm in a pronated position than in a supinated position. The greater length of the biceps tendon in the pronated forearm position is thought to create more stress on the superior labrum.

Objective Evidence Regarding the Test

Mimori et al (1999) reported results of a prospective analysis of the Mimori pain provocation test in 32 patients who, after testing, had MRI evaluation of the shoulder; 15 of these patients were also evaluated with arthroscopy to determine the efficacy of the pain provocation test. In 22 patients, detachment of the superior labrum was confirmed with an arthrogram, and all of these patients had a positive pain provocation test; 11 of 15 patients had type II SLAP lesions at the time of arthroscopy and all of them had a positive Mimori pain provocation test; sensitivity was 100% and specificity was 90%. No additional research is available for this test. In the same study, the crank test (pages 119–120) detected detachment of the superior labrum, with a sensitivity of 83% and a specificity of 100%. This study supports the use of both the pain provocation and crank test in patients with suspected SLAP lesions.

ADDITIONAL
SHOULDER
EVALUATION
TECHNIQUES

CHAPTER

14 | Muscular Strength Testing

INTRODUCTION

The most clinically relevant method used to assess strength of the shoulder girdle is manual muscle testing (MMT). Since its development in the early 1900s during the study of muscle function in patients with poliomyelitis, MMT has become a standard practice during the physical evaluation of patients with both neurologic and orthopedic injuries (Daniels & Worthingham, 1980). Although beneficial in nearly all aspects of rehabilitative evaluation, MMT has some limitations in reliability. The technique of MMT has been found to be reliable within one grade between two examiners (Aitkens et al, 1989; Lilienfeld et al, 1954); however, Frese et al (1987) reported low intertester reliability in 110 patients for the middle trapezius and gluteus medius musculature. They concluded that caution must be used when interpreting the results of MMT between two or more examiners. It is beyond the scope of this text to completely review all aspects of MMT. This chapter describes several studies that have objectively identified positions for testing muscles in the shoulder complex, with particular emphasis on the rotator cuff (Kelly et al, 1996). The reader is referred to more detailed texts dedicated to MMT (Daniels and Worthington, 1980; Kendall and McCreary, 1983) for comprehensive descriptions and theories on the technique itself. Table 14-1 lists specific muscles and their respective neural derivations and actions.

During a comprehensive musculoskeletal evaluation, MMT of the axioscapular, scapulohumeral, and scapulothoracic muscles is indicated, with specific reference to the muscles of the rotator cuff. Testing the muscles in the distal portion of the upper extremity and trunk is also indicated, as a result of the kinetic chain function of the body and the importance of the transfer of muscle force from the lower extremity and trunk during functional activities (Marshall & Elliott, 2000). Use of concepts such as total arm strength and kinetic chain during rehabilitation requires knowledge of muscular strength and the endurance of the segments proximal and distal to the

glenohumeral joint (Ellenbecker & Mattalino, 1996; Davies & Ellenbecker, 1993).

MANUAL MUSCLE TESTING OF THE ROTATOR CUFF

Kelly et al (1996) used electromyography (EMG) to determine the optimal position for testing the muscles of the rotator cuff in human subjects. Four criteria were used to establish which position was optimal for each rotator cuff muscle: maximal activation of the muscle, minimal contribution from shoulder synergists, minimal provocation of pain, and good test-retest reliability.

Supraspinatus

Kelly et al (1996) found the optimal muscle testing position for the supraspinatus to be at 90 degrees of elevation, with the patient seated. The scapular plane position was used (in this research this represented 45 degrees of horizontal adduction from the coronal plane) with external rotation of the humerus such that the forearm was placed in neutral position and the thumb was pointing upward (Figure 14-1). This position was termed the *full can testing position*. Another position used to assess the strength of the supraspinatus muscle-tendon unit is the empty can test (Figure 14-2). This test position has been advocated by Jobe and Bradley (1989), and indwelling EMG has documented high levels of supraspinatus muscular activation (Malanga et al, 1997). See the discussion by Itoi et al (1999) comparing the empty can and full can tests on pages 97–99 in this text.

Infraspinatus

According to Kelly et al (1996), the optimal position to test for infraspinatus strength is with the patient in a seated position, with 0 degrees of glenohumeral joint elevation and in 45 degrees of internal rotation from neutral (Figure 14-3). This position is similar to that used in the Neer drop test (pages 102–103) to evaluate for severe functional loss of the infraspinatus muscle. Jenp

TABLE 14-1   Muscles About the Shoulder: Actions and Neural Derivation

Action	Muscles Acting	Nerve Supply	Nerve Root Derivation
Forward flexion	1. Deltoid (anterior fibers)	Axillary (circumflex)	C5-C6 (posterior cord)
	2. Pectoralis major (clavicular fibers)	Lateral pectoral	C5-C6 (lateral cord)
	3. Coracobrachialis	Musculocutaneous	C5-C7 (lateral cord)
	4. Biceps (when strong contraction required)	Musculocutaneous	C5-C7 (lateral cord)
Extension	1. Deltoid (posterior fibers)	Axillary (circumflex)	C5-C6 (posterior cord)
	2. Teres major	Subscapular	C5-C6 (posterior cord)
	3. Teres minor	Axillary (circumflex)	C5-C6 (posterior cord)
	4. Latissimus dorsi	Thoracodorsal	C6-C8 (posterior cord)
	5. Pectoralis major (sternocostal fibers)	Lateral pectoral / Medial pectoral	C5-C6 (posterior cord) / C8, T1 (medial cord)
	6. Triceps (long head)	Radial	C5-C8, T1 (posterior cord)
Horizontal adduction	1. Pectoralis major	Lateral pectoral	C5-C6 (lateral cord)
	2. Deltoid (anterior fibers)	Axillary (circumflex)	C5-C6 (posterior cord)
Horizontal abduction	1. Deltoid (posterior fibers)	Axillary (circumflex)	C5-C6 (posterior cord)
	2. Teres major	Subscapular	C5-C6 (posterior cord)
	3. Teres minor	Axillary (circumflex)	C5-C6 (brachial plexus trunk)
	4. Infraspinatus	Suprascapular	C5-C6 (brachial plexus trunk)
Abduction	1. Deltoid (posterior fibers)	Axillary (circumflex)	C5-C6 (posterior cord)
	2. Supraspinatus	Suprascapular	C5-C6 (brachial plexus trunk)
	3. Infraspinatus	Suprascapular	C5-C6 (brachial plexus trunk)
	4. Subscapularis	Subscapular	C5-C6 (posterior cord)
	5. Teres minor	Axillary (circumflex)	C5-C6 (posterior cord)
	6. Long head of biceps (if arm laterally rotated first, trick movement)	Musculocutaneous	C5-C7 (lateral cord)
Adduction	1. Pectoralis major	Lateral pectoral	C5-C6 (lateral cord)
	2. Latissimus dorsi	Thoracodorsal	C6-C8 (posterior cord)
	3. Teres major	Subscapular	C5-C6 (posterior cord)
	4. Subscapularis	Subscapular	C5-C6 (posterior cord)
Medial rotation	1. Pectoralis major	Lateral pectoral	C5-C6 (lateral cord)
	2. Deltoid (anterior fibers)	Axillary (circumflex)	C5-C6 (posterior cord)
	3. Latissimus dorsi	Thoracodorsal	C6-C8 (posterior cord)
	4. Teres major	Subscapular	C5-C6 (posterior cord)
	5. Subscapularis (when arm is by side)	Subscapular	C5-C6 (posterior cord)
Lateral rotation	1. Infraspinatus	Suprascapular	C5-C6 (brachial plexus trunk)
	2. Deltoid (posterior fibers)	Axillary (circumflex)	C5-C6 (posterior cord)
	3. Teres minor	Axillary (circumflex)	C5-C6 (posterior cord)
Elevation of scapula	1. Trapezius (upper fibers)	Accessory / C3-C4 nerve roots	Cranial nerve XI / C3-C4
	2. Levator scapulae	C3-C4 nerve roots / Dorsal scapular	C3-C4 / C5
	3. Rhomboid major	Dorsal scapular	(C4), C5
	4. Rhomboid minor	Dorsal scapular	(C4), C5
Depression of scapula	1. Serratus anterior	Long thoracic	C5-C6, (C7)
	2. Pectoralis major	Lateral pectoral	C5-C6 (lateral cord)
	3. Pectoralis minor	Medial pectoral	C8, T1 (medial cord)
	4. Latissimus dorsi	Thoracodorsal	C6-C8 (posterior cord)
	5. Trapezius (lower fibers)	Accessory / C3-C4 nerve roots	Cranial nerve XI / C3-C4

From Magee DJ: *Orthopedic physical assessment*, ed 4, Philadelphia, 2002, WB Saunders.

TABLE 14-1   **Muscles About the Shoulder: Actions and Neural Derivation—cont'd**

ACTION	MUSCLES ACTING	NERVE SUPPLY	NERVE ROOT DERIVATION
Protraction (forward movement) of scapula	1. Serratus anterior 2. Pectoralis major 3. Pectoralis minor 4. Latissimus dorsi	Long thoracic Lateral pectoral Medial pectoral Thoracodorsal	C5-C6, (C7) C5-C6 (lateral cord) C8, T1 (medial cord) C6-C8 (posterior cord)
Retraction (backward movement) of scapula	1. Trapezius 2. Rhomboid major 3. Rhomboid minor	Accessory Dorsal scapular Dorsal scapular	Cranial nerve XI (C4), C5 (C4), C5
Lateral (upward) rotation of inferior angle of scapula	1. Trapezius (upper and lower fibers) 2. Serratus anterior	Accessory C3-C4 nerve roots Long thoracic	Cranial nerve XI C3-C4 C5-C6, (C7)
Medial (downward) rotation of inferior angle of scapula	1. Levator scapulae 2. Rhomboid major 3. Rhomboid minor 4. Pectoralis minor	C3-C4 nerve roots Dorsal scapular Dorsal scapular Dorsal scapular Medial pectoral	C3-C4 (C4), C5 (C4), C5 (C4), C5 C8, T1 (medial cord)
Flexion of elbow	1. Brachialis 2. Biceps brachii 3. Brachioradialis 4. Pronator teres 5. Flexor carpi ulnaris	Musculocutaneous Musculocutaneous Radial Median Ulnar	C5-C6, (C7) C5-C5 C5-C6, (C7) C6-C7 C7-C8
Extension of elbow	1. Triceps 2. Anconeus	Radial Radial	C6-C8 C7-C8, (T1)

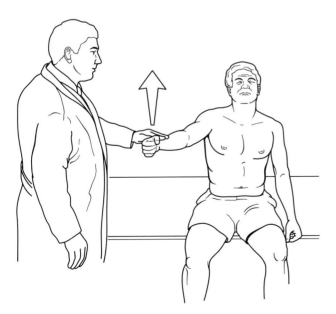

Figure 14-1 Full can test. (Adapted from Kelly BT, Kadrmas WR, Speer KP: The manual muscle examination for rotator cuff strength. An electromyographic investigation, *Am J Sports Med* 24(5):585, 1996.)

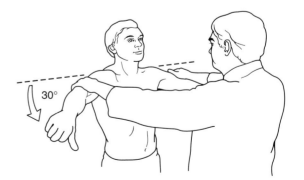

Figure 14-2 Empty can test. (Adapted from Jobe FW, Bradley JP: The diagnosis and nonoperative treatment of shoulder injuries in athletes, *Clin Sports Med* 8(3):424, 1989.)

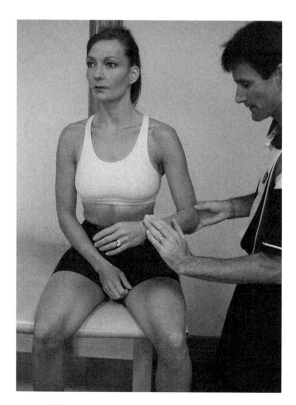

Figure 14-3 Infraspinatus MMT position.

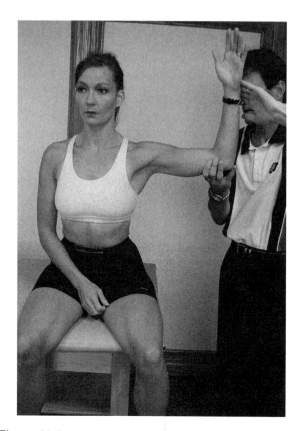

Figure 14-4 Patte test: MMT in 90 degrees of external rotation with 90 degrees of scapular plane elevation.

et al (1996) recommended an alternative position for testing infraspinatus strength in which the shoulder is in 90 degrees of elevation in the sagittal plane, with the arm in half maximal external rotation.

Teres Minor

Kelly et al (1996) did not report on the teres minor muscle; however, both Walch et al (1998) and Leroux et al (1995) have recommended the use of the Patte test (Patte et al, 1988) to isolate the teres minor. In this test, the glenohumeral joint is abducted 90 degrees in the scapular plane with 90 degrees of external rotation (Figure 14-4).

Subscapularis

Kelly et al (1996) reported the optimal position for subscapularis muscular activation to be in the Gerber lift-off position (Figure 14-5). This position is consistent with Gerber and Krushell (1991) but in contrast to Stefko et al (1997), who found the highest isolated muscular activity with the dorsal aspect of the hand placed up near the inferior border of the ipsilateral scapula (see

pages 99–101 for additional discussion of the Gerber lift-off test).

ALTERNATIVE FORMS OF STRENGTH EVALUATION FOR THE SHOULDER

Because of the limitations of MMT, particularly in the evaluation of muscular strength in individuals with only subtle muscular weakness or muscular imbalance, clinicians often use alternative forms of muscular strength testing. These alternatives can include augmentation of MMT positions with hand-held dynamometers to assess isometric muscular performance, as well as the use of isokinetic dynamometers to evaluate dynamic muscular performance characteristics. A review of the basic theory, rationale for use, and interpretation of isokinetics is indicated to facilitate optimal dynamic evaluation of the shoulder complex.

Rationale for Use of Isokinetics in Upper Extremity Strength Assessment

Unlike the lower extremity, where most functional and sport-specific movements occur in a closed kinetic chain environment, the upper extremity almost exclusively func-

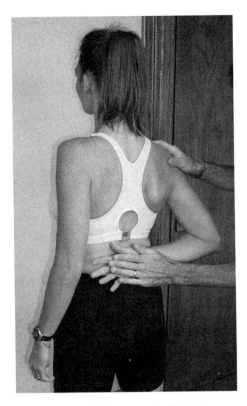

Figure 14-5 Gerber lift-off MMT.

methodology for the upper extremity. MMT provides a static alternative for the assessment of muscular strength, using well-developed patient positions and stabilization (Daniels & Worthingham, 1980; Kendall & McCreary, 1983). Despite the detailed description of manual assessment techniques, the reliability of MMT is compromised as a result of clinician size/strength differences and the subjective nature of the grading system (Frese et al, 1987).

Ellenbecker (1996) compared isokinetic testing of the shoulder internal and external rotators with MMT in 114 subjects exhibiting manually assessed, symmetric normal grade (5/5) strength. Isokinetic testing found 13% to 15% bilateral differences in external rotation and 15% to 28% bilateral differences in internal rotation. Of particular significance was the large variability in the size of this mean difference between extremities, despite bilaterally symmetric MMT. The use of MMT is an integral part of a musculoskeletal evaluation. MMT provides a time-efficient, gross screening of muscular strength of multiple muscles using a static, isometric muscular contraction, particularly in situations of neuromuscular disease or in patients with large muscular strength deficits. Limitations of MMT appear to be most evident where only minor impairment of strength is present, as well as in the identification of subtle, isolated strength deficits. Differentiation of agonist/antagonist muscular strength balance is also complicated when using manual techniques, as opposed to using isokinetic instrumentation (Ellenbecker, 1996).

Use of Isokinetic Testing for the Shoulder Complex

Initial testing and training using isokinetics for rehabilitation and testing of the shoulder typically involve the modified-base position, which is obtained by tilting the dynamometer approximately 30 degrees from the horizontal base position (Davies, 1992). The patient's glenohumeral joint is placed in 30 degrees abduction and 30 degrees forward flexion into the plane of the scapula or scaption, and with a 30-degree diagonal tilt of the dynamometer head from the transverse plane (Figure 14-6). This position has also been termed the *30/30/30 internal/external rotation position* by Davies (1992). The modified base position places the shoulder in the scapular plane 30 degrees anterior to the coronal plane (Saha, 1983). The scapular plane is characterized by enhanced bony congruity and a neutral glenohumeral position, which results in a mid-range position for the anterior capsular ligaments and enhances the length-tension relationship of the scapulohumeral musculature (Saha, 1983). The modified base position does not place the suprahumeral structures in an impingement situation and is well tolerated by patients (Davies, 1992).

tions in an open kinetic chain format (Ellenbecker & Davies, 2001). The throwing motion, volleyball spike, tennis serve, and tennis groundstrokes are all examples of open kinetic chain activities for the upper extremity. The use of open kinetic chain muscular strength, power, and endurance assessment methodology allows for isolation of particular muscle groups, as opposed to closed-chain methods, which use multiple joint axes, planes, and joint and muscle segments. Traditional isokinetic upper extremity test patterns are open chain with respect to the shoulder. The velocity spectrum (1 degree per second to approximately 600 degrees per second) currently available on commercial isokinetic dynamometers provides specificity with regard to testing the upper extremity by allowing the clinician to assess muscular strength, power, and endurance at faster, more functional speeds. Admittedly, most functional activities have angular velocities far exceeding the capabilities of isokinetic dynamometers; however, the velocities in the upper extremity are a summation of numerous joint movements and muscular forces (Marshall & Elliott, 2000).

The dynamic nature of upper extremity movements is a crucial factor in directing the clinician to optimal testing

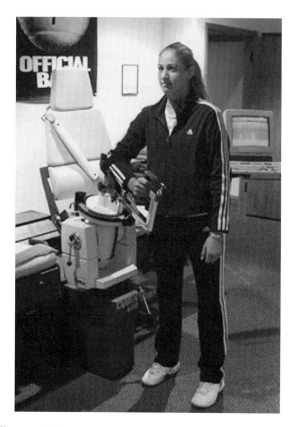

Figure 14-6 Modified base isokinetic dynamometer position used for testing and training glenohumeral joint internal and external rotation.

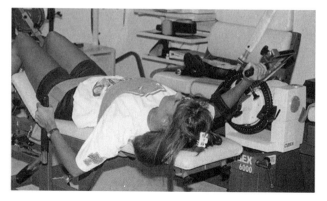

Figure 14-7 The Cybex isokinetic dynamometer position used for testing the glenohumeral joint in 90 degrees of abduction in the coronal plane.

Isokinetic testing using the modified base position requires consistent application of the patient to the dynamometer. Studies have demonstrated significant differences in internal and external rotation strength, with varying degrees of abduction, flexion, and horizontal abduction/adduction of the glenohumeral joint (Hageman et al, 1989; Soderberg & Blaschak, 1987; Walmsley & Szybbo, 1987). The modified base position uses a standing patient position on many dynamometer systems, which can lead to compromises in both glenohumeral joint isolation and test-retest reliability. Despite these limitations, valuable data can be obtained early in the rehabilitative process using this neutral modified base position, which is a safe, comfortable position for most patients with most pathologies and postsurgical considerations (Davies, 1992; Ellenbecker & Davies, 2001).

Knops et al (1999) conducted a test-retest reliability study of the modified neutral position for internal/external rotation of the glenohumeral joint. This position places the arm in a 30/30/30 position. Velocity spectrum testing at 60/180/300 degrees per second was performed,

with intraclass correlation coefficients (ICCs) applied to determine the degree of test-retest reliability. There was high test-retest reliability, with ICCs ranging between 0.91 and 0.96. This is one of the first studies to demonstrate reliability of this frequently used position in the clinical setting.

Internal and external rotation strength is also frequently assessed using isokinetic testing with 90 degrees of glenohumeral joint abduction (Figure 14-7). Specific advantages of this test position include greater stabilization in either a seated or supine test position on most dynamometers and placement of the shoulder in an abduction angle corresponding to the overhead throwing position used in many sport activities (Elliott et al, 1986). Initial tolerance of the patient to the modified base position (30/30/30) is required as a precursor to use of the 90-degree abducted position. Ninety-degree abducted isokinetic testing can be performed in either the coronal or scapular plane. Benefits of the scapular plane are similar to those discussed in the modified position and include protection of the anterior capsular glenohumeral ligaments and a theoretical length-tension enhancement of the posterior rotator cuff (Greenfield et al, 1990). Changes in length-tension relationships and the line of action of scapulohumeral and axiohumeral musculature are reported in 90 degrees of glenohumeral joint abduction compared with a more neutral adducted glenohumeral joint position (Davies, 1992). Use of the 90-degree abducted position of isokinetic strength assessment addresses more specifically muscular function required for overhead activities (Bassett et al, 1994).

Primary emphasis is placed on assessment of internal and external rotation strength of the shoulder during rehabilitation. Rationale for this apparently narrow focus is provided by an isokinetic training study by Quincy et al

(2000). Six weeks of isokinetic training of the internal and external rotators produced statistically significant improvements in not only internal and external rotation strength but also in flexion/extension and abduction/adduction strength. Isokinetic training of shoulder flexion/extension and abduction/adduction produced improvements only in the position of training with no overflows. The overflow of strength caused by training the internal and external rotators provides the rationale for the primary emphasis on strength development and assessment in rehabilitation. Additional research has identified the internal/external rotation movement pattern as the preferable testing pattern in patients with rotator cuff tendinosis (Holm et al, 1996).

Interpretation of Glenohumeral Joint Internal and External Rotation Testing

Bilateral Comparisons

Similar to isokinetic testing of the lower extremity, assessment of an extremity's strength, power, and endurance relative to the contralateral side forms the basis for standard data interpretation. This practice is more complicated in the upper extremity because of limb dominance, particularly in the unilaterally dominant sport athlete. In addition to the complexities added by limb dominance, isokinetic descriptive studies demonstrate disparities in the degree of limb dominance, as well as the presence of strength dominance only in specified muscle groups (Alderink & Kluck, 1986; Chandler et al, 1992; Cook et al, 1987; Ellenbecker, 1991, 1992; Ellenbecker & Mattalino, 1999a; Hinton, 1988).

In general, a maximum limb dominance of the internal and external rotators of 5% to 10% is assumed in non-athletic and recreational level upper extremity sport athletes (Davies, 1992). Ellenbecker and Bleacher (1999) measured 38 active adult females between the ages of 18 and 45 and found significantly greater internal rotation strength ($P < 0.01$), with no significant difference in external rotation strength. Testing was performed using the NORM isokinetic dynamometer (Cybex, Inc., Ronkonkoma, NY), with subjects seated with stabilization straps and the shoulder in the scapular plane and at 45 degrees of glenohumeral joint abduction.

Several studies have been performed to determine the degree of unilateral strength dominance in unilaterally dominant upper extremity sport athletes. Significantly greater internal rotation strength has been identified in the dominant arm in professional (Ellenbecker & Mattalino, 1999a; Brown et al, 1988), collegiate (Cook et al, 1987), and high school (Hinton, 1988) baseball players, as well

as in elite level junior (Chandler et al, 1992; Ellenbecker, 1991) and adult (Ellenbecker, 1991) tennis players. No difference between extremities was demonstrated in concentric external rotation in professional (Ellenbecker & Mattalino, 1999a; Wilk et al, 1993) and collegiate (Cook et al, 1987) baseball pitchers, as well as in elite junior (Chandler et al, 1992; Ellenbecker, 1992) and adult (Ellenbecker, 1991) tennis players. This selective strength development in the internal rotators produces significant changes in agonist/antagonist muscular balance. In all the aforementioned activities, the internal rotators are the primary muscle group used during the acceleration phase of the throwing or overhead activity, thereby demonstrating specificity of muscular adaptation. Identification of this muscular imbalance using isokinetic testing has implications for rehabilitation and injury prevention.

Unilateral Strength Ratios (Agonist/Antagonist)

Assessment of muscular strength balance of the internal and external rotators is of vital importance when interpreting upper extremity strength tests. Alteration of this external/internal ratio (ER/IR) has been reported in patients with glenohumeral joint instability and impingement (Leroux et al, 1994; Warner et al, 1990). The initial description of the ER/IR ratio on normal subjects was published by Ivey et al (1985) and Davies (1992) for both males and females. An ER/IR ratio of approximately 66% is targeted in normal subjects. One unique aspect of the ER/IR ratio is that it appears to remain approximately 66% throughout the velocity spectrum. The ER/IR ratio is one of the few unilateral strength ratios in the body to demonstrate this unique, consistent relationship at all velocities.

There have been widespread reports of alteration of the ER/IR ratio resulting from selective muscular development of the internal rotators without concomitant external rotation strength (Alderink & Kluck, 1986; Chandler et al, 1992; Cook et al, 1987; Ellenbecker, 1991, 1992; Ellenbecker & Mattalino, 1999a; Hinton, 1988). This alteration has provided clinicians objective rationale for the global recommendation of preventive posterior rotator cuff external rotation (ER) strengthening programs for athletes in high-level overhead activities (Wilk & Arrigo, 1993). Clinicians have advocated biasing this ratio in favor of the external rotators for both prevention of injury in throwing and racquet sport athletes, as well as after insult or surgery to the glenohumeral joint (Davies, 1992; Wilk & Arrigo, 1993; Ellenbecker & Davies, 2001). Examples of ER/IR ratios are presented with respect to population and apparatus specificity in Tables 14-2 through 14-4 (Ellenbecker & Roetert, 2003; Ellenbecker & Mattalino, 1999a; Wilk).

TABLE 14-2   **Isokinetic External Rotation/Internal Rotation Ratios in Elite Junior Tennis Players***

	DOMINANT ARM		NONDOMINANT ARM	
	PEAK TORQUE (%)	WORK (%)	PEAK TORQUE (%)	WORK (%)
Male, 210°/sec	69	64	81	81
Male, 300°/sec	69	65	82	83
Female, 210°/sec	69	63	81	82
Female, 300°/sec	67	61	81	77

From Ellenbecker & Roetert: *J Science & Medicine in Sport*, 2003.

*A Cybex 6000 series Isokinetic Dynamometer and 90° of glenohumeral joint abduction were used. Data are expressed as ER/IR ratios representing the relative muscular balance between the external and internal rotators.

TABLE 14-3   **Unilateral External Rotation/Internal Rotation Ratios in Professional Baseball Pitchers**

SPEED	DOMINANT ARM	NONDOMINANT ARM
210°/sec		
Torque	64	74
Work	61	66
300°/sec		
Torque	65	72
Work	62	70

Data from Ellenbecker TS, Mattalino AJ: Concentric isokinetic shoulder internal and external rotation strength in professional baseball pitchers, *J Orthop Sports Phys Ther* 25:323-328, 1997.

TABLE 14-4   **Unilateral External Rotation/Internal Rotation Ratios in Professional Baseball Pitchers**

SPEED	DOMINANT ARM	NONDOMINANT ARM
180°/sec		
Torque	65	64
300°/sec		
Torque	61	70

Data from Wilk KE, Andrews JR, Arrigo CA, et al: The strength characteristics of internal and external rotator muscles in professional baseball pitchers, *Am J Sports Med* 21:61-66, 1993.

Normative Data Utilization

Use of normative or descriptive data can help clinicians further analyze isokinetic test data. Care must be taken to use normative data that are both population and apparatus specific (Davies, 1992). Tables 14-5 through 14-7 present data from large samples of specific athletic populations on two dynamometer systems. Data are presented using body weight as the normalizing factor.

Another application for normative data is to normalize the isokinetic parameters to the patient's body weight when bilateral injury is present. Bilateral comparisons and unilateral strength ratios may often be within normal limits; however, if the patient has torque- and work-to-body-weight ratios that are lower than normative data, this may indicate that the patient may not be fully rehabilitated from a muscular standpoint.

Additional Glenohumeral Joint Testing Positions

Adduction/Abduction

Isokinetic evaluation of shoulder abduction/adduction strength is an additional pattern frequently evaluated because of the key role played by the abductors in the Inman force couple (Inman et al, 1944) and the functional relationship of the adductors to throwing velocity (Bartlett et al, 1989; Pedegana et al, 1982). Specific factors important in this testing pattern are the limitation of range of motion to approximately 120 degrees to avoid glenohumeral joint impingement and consistent use of gravity correction (Davies, 1992). No formal research specifically addressing the test-retest reliability of the shoulder abduction/adduction isokinetic testing pattern has been published.

Interpretation of abduction/adduction isokinetic tests follows traditional bilateral comparison, normative data comparison, and unilateral strength ratios. Ivey et al (1985) reported abduction/adduction (AB/ADD) ratios of 50% bilaterally in normal adult females. Similar findings were reported by Alderink & Kluck (1986) in high school and collegiate baseball pitchers. Wilk et al (1991, 1992) reported dominant arm AB/ADD ratios of 85% to 95% using a Biodex dynamometer. Their analysis used a windowing technique, which removed impact artifact after free limb acceleration and end stop impact from the data. Upper extremity testing, using long input adapters and fast isokinetic testing velocities, can produce torque

TABLE 14-5   **Isokinetic Peak Torque–to–Body Weight Ratios and Single Repetition Work–to–Body Weight Ratios in Elite Junior Tennis Players***

	DOMINANT ARM		NONDOMINANT ARM	
	PEAK TORQUE (%)	WORK (%)	PEAK TORQUE (%)	WORK (%)
EXTERNAL ROTATION (ER)				
Male, 210°/sec	12	20	11	19
Male, 300°/sec	10	18	10	17
Female, 210°/sec	8	14	8	15
Female, 300°/sec	8	11	7	12
INTERNAL ROTATION (IR)				
Male, 210°/sec	17	32	14	27
Male, 300°/sec	15	28	13	23
Female, 210°/sec	12	23	11	19
Female, 300°/sec	11	15	10	13

*A Cybex 6000 series Isokinetic Dynamometer and 90° of glenohumeral joint abduction were used. Data are expressed in foot-pounds per unit of body weight for ER and IR.
From Ellenbecker & Roetert: *J Science and Medicine in Sport*, 2003.

TABLE 14-6   **Isokinetic Peak Torque–to–Body Weight Ratios from 150 Professional Baseball Pitchers***

	INTERNAL ROTATION		EXTERNAL ROTATION	
SPEED	DOMINANT ARM	NONDOMINANT ARM	DOMINANT ARM	NONDOMINANT ARM
180°/sec	27%	17%	18%	19%
300°/sec	25%	24%	15%	15%

From Wilk KE, Andrews JR, Arrigo CA, et al: The strength characteristics of internal and external rotator muscles in professional baseball pitchers, *Am J Sports Med* 21:61-66, 1993.
*Data were obtained on a Biodex Isokinetic Dynamometer.

TABLE 14-7   **Isokinetic Peak Torque–to–Body Weight and Work–to–Body Weight Ratios from 147 Professional Baseball Pitchers***

	INTERNAL ROTATION		EXTERNAL ROTATION	
SPEED	DOMINANT ARM	NONDOMINANT ARM	DOMINANT ARM	NONDOMINANT ARM
210°/sec				
Torque	21%	19%	13%	14%
Work	41%	38%	25%	25%
300°/sec				
Torque	20%	18%	13%	13%
Work	37%	33%	23%	23%

Data from Ellenbecker TS, Mattalino AJ: Concentric isokinetic shoulder internal and external rotation strength in professional baseball pitchers, *J Orthop Sports Phys Ther* 25:323-328, 1997.
*Data were obtained on a Cybex 350 Isokinetic Dynamometer.

artifact that significantly changes the isokinetic test result. Wilk recommends windowing the data by removing all data obtained at velocities outside 95% of the pre-set angular testing velocity.

Flexion/Extension and Horizontal Abduction/Adduction

Additional isokinetic patterns used to obtain more detailed profiles of shoulder function are flexion/extension and horizontal AB/ADD. Both of these motions are generally tested in a less functional supine position to improve stabilization. Normative data related to these testing positions are less prevalent in the literature. Test-retest research is available for shoulder extension/flexion testing and demonstrates ICCs between 0.75 and 0.91 (Moffroid et al, 1969). No formal test-retest data are currently available for shoulder horizontal AB/ADD.

Flexion/extension ratios reported on normal subjects by Ivey et al (1985) are 80% (4:5). Ratios on athletes with shoulder extension dominant activities are reported at 50% for baseball pitchers (Alderink & Kluck, 1986) and 75% to 80% for highly skilled adult tennis players (Ellenbecker, 1991). Further development of normative data is needed to more clearly define strength in these upper extremity patterns. Body position and gravity compensation are key factors affecting proper data interpretation.

Scapulothoracic Testing: Protraction/Retraction

In addition to the supraspinatus/deltoid force couple, the serratus anterior/trapezius force couple is crucial in a thorough evaluation of upper extremity strength. Gross MMT and screening that attempt to identify scapular winging are commonly used in the clinical evaluation of the shoulder complex. Davies and Hoffman (1993) have published normative data on 250 shoulders, regarding isokinetic protraction/retraction testing. A nearly 1:1 relationship of protraction/retraction strength was reported. Testing and training the serratus anterior, trapezius, and rhomboid musculature enhance scapular stabilization and strengthen primary musculature involved in the scapulohumeral rhythm. Nearly all disciplines of rehabilitative medicine emphasize promotion of proximal stability to enhance distal mobility.

Additional Isokinetic Testing Concepts

Concentric versus Eccentric Considerations

Dynamic strength assessment has had a significant effect, primarily in research investigations. The extrapolation of research-oriented isokinetic principles to patient populations has been a gradual process. Use of eccentric testing in the upper extremity is clearly indicated based on the prevalence of functionally specific eccentric work. Maximal eccentric functional contractions of the posterior rotator cuff during the follow-through phase of the throwing motion and tennis serve provide rationales for eccentric testing and training in rehabilitation and preventative conditioning (Davies, 1992). Kennedy et al (1993) found mode-specific differences between the concentric and eccentric strength characteristics of the rotator cuff. Ellenbecker et al (1988), Mont et al (1994), and Treiber et al (1998) demonstrated the applications of eccentric training of the rotator cuff muscles, its effects on muscular strength, and its carryover to functional performance. Further research regarding eccentric muscular training is necessary before widespread use of eccentric isokinetics can be applied to patient populations.

Basic characteristics of eccentric isokinetic testing, such as greater force production compared with concentric contractions at the same velocity, are reported in the internal and external rotators (Ellenbecker et al, 1988; Davies & Ellenbecker, 1992). This enhanced force generation is generally explained by the contribution of the series elastic (noncontractile) elements of the muscle-tendon unit to force generation in eccentric conditions. An increase in postexercise muscle soreness, particularly of latent onset, is common after periods of eccentric work. Therefore eccentric testing would not be the mode of choice during early inflammatory stages of an overuse injury (Davies & Ellenbecker, 1992). Many clinicians recommend the use of dynamic concentric testing before performing an eccentric test. Both concentric and eccentric isokinetic training of the rotator cuff has produced objective concentric and eccentric strength improvements in elite tennis players (Ellenbecker et al, 1988).

Isokinetic Fatigue Testing

Isokinetic dynamometers have also been extensively used in the measurement of muscular fatigue (Ellenbecker & Roetert, 1999; Kannus et al, 1992). Isokinetic muscular fatigue tests typically consist of measuring the number of repetitions of maximum effort that are required to reach a 50% reduction in torque, work, or power from the beginning to the end of a certain time period or number of contractions. Relative fatigue ratios consist of comparing the work in the last half of a preset number of muscular contractions with the work performed in the first half (Kannus et al, 1992; Davies, 1992).

Relative fatigue ratios have been studied in elite tennis players and have produced clinically applicable information. Ellenbecker and Roetert (1999) measured the relative fatigue response in the internal and external rotators of 72 elite junior tennis players using 20 maximal effort concentric testing repetitions at 300 degrees per second in the supine position, with 90 degrees of glenohumeral joint abduction. The external rotators fatigued to a level of 69%, and the internal rotators fatigued only to a level of 83%. These percentages are significant because of the substantial contribution the external rotators play in humeral deceleration during overhead throwing and serving activities (Elliott et al, 1986), as well as dynamic stabilization of the humeral head in the glenoid (Bassett et al, 1994). That the external rotators appear to fatigue more quickly and to a greater extent than the internal rotators further supports the current concepts of preventive conditioning and balancing of the shoulder external rotators in unilaterally dominant upper extremity athletes.

A similar study was performed on swimmers by Beach et al (1992). They tested collegiate swimmers at 240 degrees per second using 50 repetitions. Relative fatigue ratios for external rotation were 80%, with internal rotation fatigue ratios of 105% in the collegiate swimmers. The authors also found a significant correlation between isokinetic fatigue ratios and shoulder pain among this swimming population.

These studies demonstrate the important role fatigue testing plays, both in guiding and providing rationale for the high-repetition training programs used in rehabilitation and in providing a clinically acceptable method for assessing muscular fatigue.

Relationship of Isokinetic Testing to Functional Performance in the Upper Extremity

Dynamic muscular strength assessment is used to evaluate the underlying strength, power, endurance, and balance of strength in specific muscle groups. This information is used to determine the specific anatomic structures that require strengthening, as well as to demonstrate the efficacy of treatment procedures. Isokinetic testing of the shoulder internal and external rotators has been used as one aspect in demonstrating functional outcome after rotator cuff repair on select patient populations (Gore et al, 1986; Rabin & Post, 1990; Walker et al, 1987; Walmsley & Hartsell, 1992; Kirschenbaum et al, 1993), as well as after arthroscopic thermal capsulorrhaphy to treat unidirectional glenohumeral joint instability (Ellenbecker & Mattalino, 1999b).

Isokinetic testing is also used to determine the relationship of muscular strength to functional performance. Several studies have tested upper extremity muscle groups and correlated their respective levels of strength to sport-specific functional tests. Pedegana et al (1982) found a statistically significant correlation between elbow extension, wrist flexion, shoulder extension, shoulder flexion, and shoulder external rotation strength measured isokinetically and throwing speed in professional pitchers. In a similar study, Bartlett et al (1989) found the shoulder adductors to correlate to throwing speed.

Ellenbecker et al (1988) found that 6 weeks of concentric isokinetic training of the rotator cuff resulted in a statistically significant improvement in serving velocity in collegiate tennis players. In a similar study, Mont et al (1994) found serving velocity improvements after both concentric and eccentric internal and external rotation training. Treiber et al (1998) used isokinetic testing to document strength changes before and after a 4-week training program using isotonic dumbbell or Thera-Band internal and external rotation strengthening. In addition to documenting strength improvements with isokinetic testing, an increase in tennis serve velocity was measured in the experimental group.

The complex biomechanical sequences of segmental velocities and interrelationship between the kinetic chain link with the lower extremities and trunk make it difficult to identify a direct relationship between an isolated structure and a complex functional activity. Isokinetic testing can provide a reliable, dynamic measurement of isolated joint motions and muscular contributions that can assist the clinician in assessing underlying muscular strength and strength balance.

Closed Kinetic Chain Upper Extremity Testing

Another method used to assess neuromuscular control of the shoulder has been the use of closed chain upper extremity tests. Although widespread use of closed chain training techniques has been reported in the physical medicine and rehabilitation literature (Ellenbecker et al, 2000b), limited evaluation methods for the upper extremity currently exist to properly assess closed-chain function.

One of the gold standards in physical education for gross assessment of upper extremity strength has been the push-up. This test has been used to generate sport-specific normative data in normal populations (Ellenbecker et al, 2000b; Roetert & Ellenbecker, 1998), but it is not typically considered appropriate for use in patient populations with shoulder dysfunction. Positional demands placed on the anterior capsule and increased joint loading limit the effectiveness of this test in musculoskeletal rehabilitation. Modification of the push-up has been reported and used clinically as an acceptable alternative to assess closed-chain function in the upper extremities.

Davies has developed the closed kinetic chain (CKC) upper extremity stability test in an attempt to assess more accurately the functional ability of the upper extremity (Ellenbecker & Davies, 2000; Ellenbecker et al, 2000b; Goldbeck & Davies, 2000). The test is initiated in the starting position of a standard push-up for males and modified (off knees) push-up for females. Two strips of tape are placed parallel to each other, 3 feet apart on the floor (Figure 14-8). The subject or patient then moves both hands back and forth, touching each line alternatively as many times as possible in 15 seconds. Each touch of the line is counted and tallied to generate the CKC upper extremity stability test score. Normative data have been established, with men averaging 18.5 touches in 15 seconds, and females averaging 20.5 touches. The CKC upper extremity stability test has been subjected to a test-retest reliability test, with an ICC generated at

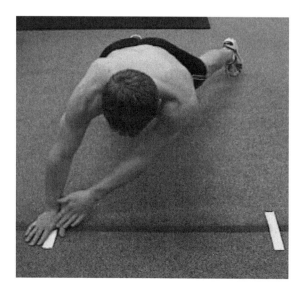

Figure 14-8 Davies closed kinetic chain test.

0.927, indicating high clinical reliability between sessions (Goldbeck & Davies, 2000).

Ellenbecker and Roetert (1996) and Ellenbecker and Mattalino (1997) have used other methods of CKC testing for the upper extremity. The unilateral CKC stance stability test consists of 20-second testing over a Fastex (Cybex International, Medway, MA) or Biodex Stability System (Shirley, NY) to measure postural sway or perturbation. The subject assumes a unilateral upper extremity stance with a standardized trunk-extremity angle of 80 degrees and feet placed 1 foot apart. The contralateral extremity is placed in the lumbar spine to minimize compensation. The subject is instructed to remain as still as possible, with the eyes closed, during the 20-second test, in which the amount of postural sway or movement is measured (Ellenbecker & Roetert, 1996; Ellenbecker & Mattalino, 1997).

Ellenbecker and Roetert (1996) used this test to measure upper extremity closed-chain stance stability in 19 professional baseball players and 75 elite junior tennis players. Results of the bilateral comparisons of these players showed no significant differences between extremities. By contrast, previous open kinetic chain testing on athletes in this population found significantly greater dominant arm strength when compared with the nondominant extremity (Ellenbecker, 1991, 1992; Wilk et al, 1993; Ellenbecker & Mattalino, 1999a). Ellenbecker and Mattalino (1997) tested patients undergoing rehabilitation for glenohumeral joint impingement and instability, and compared bilateral CKC function using the unilateral stance stability test and traditional open kinetic chain isokinetic glenohumeral rotational testing. There was no statistically significant correlation between results of the bilateral comparisons of the open and CKC tests. The presence of a significant deficit in isokinetically measured open kinetic chain external rotation did not necessarily correlate to a deficit in CKC function. This research indicates that CKC upper extremity testing may provide unique information on upper extremity function; however, further research is needed to better understand its role and relationship to other more traditional methods of upper extremity evaluation.

CHAPTER
15 | Shoulder Rating Scales

INTRODUCTION

The use of rating scales that assess the glenohumeral joint and upper extremity in general is an important part of the evaluation process. The use of such scales can vary from the multitude of developed rating systems or scales to the simple application of the visual analog scale rating a patient's pain or symptoms from 0 to 10 or 0 to 100. This chapter outlines some of the most common shoulder rating scales and describes applicable research that has validated the instruments.

In general, health questionnaires such as rating scales can be divided into two categories: generic and joint- or disease-specific. An example of a generic health status questionnaire is the Short Form–36 (SF-36) (Ware et al, 1993). Generic questionnaires assess unexpected health effects using a common instrument such as the SF-36 across different patient groups. Beaton and Richards (1998) compared the sensitivity to change in five shoulder joint–specific questionnaires and the SF-36 in a large sample of patients with shoulder pain. The shoulder-specific questionnaires were more sensitive to change than the SF-36. Despite this finding, use of the SF-36 can provide valuable insight about the general health effects that shoulder pain and disability caused by shoulder injury or surgery can have on patients undergoing rehabilitation. Gartsman et al (1998) used the SF-36 on 544 patients with glenohumeral joint instability (149), rotator cuff tears (111), adhesive capsulitis (100), glenohumeral osteoarthritis (67), and impingement (117) before and after treatment. Compared with the normative data in the United States, these patients had significant decreases in health ratings for Physical Functioning, Role-Physical, Bodily Pain, Social Functioning, Role-Emotional, and the Physical Component Summary as measured by the SF-36 survey instrument. Patients with shoulder pathology perceived their general health in the same category as published standards for patients with congestive heart failure, acute myocardial infarction, diabetes mellitus, and clinical depression. This finding supports the use of a generic-type scale to lend valuable insight into the general health

status and perception of health status in patients undergoing treatment for shoulder pathology.

SHOULDER-SPECIFIC RATING SCALES

This chapter describes several joint- or shoulder-specific rating scales that are commonly used and recommended for patients after either injury or surgical procedures to the shoulder. Unlike the knee joint, where one or two joint-specific rating scales have become gold standards for evaluation, the shoulder has no single universally accepted scale or instrument. Given the wide variety in use, this chapter discusses several popular instruments and includes examples of each instrument to facilitate application by the reader.

CONSTANT-MURLEY SCORING SYSTEM

This system was originally described by Constant and Murley (1987) as a simple clinical method of shoulder functional assessment that combines individual parameter assessments with an overall rating on a 100-point scoring system; 35% of the Constant-Murley system is subjective and 65% is objective. The subjective portions of the scoring system include the degree of pain the patient is experiencing, as well as the patient's ability to perform simple activities of daily living. The objective parameters include actual measurements of active range of motion in flexion, abduction, and combined internal and external rotation with a goniometer. Strength testing is carried out with the use of a spring balance to test shoulder power in 90 degrees of abduction. In patients with less than 90 degrees of abduction, strength testing occurs at a point in the range of motion near the maximum. The amount of weight or force that can be lifted in the scapular plane is recorded with a value between 0 and 25 based on the amount lifted or pounds of force measured depending on the method used.

Constant and Murley (1987) developed age- and gender-specific scoring ranges in 900 normal individuals. The Constant-Murley system is used extensively in Europe and is one of the most commonly used outcome measures in many short- and long-term follow-up studies evaluating the efficacy of various shoulder surgical procedures. The European Shoulder and Elbow Society requires that the results of clinical data be reported using the Constant-Murley score.

Ianotti et al (1996) used the Constant-Murley scoring system to determine the postoperative function of patients after the repair of full-thickness rotator cuff tears. In their study, a preoperative Constant score of 35 points was reported among the 40 patients with a rotator cuff tear. The authors used the categories of *excellent* for Constant scores of 90 to 100, *good* for scores of 80 to 89, *fair* for scores ranging between 70 and 79, and *poor* for scores less than 70 points. They grouped the good and excellent scores together and characterized this group as *satisfied* or *satisfactory outcomes* (Constant score greater than 80 points) and *unsatisfactory* as scores less than 80 points.

Patients were evaluated 2 years after open repair of a full-thickness rotator cuff tear; 60% of shoulders had excellent Constant scores, with 28% having good scores. The authors concluded that 88% of patients undergoing a full-thickness rotator cuff tear had a satisfactory outcome. Many other studies have used the Constant-Murley system; however, the study of Ianotti et al (1996) is presented here as an example of the application of one scoring system used in clinical and research follow-up evaluation.

MODIFIED ROWE SCALE

The Rowe scale was originally developed as a tool to assess outcome after open anterior stabilization procedures. The three main headings in the Rowe scale are *Stability, Motion,* and *Function*. A total of 100 possible points are allotted for this scale. The scale is heavily weighted toward the Stability category. The allotment of 50 possible points for a stable shoulder is a major component of this shoulder rating scale. The presence of instability in virtually any form significantly detracts from the composite score, making the scale an excellent choice to use in patients after glenohumeral joint stability procedures (both open and arthroscopic), as well as in nonoperative rehabilitation of the unstable shoulder.

Table 15-1 lists the components of the modified Rowe scale, which was developed to address slightly higher demands that athletes and more active individuals have. Ellenbecker et al (2003a, 2003b) used the modified Rowe scale in a long-term follow-up study of patients after arthroscopic thermal capsulorrhaphy and in the baseline assessment of uninjured elite unilaterally dominant overhead athletes.

UCLA RATING SCALE

The UCLA rating scale is a similar instrument to the modified Rowe scale that combines the components of pain, function, range of motion, manually assessed muscle strength, and patient satisfaction (Ellman et al, 1986). Objective portions of this scale include active range of motion of forward flexion measured in degrees. This measurement accounts for as much as 5 points if it is greater than or equal to 150 degrees; muscle strength in forward flexion is assessed manually and accounts for 5 points if it is normal. The patient provides a subjective assessment of pain, functional use, and overall satisfaction with the surgical procedure that accounts for a total of 35 points. Box 15-1 shows the component parts of the UCLA rating scale, as well as the allotment of points for each section.

Roddey et al (2000) studied the self-report sections of the UCLA, simple shoulder test (SST), and shoulder pain and disability index (SPADI) in 192 patients with shoulder dysfunction. All three scales demonstrated good internal consistency; however, the authors could not validate or invalidate the use of the UCLA rating scale for either group or individual comparison. Further research is needed to determine the validity and reliability of this scale in the clinical setting.

Soldatis et al (1997) used the Rowe, American Shoulder Elbow Surgeons (ASES), UCLA, Constant-Murley, and SST to determine the presence and severity of shoulder symptoms in healthy college athletes at mid-season. Athletes were chosen from men's baseball, basketball, and football; and women's volleyball, basketball, swimming, and tennis. In general, shoulder pain was the most frequent symptom reported in 47% of all participants. The UCLA rating system was deemed the most "sensitive" for evaluating healthy college athletes in this study. The authors concluded that the ideal scoring system for shoulders has yet to be developed, but these shoulder rating systems can be used as a reference in the evaluation and treatment of athletes.

MODIFIED AMERICAN SHOULDER ELBOW SURGEON RATING SCALE

The self-reported portion of the ASES rating scale consists of 15 questions that are answered using a score ranging from normal (3), which indicates an ability to perform that activity without any problem, to (0), which indicates an activity that cannot be performed at all. Figure 15-1 contains the self-reported questions from the modified ASES rating scale (Barrett et al, 1987), which evolved from the Neer rating scale. Beaton and Richards (1998) used the self-reported section of the modified ASES

TABLE 15-1   Modified Rowe Scale

Scoring System	Units	Excellent (100-90)	Good (89-75)	Fair (74-51)	Poor (50 or Less)
STABILITY					
No recurrence or subluxation	50	No recurrences	No recurrences	No recurrences	Recurrence of dislocation
Apprehension when placing arm in certain positions	30	No apprehension when placing arm in complete elevation and ER	Mild apprehension when placing arm in elevation and ER	Moderate apprehension during elevation and ER	Marked apprehension during elevation or extension
Subluxation (not requiring reduction)	10	No subluxation	No subluxation	No subluxation	
Recurrent dislocation	0				
MOTION					
100% of normal ER, IR, and elevation	20	100% of normal ER, complete elevation and IR	75% of normal ER, complete elevation and IR	50% of normal ER, 75% elevation and IR	No ER; 50% of elevation (can get hand only to face); 50% IR
75% of normal ER, normal elevation, and IR	15				
50% of normal ER, 75% of normal elevation and IR	5				
50% of normal elevation and IR, no ER	0				
FUNCTION					
No limitation in work or sports; little or no discomfort	30	Performs all work and sports; no limitation in overhead activities; shoulder strong in lifting, swimming, tennis, throwing; no discomfort	Mild limitation in work and sports; shoulder strong; minimum discomfort	Moderate limitation doing overhead work and heavy lifting; unable to throw, serve hard in tennis, or swim; moderate disabling pain	Marked limitation; unable to perform overhead work and lifting; cannot throw, play tennis, or swim; chronic discomfort
Mild limitation and minimum discomfort	25				
Moderate limitation and discomfort	10				
Marked limitation and pain	0				

ER, External rotation; *IR*, internal rotation.

Total units possible: 100.

From Rowe CR, Patel D, Southmayd WW: The Bankart procedure: a long term end-result study, *J Bone Joint Surg* 60A:1-16, 1978.

Box 15-1 UCLA Rating Scale: Functional/Reaction Measures

PAIN

Present all of the time and unbearable; strong medication frequently	1
Present all of the time but bearable; strong mediation occasionally	2
None or little at rest, present during light activities; salicylates frequently	4
Present during heavy or particular activities only; salicylates occasionally	6
Occasional and slight	8
None	10

FUNCTION

Unable to use limb	1
Only light activities possible	2
Able to do light housework or most of activities of daily living	4
Most housework, shopping, and driving possible; able to fix hair and dress and undress, including fastening brassiere	6
Slight restriction only; able to work above shoulder level	8
Normal activities	10

ACTIVE FORWARD FLEXION

150 degrees or more	5
120 to 150 degrees	4
90 to 120 degrees	3
45 to 90 degrees	2
30 to 45 degrees	1
Less than 30 degrees	0

STRENGTH OF FORWARD FLEXION (MMT)

Grade 5 (normal)	5
Grade 4 (good)	4
Grade 3 (fair)	2
Grade 2 (poor)	2
Grade 1 (muscle contraction)	1
Grade 0 (nothing)	0

SATISFACTION OF THE PATIENT

Satisfied and better	5
Not satisfied and worse	0

MAXIMUM SCORE: 35 POINTS

From Ellman H, Hander G, Bayer M: Repair of the rotator cuff: end-result study of factors influencing reconstruction, *J Bone Joint Surg* 68A: 1136-1144, 1986.

rating scale in addition to four other joint-specific scales and the SF-36 in 99 patients with shoulder dysfunction. They found acceptable levels of reliability and responsiveness using the modified ASES rating scale; they also found the ASES scale and the other four joint-specific scales to be more sensitive to change in patients with shoulder pain than the generic SF-36 questionnaire. The modified ASES shoulder rating scale has also been used in the follow-up evaluation of patients after arthroscopic thermal capsulorrhaphy for treatment of unidirectional instability, as well as in the baseline evaluation of unilaterally dominant elite upper extremity athletes (Ellenbecker, 2000b, 2003a).

SIMPLE SHOULDER TEST

Matsen et al (1994) developed a brief questionnaire to facilitate and standardize patient reporting of functional status of their injured shoulder. The SST is comprised of a minimal data set of 12 questions that were derived from the basic complaints of patients entering the University of Washington Shoulder Service for treatment (Figure 15-2). Before developing the SST for patients, a pool of 60- and 70-year-old healthy individuals were tested to ensure that healthy older individuals could perform these functions.

The 12 questions in the SST can be answered with a yes or no response. It is important that the patient answer the questions without assistance to ensure that the answer reflects the patient's assessment of function. The SST is designed to represent the functional status of the shoulder rather than degrees of motion or pounds of force that are assessed with other more traditionally applied measures. Matsen et al (1994) added questions to the SST for certain athletic patient populations (e.g., does your shoulder allow you to serve with your usual speed and control?). These questions can be added, but the initial data set should be kept intact to facilitate administration of the SST in the clinical setting.

Figure 15-3 lists the questions for the SST and the normal responses from a group of 80 healthy subjects 60 to 70 years old without shoulder complaints during clinical examination of their shoulders and with normal ultrasound evaluation of the glenohumeral structures (Matsen et al, 1994). The test-retest reliability of the SST has been measured by Matsen et al (1994), with 70 patients completing the test on two separate occasions. A total of 63% of the patients had identical responses on retesting; 90% of the patients answered all but one of the questions identically between sessions. The simplicity of the SST facilitates communication of results to patients and is recommended for both clinical and research applications (Matsen et al, 1994).

THE SHOULDER PAIN AND DISABILITY INDEX

The SPADI is a self-administered questionnaire that consists of two dimensions, pain and function or functional activities (Heald et al, 1997). Box 15-2 lists the five

MODIFIED AMERICAN SHOULDER & ELBOW SURGEONS RATING SCALE

Please rate your ability to do the following daily activities using the following scale:

0 = unable   1 = very difficult   2 = somewhat difficult   3 = not difficult at all

Get dressed, including
putting on your coat   _____

Wash back/do up bra   _____

Manage toileting   _____

Comb hair   _____

Reach a high shelf   _____

Lift heavy objects   _____

Do usual work   _____

Do usual sport   _____

Sleep on your painful side   _____

Throw a ball overhand   _____

Open a jar of food   _____

Cut with a knife   _____

Use a phone   _____

Do up buttons   _____

Carry shopping bag   _____

Figure 15-1 Modified American Shoulder Elbow Surgeons (ASES) rating scale.

questions from the pain dimension and the eight questions from the functional activity dimension.

Heald et al (1997) administered the SPADI to 103 patients undergoing outpatient rehabilitation for shoulder pain. Scores of patients who completed the SPADI at both the initial and final treatments were analyzed to determine the responsiveness of the index. The SPADI was more responsive in this patient population than the sickness impact profile (SIP), which is a generic rating instrument. Evidence to support the construct validity of the SPADI was moderately strong; however, it was suggested that the SPADI may not readily measure occupational and recreational disability.

Roach et al (1991) measured test-retest reliability of the SPADI in a group of 23 subjects for both the total

scores and the pain and disability dimensions. Williams et al (1995) also studied the SPADI and examined the construct validity using a population of 102 patients with shoulder involvement. Their research supported the construct validity of this instrument, suggesting that the SPADI is another valuable tool that can be used clinically during the examination and treatment of patients with shoulder pathology.

ATHLETIC SHOULDER OUTCOME RATING SCALE

After reviewing the list of questions used in the SPADI and other rating scales, it is apparent that the level of questions in most scales is not applicable to the demands and intensities inherent in upper extremity sport

UNIVERSITY OF WASHINGTON SHOULDER INFORMATION FORM

SIMPLE SHOULDER TEST

Please answer these questions about your shoulder.   Date: _____

	Yes	No
1. Is your shoulder comfortable with your arm at rest by your side?	☐	☐
2. Does your shoulder allow you to sleep comfortably?	☐	☐
3. Can you reach the small of your back to tuck in your shirt with your hand?	☐	☐
4. Can you place your hand behind your head with the elbow straight out to the side?	☐	☐
5. Can you place a coin on a shelf at the level of your shoulder without bending your elbow?	☐	☐
6. Can you lift 1 pound (a full pint container) to the level of your shoulder without bending your elbow?	☐	☐
7. Can you lift 8 pounds (a full gallon container) to the level of the top of your head without bending your elbow?	☐	☐
8. Can you carry 20 pounds (a bag of potatoes) at your side with the affected extremity?	☐	☐
9. Do you think you can toss a softball underhand 10 yards with the affected extremity?	☐	☐
10. Do you think you can thow a softball overhand 20 yards with the affected extremity?	☐	☐
11. Can you wash the back of your opposite shoulder with the affected extremity?	☐	☐
12. Would your shoulder allow you to work full time at your regular job?	☐	☐

Are there other important things you cannot do as a result of your shoulder problem?

Previous doctors you have seen about your shoulder problem:

Previous tests you have had concerning your shoulder problem:

Previous nonmedical treatment you have had for your shoulder problem:

How many cortisone, steroid, or other types of injections have you had in your shoulder?

Previous shoulder surgeries (please list which shoulder, procedure, and date):

Are there any other aspects of your shoulder problems that we should know about?

Any family history of shoulder problems?

Figure 15-2 Simple shoulder test. (Adapted from Matsen FA III, Lippitt SB, Sidles JA, et al: *Practical evaluation and management of the shoulder*, Philadelphia, 1994, WB Saunders, p. 15, with permission.)

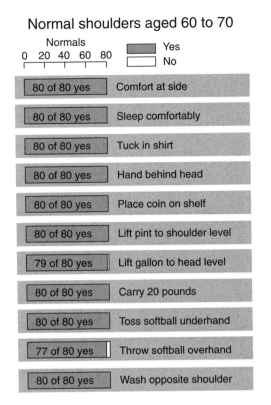

Figure **15-3** Normal responses to the SST in persons 60 to 70 years old.

Box 15-2 Shoulder Pain and Disability Index (SPADI)

PAIN DIMENSION—HOW SEVERE IS YOUR PAIN:

1. At its worst?
2. When lying on the involved side?
3. Reaching for something on a high shelf?
4. Touching the back of your neck?
5. Pushing with the involved arm?

DISABILITY DIMENSION—HOW MUCH DIFFICULTY DO YOU HAVE:

1. Washing your hair?
2. Washing your back?
3. Putting on an underskirt or pullover sweater?
4. Putting on a shirt that buttons down the front?
5. Putting on your pants?
6. Placing an object on a high shelf?
7. Carrying a heavy object (e.g., 10 pounds)?
8. Removing something from your back pocket?

To answer each of the questions, patients place a mark on a 10-cm visual analog scale for each question. The ends of each line have the verbal anchors of "no pain at all" and "worst pain imaginable" for the pain dimension and for the functional disability dimension "no difficulty" and "so difficult it required help." The scores from both dimensions are averaged to derive a total score.

Data from Heald SL, Riddle DL, Lamb RL: The shoulder pain and disability index: the construct validity and responsiveness of a region specific disability measure, *Phys Ther* 77(10):1079-1089, 1997.

participation. Tibone and Bradley (1993) stated: "to adequately determine the overall results, a different set of parameters is required for evaluation of outcome in the athletic shoulder." They formulated a rating system to evaluate overall results in the athletic shoulder. Their outcome instrument contains major subjective headings—pain, strength and endurance, stability, intensity, and performance—with objective information, specifically regarding range of motion, also factored into the rating system (Figure 15-4). Range of motion is measured with a goniometer to determine active external rotation in a standing position with 90 degrees of abduction, as well as total active elevation in the scapular plane. Internal rotation is not measured because Tibone and Bradley (1993) believe that overhead athletes often have internal rotation range of motion losses, and including internal rotation active range of motion might lead to unfair loss of points after injury or surgery. Overall results are graded such that an excellent score consists of 90 to 100 points, good scores range from 70 to 89, fair scores range from 50 to 69, and a poor score is less than 50. Neither test-retest reliability nor responsiveness or validity was measured in this study. The type of questions inherent in this questionnaire more

adequately address both the demands and intensities required in the glenohumeral joint of the overhead athlete. Further research using this instrument is needed to establish its accuracy and effectiveness.

SINGLE ASSESSMENT NUMERIC EVALUATION METHOD

One of the limiting factors of most subjective rating scores and rating systems is the amount of time it takes patients, clinicians, and researchers to perform the necessary functions involved in that particular scale or scoring system. Williams et al (1999) developed the single assessment numeric evaluation (SANE) method. This method uses a single question that is easily processed and applied: "How would you rate your shoulder today as a percentage of normal?" Patients are instructed to provide SANE ratings in whole numbers. This method provides a rapid and easy method to obtain the patient's perception of shoulder function and overall status. This method is an excellent example of a self-administered, patient-based method for evaluating patient outcome. It differs from the clinical data, which require a more objective process (Williams et al, 1999).

ATHLETIC SHOULDER OUTCOME RATING SCALE

Name_____ Age_____ Sex_____

Dominant hand (R)_____ (L)_____ (Ambidextrous)_____

Date of examination_____

Surgeon_____

Type of sport_____

Position played_____

Years played_____

Prior injury_____

Activity Level

1. Professional (major league)
2. Professional (minor league)
3. College
4. High school
5. Recreational (full time)
6. Recreational (occasionally)

Diagnosis

1. Anterior instability
2. Posterior instability
3. Multidirectional instability
4. Recurrent dislocations
5. Impingement syndrome
6. Acromioclavicular separation
7. Acromioclavicular arthrosis
8. Rotator cuff repair (partial)
9. Rotator cuff tear (complete)
10. Biceps tendon rupture
11. Calcific tendinitis
12. Fracture

SUBJECTIVE (90 points)

	Points
I Pain	
• No pain with competition	10
• Pain after competing only	8
• Pain while competing	6
• Pain preventing competing	4
• Pain with ADLs	2
• Pain at rest	0
II Strength/Endurance	
• No weakness, normal competition fatigue	10
• Weakness after competition, early competition fatigue	8
• Weakness during competition, abnormal competition fatigue	6
• Weakness or fatigue preventing competition	4
• Weakness or fatigue with ADLs	2
• Weakness or fatigue preventing ADLs	0
III Stability	
• No looseness during competition	10
• Recurrent subluxations while competing	8
• Dead-arm syndrome while competing	6
• Recurrent subluxations prevent competition	4
• Recurrent subluxations during ADLs	2
• Dislocation	0
IV Intensity	
• Preinjury versus postinjury hours of competition (100%)	10
• Preinjury versus postinjury hours of competition (less than 75%)	8
• Preinjury versus postinjury hours of competition (less than 50%)	6
• Preinjury versus postinjury hours of competition (less than 25%)	4
• Preinjury and postinjury hours of ADLs (100%)	2
• Preinjury and postinjury hours of ADLs (less than 50%)	0

Figure 15-4 Athletic shoulder outcome rating scale. (Adapted from Matsen FA, Fu FH, eds: *The shoulder: a balance of mobility and stability*, Rosemont, IL, 1993, American Academy of Orthopaedic Surgery, pp. 526–527, with permission.)

To test the effectiveness of the SANE method, Williams et al (1999) used the SANE score during 209 follow-up evaluations of 163 military cadets after surgical procedures for glenohumeral joint dislocations, chronic subluxations, and acromioclavicular joint separations. The Rowe and ASES scales were used in addition to the SANE method for all patients at various times during follow-up evaluations. Results showed statistically significant ($P < 0.001$) correlations between the overall results of the Rowe scale and SANE score ($r = 0.77$), as well as between the ASES and SANE scores ($r = 0.69$). The authors recommend the use of the SANE method during follow-up evaluation to obtain patient-based information on perception of shoulder function. One obvious weakness of this method noted by the authors is the inability to determine "why" patients rate their shoulder at a certain level. The authors did not recommend that this rating method replace other rating scales, but they did recommend its use as a convenient adjunct to clinical evaluation methods and other rating scales. Further research on other subject populations is needed to better understand the global effectiveness of this subjective rating method.

APPLICATION OF SHOULDER RATING SCALES TO CLINICAL PRACTICE

The myriad of shoulder rating scales described in this chapter demonstrates the variety of instruments currently available to clinicians both when measuring the baseline status and when documenting progress after a series or completion of rehabilitative interventions. I recommend the use of one or a series of shoulder rating scales specific to the individual patient (i.e., modified Rowe scale for instability patients) based on the intended population, both at initial patient examination and at the completion of physical therapy (i.e., discharge) to document patient progression. The postoperative use of shoulder rating scales at predetermined periods can provide important insight into the function and subjective level of pain and limitation that patients experience at various times after surgery (Ellenbecker et al, 2003a). The use of these scales adds an additional variable to the traditional examination of patients (range of motion and strength) with shoulder injury.

SUMMARY

Additional shoulder-specific rating scales, such as the instruments used by the Hospital for Special Surgery in New York (Altchek et al, 1990) and the rating scale designed by Neer et al (1982), can also be used in specific patient populations after the surgical procedures for which the instruments were initially intended and applied in research. This chapter described some of the most commonly applied instruments, along with research demonstrating either the effectiveness of the instrument or examples of applications of each instrument, to facilitate their use and application in both clinical and research arenas. Further research will better identify the effectiveness of each rating system, as well as new and more sensitive shoulder rating scales that may produce a more "universally accepted" upper extremity rating system for both clinical and research application.

Proprioceptive Testing of the Glenohumeral Joint

INTRODUCTION AND DEFINITIONS

Review of the orthopedic and musculoskeletal rehabilitation literature identifies many different versions of definitions for the terms associated with joint proprioception and neuromuscular control. In Goetz's *Textbook of Clinical Neurology*, proprioception is defined as any postural, positional, or kinetic information provided to the central nervous system by sensory receptors in muscles, tendons, joints, or skin (Goetz, 1999). Other texts define proprioception as "awareness of the position and movements of our limbs, fingers, and toes derived from receptors in the muscles, tendons, and joints" (Adams et al, 1997). Sherrington (1906) classically defined proprioception as afferent information arising from the proprioceptive field and identified mechanoreceptors or proprioceptors as being the source of the origination of this afferent information.

These original definitions of the term *proprioception* continue to be used today; however, a more advanced definition of the sensory involvement that encompasses human proprioceptive function is clearly needed. In a classic monograph entitled *Physiologie des Muskelsinnes*, Goldsheider (1898) proposed that muscle sense be divided into four distinct and separate sensory functions: sensation of passive movements, sensation of active movements, sensation of position, and appreciation or sensation of heaviness and resistance. These original classifications have been expanded to decrease confusion. The sensation of passive movements is considered a product of sensations induced by external forces that results in a change in limb position with noncontracting muscles. The sensation of active movement (or *kinesthesia* as it is now better known) encompasses the appreciation of change in position of a limb with contracting muscles. The appreciation of a limb's position in space has been termed *stagnosia*. In the presence of tension, the appreciation of force applied during a voluntary contraction has been termed *dynamaesthesia* (Roland and Ladegaard-Pedersen, 1977).

Although these expanded definitions provide additional information regarding human proprioception, adaptations of them have been suggested and are used in this chapter. *Proprioception* can be defined as afferent information received, including joint position sense, kinesthesia, and sensation of resistance. *Joint position sense* can be defined as the ability to appreciate and recognize where a joint or limb is in space. *Kinesthesia* can be defined as the ability to sense or recognize joint motion or movement. *Sensation to resistance* can be defined as the ability to sense force or tension generated through a joint. The appropriate efferent response to these afferent proprioceptive inputs has been termed *neuromuscular control*.

AFFERENT NEUROBIOLOGY OF THE GLENOHUMERAL JOINT

Afferent proprioceptive function of the human glenohumeral joint includes both the muscular-based afferent receptors in human active and passive movement and joint position detection (Roland and Ladegaard-Pedersen, 1977). In 1898, Goldsheider proposed that sensation of passive movements was solely the product of joint-based receptors. This view is still widely accepted today with passive movements.

Until the 1970s it was thought that, regarding sensory feedback of active human movements, after voluntary movement was initiated by the cerebral cortex, only low-level control was presented by the receptors in the muscles and tendons. Sensory information from the muscles and tendons was sent to the spinal cord and some subcortical extrapyramidal parts of the brain such as the cerebellum, but it played no role as contributors to conscious sensation, which remained in the province of the joint receptors (Roland and Ladegaard-Pedersen, 1977). In the early 1970s, however, Goodwin et al (1972) and Eklund (1972) independently showed the qualitative role that muscular receptors play in sensations of active movement.

AFFERENT MECHANORECEPTOR CLASSIFICATION

Mechanoreceptors are sensory neurons or peripheral afferents located within joint capsular tissues, ligaments, tendons, muscle, and skin (Grigg, 1994; Wyke, 1972).

Deformation or stimulation of the tissues in which the mechanoreceptor's lie produces a gated release of sodium, eliciting an action potential (Myers & Lephart, 2000). Four primary types of afferent mechanoreceptors have been classified and are commonly present in non-contractile capsular and ligamentous structures in human joints.

Type I articular receptors are traditionally globular or ovoid corpuscles with a very thin capsule. They are numerous in the capsular tissues in all the limb joints, as well as the apophyseal joints of the vertebral column. Wyke (1972) reported that the population of type I receptors appears more dense in proximal joints than in distal joints. Type I receptors are typically located in the superficial layers of the joint capsule.

Physiologically, type I receptors are low-threshold, slowly adapting mechanoreceptors. A portion of the type I receptors is always active in every joint position (Wyke, 1972). The resting discharge of the type I receptors allows the body to know where the limb is placed and receives constant output on limb position in virtually any joint position. The type I receptor is categorized as both a static and dynamic mechanoreceptor (Wyke, 1972) whose discharge pattern signals static joint position; intraarticular pressure changes; and the direction, amplitude, and velocity of joint movements.

Type II mechanoreceptors are elongated, conical corpuscles with thick multilaminated connective tissue capsule. They are present in the fibrous capsules of all joints but are reported to be more numerous in distal joints than in the proximal joints (Wyke, 1972). Type II corpuscles are located in the deeper layers of the fibrous joint capsule, particularly at the border between the fibrous capsule and the subsynovial fibroadipose tissue, often alongside articular blood vessels. Type II mechanoreceptors are low-threshold, rapidly adapting receptors and are entirely inactive in immobile joints (Wyke, 1972). They become activated for brief moments (1 second or less) at the onset of joint movement. The type II receptor is considered a dynamic mechanoreceptor whose brief, high-velocity discharges signal joint acceleration and deceleration with both active and passive joint movements.

Type I and II mechanoreceptors are the primary receptors located in the joint capsule. Type III receptors are primarily confined to the joint intrinsic and extrinsic ligamentous structures (Wyke, 1972). The type III receptor is predominantly found in the superficial surfaces of the joint ligaments, near their bony attachments. Research delineating the type III mechanoreceptor classifies this receptor as a high-threshold, slowly adapting structure,

similar in nature to the Golgi tendon organ. These receptors are completely inactive in immobile joints and become active or stimulated toward the extreme ends of joint ranges of motion only where the ligamentous structures become taut. Wyke (1967) also reported that the type III receptors become activated with longitudinal traction to the limbs, activating the receptors centripetally at a high velocity only if extreme joint displacement or joint traction is maintained.

Unlike types I, II, and III receptors, type IV receptors are noncorpuscular and are represented by plexuses of small unmyelinated nerve fibers or free nerve endings. These receptors are typically distributed throughout the fibrous joint capsule, adjacent periosteum, and articular fat pads. They represent the pain receptor system of articular tissues and are entirely inactive in normal circumstances. Marked mechanical deformation or chemical irritation, such as exposure of the nerve endings to agents including histamine, bradykinin, and other inflammatory exudates produced by damaged or necrotic tissues, can stimulate activation of the type IV receptor (Wyke, 1967, 1972; Myers & Lephart, 2000).

AFFERENT JOINT RECEPTORS IN THE HUMAN GLENOHUMERAL JOINT

The classification system for the four primary types of mechanoreceptors found in human noncontractile capsular and ligamentous tissues provides generalized information regarding the location of these receptors in the human body. Vangsness et al (1995) studied the neural histology of the human shoulder joint, including the glenohumeral ligaments, labrum, and subacromial bursa. They found two types of slowly adapting Ruffini end organs and rapidly adapting pacinian corpuscles in the superior, middle, and inferior glenohumeral ligaments. The Ruffini end organs were more common than the pacinian corpuscles. Shimoda (1955) and Kikuchi (1968) reported that the type II pacinian corpuscles were found more commonly in the human glenohumeral joint capsular ligaments than in the human knee. Analysis of the coracoclavicular and acromioclavicular ligaments showed equal distribution of type I and II mechanoreceptors. Morisawa et al (1994) identified types I, II, III, and IV mechanoreceptors in human coracoacromial ligaments. These reviews show how the glenohumeral joint capsular ligaments aid in providing afferent proprioceptive input by their inherent distributions of both type I Ruffini mechanoreceptors and the more rapidly adapting pacinian receptors. A rapidly adapting receptor like the pacinian can identify changes in tension in the joint capsular ligaments, but quickly decreases its input after the tension becomes constant (Vangsness et al, 1994). In this way, the type II receptor has the ability to monitor acceleration and deceleration of a ligament's tension.

Several authors have studied the labrum and subacromial bursa. Vangsness et al (1994) found no evidence for mechanoreceptors in the glenoid labrum; however, they noted free nerve endings in the fibrocartilage tissue in the peripheral half. The subacromial bursa was found to have diffuse, yet copious, free nerve endings, with no evidence of larger more complex mechanoreceptors. Ide et al (1996) also studied subacromial bursa taken from three cadavers and found a copious supply of free nerve endings, most of which were located on the roof side of the subacromial arch, which is exposed to impingement-type stresses. Unlike the study by Vangsness et al (1994), Ide et al (1996) did find evidence of both Ruffini and pacinian mechanoreceptors in the subacromial bursa. Their findings suggest that the subacromial bursa receives both nociceptive stimuli and proprioception and may play a role in regulating shoulder movement. More research into the exact distribution of these important structures in the human shoulder is indicated to give clinicians additional information and enhance understanding of proprioceptive function of the shoulder.

AFFERENT RECEPTORS OF THE CONTRACTILE TISSUES OF THE HUMAN GLENOHUMERAL JOINT

In addition to the afferent structures found in the non-contractile tissues of the human shoulder (joint capsule, subacromial bursa, and intrinsic and extrinsic ligaments), significant contributions to the regulation of human movement and proprioceptive feedback are obtained from receptors located in contractile structures.

Two primary mechanisms for afferent feedback from the muscle tendon unit are the muscle spindle mechanism and the Golgi tendon organ (Myers & Lephart, 2000; Nyland et al, 1998). Research classifying muscle spindles has traditionally grouped intrafusal muscle fibers into two groups based on the type of afferent projections (Nyland et al, 1998; Barker et al, 1976). These groups consist of nuclear bag and nuclear chain fibers. Nuclear chain fibers project from large afferent axons. Nuclear bag fibers are innervated by gamma 1 (dynamic) motor neurons and are more sensitive to the rate of muscle length change, such as occurs during a rapid stretch of a muscle during an eccentric contraction or passive stretch (Nyland et al, 1998). Intrafusal nuclear chain fibers are innervated by gamma 2 (static) motor neurons and are more sensitive to static muscle length. The combination of the nuclear chain and nuclear bag fibers allows the afferent communication from

the muscle tendon unit to remain sensitive over a wide range of motion, during both reflex and voluntary activation.

Muscle spindles provide much of the primary information for motor learning in terms of muscle length and joint position. Upper levels of the central nervous system can bias the sensitivity of muscle spindle input and sampling (Nyland et al, 1998). Muscle spindles do not occur in similar densities in all muscles in the human body. Spindle density most likely is related to muscle function, with greater densities of muscle spindles being reported in muscles that initiate and control fine movements or maintain posture. Muscles that cross the front of the shoulder, such as the pectoralis major and biceps, have a large number of muscle spindles per unit of muscle weight (Voss, 1971). Muscles with attachment to the coracoid, such as the biceps, pectoralis minor, and coracobrachialis, also have high spindle densities. Lower spindle densities have been reported for the rotator cuff muscle tendon units, with the subscapularis and infraspinatus having greater densities than the supraspinatus and teres minor (Voss, 1971). This lower rotator cuff spindle density most likely suggests synergistic mechanoreceptor activation with the scapulothoracic musculature, with glenohumeral joint movement (Nyland, 1998; Inman, 1944). This coupled or shared mechanoreceptor activation is an example of kinetic link or proximal-to-distal sequencing that occurs with predictable or programmed movement patterns in the human body (Marshall & Elliott, 2000).

The second major aspect of musculotendinous afferent activity is the Golgi tendon organ. These tendinous mechanoreceptors are present in the human shoulder and respond to tension generated with muscular contraction (Myers & Lephart, 2000; Nyland, 1998). Activation of the Golgi tendon organs relays afferent feedback regarding muscle tension and joint position. Activation of the tension-sensitive Golgi tendon organ produces a protective mechanism that causes relaxation of the agonist muscle that is undergoing tension, with simultaneous stimulation of antagonistic musculature.

EFFECTS OF GLENOHUMERAL JOINT INSTABILITY ON PROPRIOCEPTION

Several studies have addressed the influence of glenohumeral joint instability on proprioception. One of the most common clinical maladies addressed by clinicians is anterior glenohumeral joint instability. Speer et al (1994b) studied the effects of a simulated Bankart lesion in cadavers. Coupled anterior/posterior translations were assessed in the presence of sequentially applied loads of 50 Newtons in anterior, posterior, superior, and inferior directions. The effects of a simulated Bankart lesion resulted in small (maximum of 3.4 mm) increases in anterior and inferior translations of the humeral head relative to the glenoid in all positions of elevation, and in posterior translation at 90 degrees of elevation only. Speer et al (1994b) concluded that detachment of the anterior inferior labrum from the glenoid (Bankart lesion) alone does not create large enough increases in humeral head translation to allow for anterior glenohumeral joint dislocation. Permanent stretching or elongation of the inferior glenohumeral ligament may also occur and may be necessary to produce a full dislocation of the glenohumeral joint. This elongation or permanent stretching of the ligamentous structures may lead to alterations of the intrinsic tensile relationships of the glenohumeral joint capsule and capsular ligaments. The authors concluded that capsular elongation may be responsible for the high incidence of failed anterior reconstructions to address anterior glenohumeral joint instability that do not fully restore normal capsular tension of the anterior structures.

Blaiser et al (1994) compared the proprioceptive ability of subjects without known shoulder pathology with individuals with clinically determined generalized joint laxity. Individuals with greater glenohumeral joint laxity had less sensitive proprioception compared with those with less glenohumeral joint laxity. They found enhanced proprioception at or near the end range of external rotation, when the anterior capsular structures have greater internal tension. The authors concluded that decreased joint angular reposition sense is one characteristic in individuals with increased glenohumeral joint laxity.

Smith and Brunolli (1989) examined kinesthesia after glenohumeral joint dislocation in 8 subjects and compared their inherent joint position sense with 10 normal subjects using an instrumented modification of a shoulder wheel. They reported a significant decrease in joint awareness in the involved shoulders after shoulder dislocation compared with all uninvolved shoulders tested in the study.

Lephart et al (1994) studied glenohumeral joint proprioception in 90 subjects in three experimental groups. One group consisted of 40 college-aged subjects with normal shoulders, another group of 30 patients diagnosed with anterior instability, and a third group of 20 subjects who had undergone surgical reconstruction for shoulder instability. No significant difference was found between extremities (dominant versus nondominant) in the normal subjects' kinesthesia and joint position sense; however, subjects with anterior instability had significant differences between the normal and unstable shoulder. Subjects with anterior instability had significantly longer

thresholds to detection of passive motion, as well as greater inaccuracy with joint angular replication testing than they experienced with their contralateral uninjured extremity. Lephart et al (1994) found no significant differences among kinesthesia and joint position sense in the subject's operated extremity compared with the uninjured extremity after reconstructive surgery. These patients were examined at least 6 months after open or arthroscopic repair of chronic, recurrent anterior instability. The authors concluded that these results provide evidence, consistent with the previously mentioned studies, for partial deafferentation leading to proprioceptive deficits when the capsuloligamentous structures are damaged. Reconstructive surgery in this experiment appears to restore normal joint proprioception 6 months or more after the surgical procedure.

Lephart et al (2002) tested 20 subjects diagnosed with unilateral anterior, anteroinferior, or multidirectional instability with no other concomitant pathologies. Subjects underwent testing to assess "joint angular replication" and the "threshold to detect passive motion" 6 to 24 months after arthroscopic thermal capsulorraphy. Significantly better proprioceptive function was found in the involved shoulder compared with the uninvolved shoulder, with a mean of 11 months after arthroscopic surgery using thermal energy to address glenohumeral joint instability. This study provides important objective evidence showing that no appreciable deleterious effects exist with respect to proprioceptive function of the shoulder after arthroscopic surgery with thermal capsulorraphy.

In a prospective study, Zuckerman et al (2003) evaluated proprioceptive ability in patients with traumatic anterior instability. A total of 30 consecutive patients with recurrent bouts of anterior instability were evaluated for passive position sense and detection of motion in flexion, abduction, and external rotation. A significant deficit in proprioceptive function was found in all directions in these subjects 1 week before surgical repair. All subjects underwent a standard anterior capsulorraphy and labral detachment repair followed by a standardized postoperative rehabilitation protocol. Subjects were tested 6 months after surgery using identical testing procedures. The authors reported approximately 50% improvement in proprioceptive ability, but this ability was still significantly deficient when compared with the contralateral side. One year after surgery during final evaluation, the subjects were again tested using identical procedures. No significant difference in side-to-side proprioceptive function was found. This study provides important evidence regarding the amount of time needed for the return of normal proprioceptive function and alerts clinicians that a full year may be required to attain normal values for both position sense and detection of motion. This research supports the use of rehabilitative interventions that retrain the proprioceptors of the shoulder after surgery to eliminate glenohumeral joint instability.

PRIMARY MEASUREMENT METHODS FOR ASSESSING PROPRIOCEPTION FOR THE GLENOHUMERAL JOINT

Evaluation of proprioception and neuromuscular control in the human shoulder encompasses both afferent and efferent neural function, as well as the resulting muscular activation patterns (Myers & Lephart, 2000). Proprioception consists of three major submodalities: kinesthesia, joint position sense, and sensation of resistance. Separate techniques can be used to assess each of these aspects of proprioception.

MEASUREMENT OF KINESTHESIA

Glenohumeral joint kinesthesia has been assessed using a test called the *threshold to detection of passive motion (TTDPM)*. This test assesses the subject's ability to detect a passive movement occurring typically at very slow angular velocities (Lephart et al, 1994; Myers & Lephart, 2000; Lephart & Fu, 2000). Elaborate testing devices have been used in several studies of TTDPM such as an instrumented (motorized) shoulder wheel (Smith & Brunolli, 1989) and other devices such as the one diagrammed in Figure 16-1 from the University of Pittsburgh (Lephart & Fu, 2000). Extensive research using the TTDPM test has resulted in the selection and recommendation of slow angular velocities (0.5 to 2 degrees/second) to enhance the reliability of data acquisition. In addition to the device used, blindfolds, earphones, and a pneumatic cuff are recommended to eliminate cues from the visual, auditory, and tactile realm (Lephart et al, 1994; Lephart & Fu, 2000). This ensures that only joint kinesthesia is being assessed and not simply visual or auditory responses to perceived movement.

Physiologically, the TTDPM test is designed to selectively stimulate the Ruffini or Golgi-type mechanoreceptors in the articular structures being tested. Testing is typically applied for internal and external rotation of the glenohumeral joint in varying positions of elevation in the scapular and coronal planes. Testing has been done at mid- and end-range positions of glenohumeral rotation (Lephart et al, 1994; Lephart & Fu, 2000; Myers & Lephart, 2000). As stated earlier, TTDPM in the human shoulder has been measured by Blaiser et al (1994) and was

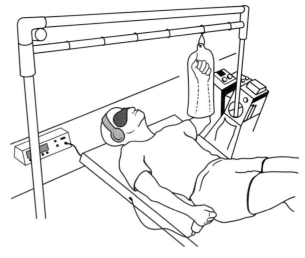

Figure 16-1 Proprioceptive testing device used for assessment of glenohumeral joint proprioception. (Reprinted with permission from Allen AA: Neuromuscular contributions to normal shoulder joint kinematics. In Lephart SM, Fu FH, eds: *Proprioception and neuromuscular control in joint stability*, Champaign, IL, 2000, Human Kinetics, p. 111.)

enhanced (smaller amount of movement before detection) at or near the end range of external rotation as compared with mid-range external rotation or internal rotation.

Warner et al (1996) reported normative data on 40 healthy college-aged individuals using the TTDPM test from both neutral rotational starting positions and 30 degrees of humeral rotation at 90 degrees of glenohumeral joint abduction. They found an average of 1.5 to 2.2 degrees for all testing conditions, with no significant difference measured between the dominant or preferred hand relative to the nondominant extremity. Allegrucci et al (1995) measured shoulder kinesthesia in healthy unilateral athletes who performed upper extremity sports. The TTDPM test was performed with the shoulder in 90 degrees of abduction at both 0 and 75 degrees of external rotation and compared bilaterally. There was greater difficulty in detecting passive motion in the dominant extremity than in the nondominant extremity. Consistent with earlier research (Blaiser et al, 1994), Allegrucci et al (1995) measured greater sensitivity to passive movement with the shoulder in 75 degrees of external rotation bilaterally, compared with the more neutral condition. These findings suggest that unilaterally dominant upper extremity athletes, such as those involved in baseball, tennis, or volleyball, may have a proprioceptive deficit on the dominant arm that may interfere with optimal afferent feedback regarding joint position. This finding provides a rationale for proprioceptive upper extremity training in athletes from this population.

MEASUREMENT OF JOINT POSITION SENSE

Joint position sense measures the ability of the subject to appreciate where the extremity is oriented in space. Testing procedures to assess joint position sense are called *joint angular replication tests*. The joint angular replication tests typically place the extremity in a particular position to allow the subject to appreciate the spatial orientation of the extremity. After this period of joint positioning, the subject's extremity is returned to a starting position. The subject then reapproximates the position initially selected as closely as possible, without any visual, auditory, or tactile cues. Researchers have used both active (Lephart et al, 1994; Lephart & Fu, 2000; Myers & Lephart, 2000; Davies & Hoffman, 1993) and passive (Voight et al, 1996) angular replication tests to assess the glenohumeral joint. Various apparatuses have been used to facilitate the accuracy of joint angular replication testing. Voight et al (1996) used an isokinetic dynamometer with 90 degrees of abduction and elbow flexion, with standard isokinetic stabilization, to perform active angular joint replication testing using a fatigue paradigm. They also used the passive mode of the isokinetic dynamometer set at 2 degrees/second to perform passive joint angular replication testing. Various authors (Lephart & Fu, 2000; Jerosch, 2000; Slobounov et al, 1999) have used complex three-dimensional spatial tracking devices to quantify arm position, using multiple positions of active joint angular replication testing.

CLINICAL MEASUREMENT OF JOINT POSITION SENSE

In the most clinically applicable research study on active joint angular reproduction, Davies and Hoffman (1993) tested subjects in a seated position using an electronic digital inclinometer (EDI, Cybex, Inc., Ronkonkoma, NY). Reference angles were chosen in the following ranges and verified with the EDI, with subsequent active angular replication by the patient and verification of extremity position with the EDI. Angles chosen were greater than and less than 90 degrees of flexion and abduction, external rotation greater than 45 degrees, external rotation less than 45 degrees, and internal rotation. Normative data developed by Davies and Hoffman on 100 male subjects without shoulder pathology showed an average of the seven measurements to be 2.7 degrees (Davies & Hoffman, 1993). This represents the average difference between the seven reference angles and the actual matched angles by the subjects over the seven measurements.

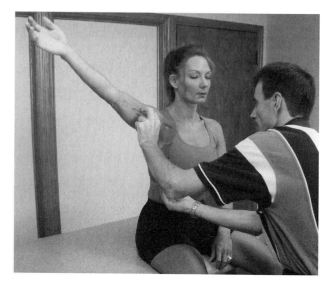

Figure 16-2 Clinical method of measuring active joint angular replication using a universal goniometer and standardized technique.

The clinically applicable method of measuring joint angular replication described by Davies and Hoffman (1993) can best be replicated in most clinics using a standard goniometer and standardized testing protocol (Figure 16-2). Although limitations exist regarding the reliability of goniometric measurement of the glenohumeral joint (see Chapter 8 for a more detailed description of joint range of motion measurement), the clinical method of using a goniometer to determine differences in joint angular replication can be performed using the positions outlined by Davies and Hoffman (1993). This method undoubtedly has limitations in regard to accuracy, but it can provide some measure of joint angular replication ability by the patient and may be of particular interest in the patient with glenohumeral joint instability. Further research using more clinically applicable methods of documenting joint angular replication and the threshold to detection of passive movement is needed before more specific guidelines can be developed.

Regardless of testing methodology, the active joint angular position replication tests primarily involve the stimulation of both joint and muscle receptors and provide a thorough assessment of afferent pathways of the human shoulder (Lephart & Fu, 2000).

EFFECTS OF MUSCULAR FATIGUE ON PROPRIOCEPTION IN THE GLENOHUMERAL JOINT

Zuckerman et al (1999) injected lidocaine into the subacromial space and glenohumeral joint to assess proprioception in young and old male subjects. They found no adverse effects from the injection of lidocaine in either location, proposing compensatory extracapsular feedback in order to ensure intact proprioception after injection. No differences in joint position sense and TTDPM testing were noted between the dominant and nondominant extremity; however, a decline in proprioception with age was found between the younger (20 to 30 years) and older (50 to 70 years) subjects.

Several studies have investigated the effect of muscular fatigue on various indices of joint proprioception and neuromuscular control. Carpenter et al (1998) tested subjects using a TTDPM test, with the shoulder in 90 degrees of abduction and 90 degrees of external rotation. By following an isokinetic fatigue protocol, subjects' detection of passive motion was marred or decreased 171% for internal rotation and 179% for external rotation. In preexercise testing, the authors found increased sensitivity moving into external rotation compared with internal rotation, but no difference between the dominant and nondominant extremity. The authors concluded that the effect of muscular fatigue on joint proprioception may play a role in injury and decrease athletic performance.

Voight et al (1996) tested subjects using an active and passive joint angular replication protocol after isokinetically induced muscular fatigue of the glenohumeral joint internal and external rotators. No significant difference in shoulder joint angular replication was found between the dominant and nondominant extremity. Significant decreases in accuracy were noted after muscular fatigue in both the active and passive joint angular replication tests. Petersen et al (1999) tested the ability of healthy subjects to discriminate movement velocity of the glenohumeral joint in the transverse plane. Subjects had a decrement in the discrimination of movement velocity after a hard isokinetic horizontal flexion/extension exercise fatigue protocol, compared with a light exercise condition.

Finally, Myers et al (1999) used an active angular replication test and neuromuscular control test to examine the effects of muscle fatigue in normal shoulders. A concentric isokinetic internal and external rotation fatigue protocol was used. Fatigue of the internal and external rotators of the shoulder decreased subjects' accuracy in detecting both mid- and end-range absolute angular error, but not their neuromuscular control using a bilaterally assessed unilateral closed-chain stability type test measuring postural sway velocity.

The consistent finding of a proprioceptive decrement after muscular fatigue in these studies has led researchers to emphasize the importance of the muscle-based receptors. Use of the active joint angular positioning tests has been reported to stimulate both joint and muscle mechanoreceptors and is considered to be a more functional assessment of afferent pathways (Lephart & Fu, 2000; Myers et al, 1999). The exact mechanism by which muscular-based proprioception is affected is not known. Muscle fatigue is thought to desensitize the muscle spindle threshold, leading to decrements in both joint position sense and neuromuscular control. Djupsjobacka et al (1994, 1995a, 1995b) reported alterations of muscle spindle output in the presence of lactic acid, potassium chloride, arachidonic acid, and bradykinin. Intramuscular concentrations of these substances are altered during muscular exertion and fatigue. This consistent relationship has provided further rationale and support for the improvement of muscular endurance of the dynamic stabilizers of the glenohumeral joint.

SUMMARY

The important role proprioception plays in normal function of the glenohumeral joint and the research documenting decrements in proprioceptive function in cases of glenohumeral joint instability and with muscular fatigue clearly provide rationales for the clinician to perform testing to determine the level of function of the proprioceptive system in the glenohumeral joint. Further research advancing clinical methods of measurement will continue to enhance the clinician's ability to measure and test for this important function.

CHAPTER 17

Analysis of Sport Technique: Tennis and Overhead Throwing Model

INTRODUCTION

Although it is beyond the scope of this text to completely review all aspects of sport technique, it is imperative to review the basic mechanism and concepts surrounding the overhead arm motion used in sport-specific activities as an essential part of the comprehensive evaluation of the patient with shoulder injury. Failure to perform this portion of the evaluation can ultimately lead to reinjury and an incomplete understanding of the injury mechanism. Although baseline information in this area is important to all clinicians working with athletes and active individuals, it is also essential to have adequate referral mechanisms in place for more complete biomechanical evaluation of sport-specific activity technique. Use of sport-specific, high-performance coaches and biomechanists is recommended, as it is uncommon for rehabilitation professionals to be proficient in activity evaluation and biomechanical modification and intervention in more than one or two sports, if at all.

This chapter briefly reviews some of the common mechanisms found in the overhead motion and provides examples of common pathomechanics often identified in individuals with shoulder injury. The overhead throwing/serving motion is the model for this chapter. It is recommended that the reader seek additional information in the areas of swimming (Toussaint et al, 2000) and golf (Farrally & Cochran, 1999) to more completely understand similar mechanisms inherent in these activities.

THE KINETIC LINK OR KINETIC CHAIN PRINCIPLE

The kinetic link principle describes how the human body can be broken down into a series of links or segments that are interrelated and ultimately affect segments both proximal and distal to that segment. Kibler (1998a, 1998b) referred to the kinetic link system as a series of sequentially activated body segments. The kinetic link principle is predicated on a concept developed and described by Hanavan (1964), who constructed a computerized form of the adult human body. This computerized form is com-

prised of conical links, including the lower extremities, torso, and upper extremities. In reference to upper extremity skill performance, work in these upper extremity segments is transmitted to the trunk and spine via a large musculoskeletal surface. A change of forces across this musculoskeletal surface results in the generation of massive amounts of energy.

Davies (1992) described how the upper extremity can be viewed as a series of links that include the trunk, scapulothoracic articulation, scapulohumeral or glenohumeral joints, and distal arm regions. Each of these links can be considered independent anatomically and biomechanically, but with reference to human function, they must be considered as a unit.

PROXIMAL-TO-DISTAL SEQUENCING

When analyzing human movement, Putnam (1993) discussed the concept of proximal-to-distal sequencing. This principle states that to produce the largest possible speed at the end of a linked chain of segments, movement must initiate in more proximal segments and proceed to the more distal segment. Also, the distal segment motion should commence at the time of maximal speed in the more proximal segment. This has been referred to by many names such as the *summation of speed principle* (Bunn, 1972), *kinetic link principle* (Kreighbaum and Barthels, 1985), and Palgenhoef's (1971) concept of *acceleration-deceleration*. This concept has been verified and illustrated by measuring the linear speeds of segment endpoints, joint angular velocities, and joint moments (Marshall & Elliott, 2000).

Several investigators have reported proximal to distal sequencing for kicking a ball, with the hip, knee, and ankle joints reaching their peak speeds in a sequence and each peak being greater than that of the proximal joint (Putnam, 1993). Most researchers feel that the proximal segment deceleration is caused by the acceleration of the distal segment (Putnam, 1993).

Proximal to distal sequencing has been reported in the upper extremity during throwing (Vaughan, 1985; Joris et al, 1985; Ishii et al, 1986), as well as in the tennis serve (Elliott et al, 1986; VanGheluwe & Hebbelinck, 1985). However, more recent analysis suggests that aspects of these upper extremity patterns (throwing, serving, and striking) have significant modifications in the traditional proximal to distal sequencing. Feltner and Dapena (1986) reported peak internal rotation velocity of the humerus after movements of the wrist and hand during overhead throwing. Sprigings et al (1994) showed that internal rotation was the largest contributor to racquet head velocity at impact despite being one of the last components in the modified sequence of proximal to distal sequencing.

APPLICATION OF THE KINETIC LINK SYSTEM TO EVALUATION OF TECHNIQUE

Groppel (1992) applied the kinetic link system to the analysis and description of optimal upper extremity sport biomechanics. He stated that initiation of the sequential activation of the kinetic link system starts at the ground as the lower extremities of the body create a ground reaction force. The sequential activation then proceeds from the legs, through the hips and trunk, and is funneled via the scapulothoracic and glenohumeral joints to the distal aspect of the upper extremity. Figure 17-1 shows the kinetic link system described and applied by Groppel (1992). The important role of both linear and angular momentum in the production of force and power in upper

extremity sport activities, such as the throwing motion and tennis serve, is clearly evident by analyzing this model. It is important to note that initiation of movement of the next segment in the kinetic chain occurs before complete deceleration of the previous segment. The angular velocity of the segmental rotation in the body's kinetic link system was originally thought to occur at increasingly faster velocities moving from the lower extremities to the upper extremities during the tennis serve (Groppel, 1992). Further biomechanical analysis, however, has demonstrated that although this sequential increase in angular velocities does occur over many of the segments, a perfect progression in angular velocity does not occur (Elliot et al, 1986).

Kibler (1998b) provided an objective analysis of force generation during a tennis serve (Table 17-1). A total of 54% of the force development during the tennis serve comes from the legs and trunk, with only 25% coming from the elbow and wrist. Nonoptimal performance and increased risk of injury occur in tennis and other sport activities when an individual attempts to use the smaller muscles and distal arm segments as a primary source for power generation (Kibler, 1994; Groppel, 1992).

EXAMPLES OF ALTERATIONS IN OPTIMAL KINETIC LINK PATTERNING

Use of the kinetic link principle is of paramount importance when analyzing sport performance or exercise movement patterns. Identification of movement patterns that do not sequentially activate all portions of the kinetic link system or omit a portion or link such as trunk rotation can lead to injury and nonoptimal performance (Kibler, 1994a, 1994b; Groppel, 1992). Examples of nonoptimal use of the kinetic link principle are depicted in Figures 17-2 and 17-3, where a segment is deleted from the sequential activation pattern or improper timing of the sequential activation is encountered, respectively.

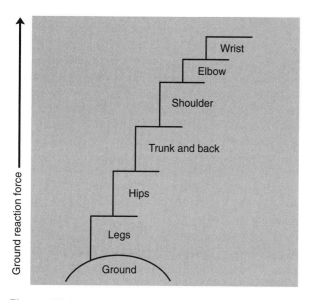

Figure 17-1 Kinetic link principle. (Adapted from Groppel JL: *High tech tennis*, ed 2, Champaign, IL, 1992, Human Kinetics Publishers.)

TABLE 17-1 Specific Segments' Contribution to Kinetic Energy and Force Production in the Tennis Serve

SEGMENT	VELOCITY M/S	KINETIC ENERGY (UNITS [%])	FORCE (UNITS [%])
Leg/trunk	2.7	197.1 (51%)	729 (54%)
Shoulder	2.2	49.1 (13%)	297 (21%)
Elbow	6.4	82 (21%)	212 (15%)
Wrist	7.8	61 (15%)	130 (10%)

From Kibler WB: Shoulder rehabilitation: principles and practice, *Med Sci Sports Exerc* 30(4): S40-S50, 1998b.

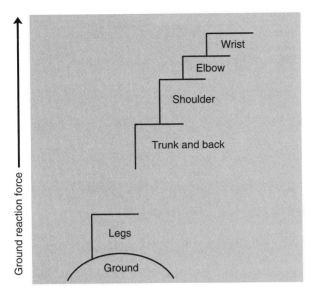

Figure **17-2** Kinetic link principle: omitting a segment from the kinetic link system. (Adapted from Groppel JL: *High tech tennis*, ed 2, Champaign, IL, 1992, Human Kinetics Publishers.)

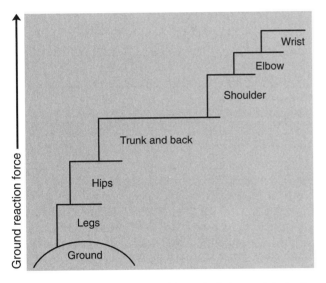

Figure **17-3** Kinetic link principle: mis-timing a link in the kinetic link system. (Adapted from Groppel JL: *High tech tennis*, ed 2, Champaign, IL, 1992, Human Kinetics Publishers.)

These two examples are common clinically when analyzing complex human movement patterns such as the tennis serve and throwing motion. It is common to have an individual perform an activity without hip rotation either from improper foot positioning or inflexibility in the hip region. Also, inappropriate timing of trunk rotation can lead to disastrous consequences in segments proximal and distal to the trunk (Marshall et al, 1993).

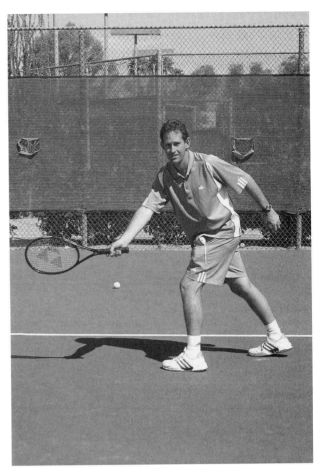

Figure **17-4** Example of a player using an excessively closed stance, resulting in an inability to utilize hip and trunk rotation.

Applying these diagrams to a functional movement pattern such as the tennis serve would involve hitting the serve with no trunk rotation, or minimal trunk rotation, because the hips are blocked from rotating by an improper stance (Figure 17-4). This movement would produce greater loads and stresses to the shoulder and elbow and possibly result in injury. If improper sequencing or timing of the rotation from the legs to the hip and trunk occurs, greater loads to the upper arm are again encountered. Figure 17-5 demonstrates how improperly timed trunk rotation can lead to a "lagging behind" phenomenon in tennis, increasing loads to the anterior aspect of the shoulder and medial elbow, and Figure 17-6 demonstrates the same phenomenon in a baseball pitcher.

Marshall et al (1993) used three-dimensional cinematography to analyze the mechanics of a highly skilled tennis player and study the torques produced during the tennis serve. Using mathematical calculations, they

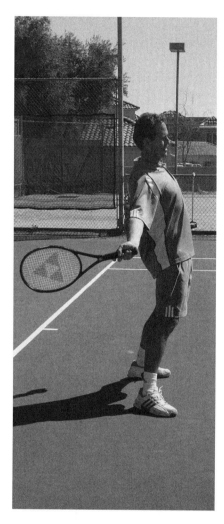

Figure 17-5 Result of early and improperly timed trunk rotation, resulting in "arm-lag."

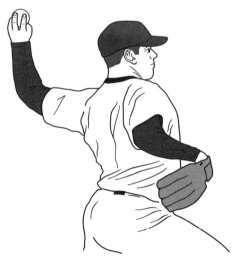

Figure 17-6 Hyperangulation concept. Shoulder is placed posteriorly or behind the scapular plane of the body.

studied the effects of delaying shoulder internal rotation (until late in the total movement) on the medial aspect of the elbow. The effects of delaying shoulder internal rotation highlight the underlying concept behind the kinetic link principle. The amount of valgus stress to the medial elbow was increased 53% immediately before ball impact when nonoptimal timing was used during the serving motion. This study graphically displays the effects of manipulation of the normal kinetic link interaction on the human body during stressful upper body sport movement and exertion.

Another important example of how the body's kinetic link system is applied during stressful musculoskeletal exertion is shown by Buckley and Kerwin (1988), again using the tennis serve. Elbow extension velocities during the tennis serve measured in elite tennis players averaged

44 radians/second (2521 degrees/second). On initial analysis, researchers would assume that the triceps (elbow extensor) musculature is contracting concentrically to produce this elbow extension velocity during the acceleration phase of the tennis serve. Jorgensen (1976) delineated that velocities beyond 20 radians/second (1146 degrees/second) are beyond the contractile velocity range of human skeletal muscle. This finding clearly confirms previous research by Quanbury et al (1975) and Robertson and Winter (1980), who reported two sources of a limb's mechanical energy: (1) muscles that are attached directly to the limb and (2) passive energy flow across a joint from an adjoining limb developed along the body's kinetic chain. These studies help to demonstrate the important role the kinetic link system plays in human movement and the importance of training the entire limb or entire kinetic link of the body when attempting to affect a specific segment or link in the kinetic link system.

CLINICAL ANALYSIS OF SPORT TECHNIQUE

In many cases, the use of video analysis using a camcorder or digital photography can assist the clinician in both identifying pathomechanics and conveying that information to the patient, parent, and/or coach. High-tech digitizing systems found in any biomechanics laboratory and some clinical centers provide the highest level of sophistication and allow for detailed analyses of human movements. However, identification of common pathomechanical features in the throwing motion and tennis strokes, as well as other sport movement patterns, can be achieved with the use of commonly available technology (Fleisig et al, 1989).

A description of the throwing motion and tennis serve and groundstrokes provides characteristic markers or patterns of performance in each specific sport activity. Although there are many variations in throwing and tennis mechanics, certain characteristics are found in most individuals that lead to optimal levels of performance. It is important to emphasize the difference between fundamentals and idiosyncrasies. *Fundamentals* can be defined as specific biomechanical movements or patterns that are characteristic of complex movement patterns such as throwing a ball or hitting a serve. *Idiosyncrasies* consist of individual variations from the normal fundamental patterns that are often recognizable and attributable to a particular player or performer. Examples of idiosyncrasies in baseball are relief pitcher Mike Fetters' violent head jerk movement, pitcher Vida Blue's high leg kick, and John McEnroe's unique stance and wind-up during his serve. Examples of both normal biomechanics and common pathomechanics are presented in these brief overviews of the sport-specific movement mechanics.

THROWING MOTION

For the purposes of evaluation, the throwing motion has been divided into four primary phases (Glousman et al, 1992): wind-up, cocking, acceleration, and follow-through (Figure 17-7). The wind-up phase begins with the initial motion of the pitcher and ends when the ball leaves the glove (Glousman et al, 1992; Fleisig et al, 1989). Little muscular activation is required in the throw-ing shoulder during this phase; therefore few injuries or episodes of pain provocation are typically described.

One essential aspect to analyze during the end of the wind-up phase is the presence of proper balance (Fleisig et al, 1989). The lead leg (left leg in a right-handed throwing athlete) is lifted and rotated around the plant leg (right leg in a right-handed throwing athlete). This rotation must be achieved in a balanced fashion and should be evaluated in reference to the shoulder, as an unstable base during this phase of throwing may have drastic consequences as the player moves into external rotation and begins the sequential segmental rotation during acceleration later in the throwing motion. The one-leg stability test (pages 37-39) is another key test to apply in the return to activity phase to ensure that the throwing or overhead athlete has ample levels of core stability to provide the stable base needed for this particular phase of the activity. A digital photo or video pause near the end of the wind-up phase with the pitcher in the balance position is one of the first checkpoints recommended (Figure 17-8).

The cocking phase is often divided into two phases (Glousman et al, 1992; Fleisig et al, 1989). The early cocking phase begins as the ball leaves the glove and continues until the lead foot contacts the ground. During the early cocking phase the arm is brought backward away from the body coupled with a forward drive of the lead leg. As the lead leg is extended forward, it strikes the mound; this is termed *foot contact*. At front foot or lead foot contact, there is another crucial marker or evaluation point. At the time the foot strikes the mound, the throwing elbow should be flexed 90 degrees and the throwing

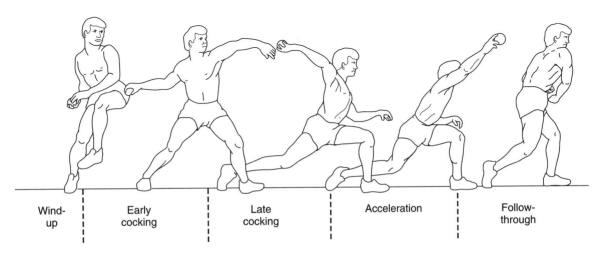

Figure 17-7 Phases of throwing. (From Glousman RE, Barron J, Jobe FW, et al: An electromyographic analysis of the elbow in normal and injured pitchers with medial collateral ligament insufficiency, *Am J Sports Med* 20(3):312, 1992.)

Wind-up   Early cocking   Late cocking   Acceleration   Follow-through

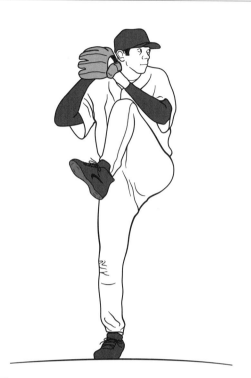

Figure **17-8** Wind-up phase: balance point position.

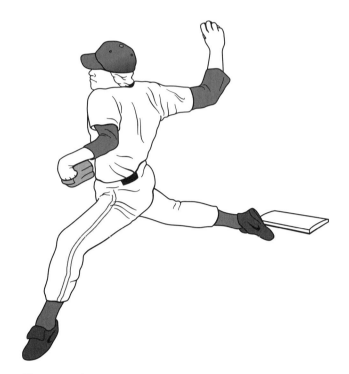

Figure **17-9** Body position at foot contact. Note elbow flexion angle and external rotation angle of the glenohumeral joint. The open stride angle (foot angled toward first base side of home plate) for a right-handed pitcher leads to an abnormal body position.

shoulder should be externally rotated to at least the neutral position (Fleisig et al, 1989) (Figure 17-9). Failure of the athlete to achieve this arm position at foot contact can lead to a "lagging" behind of the arm as the hips rotate forward in preparation for ball release. This places the arm in a "catch-up" situation, as the rest of the body is too far ahead of the arm at this point in the movement pattern (see Figure 17-6). Also, failure to flex the elbow provides a longer lever arm and more strain on the shoulder during this early stage of the throwing motion (Figure 17-10). A static photo or video pause at this position allows the clinician to evaluate and provide crucial feedback.

Additional information crucially important to the glenohumeral joint is the stride characteristics of the lower extremity during the foot contact portion of the throwing motion. Fleisig et al (2000) outlined the stride characteristics during baseball pitching. They reported stride length (distance from ankle to ankle) to range from 70% to 80% of the athlete's height. At foot contact the angle of the lead foot should be closed (angled inward) between 5 and 25 degrees, rather than pointing straight ahead toward home plate. An open stance or stride angle increases opening or early rotation of the pelvis and may lead to hyperangulation and arm lag, increasing stress on the medial elbow and shoulder (see Figures 17-6, 17-9, and 17-10). Excessively closed stride

angles block rotation of the pelvis and decrease the contribution from the lower extremity segments.

The lead foot also should land directly in front of the rear foot or in a position with a few centimeters closed stance (lead foot a few centimeters to the right of the rear foot in a right-handed thrower). Again, if the lead foot lands in a position that is too closed, pelvic rotation is impeded, forcing the pitcher to throw across the body, which minimizes contribution from the lower extremity (Fleisig et al, 2000). Consequently, landing in a "too open" position leads to early pelvic rotation and dissipation of the ground reaction forces and lower extremity contribution, and leads to arm fatigue and throwing with "too much arm" (Fleisig et al, 2000). Careful documentation of foot position using video or digital photography can provide valuable insight into possible mechanisms of arm injury stemming from lower extremity pathomechanics.

Late cocking occurs after foot contact and continues until maximal external rotation of the throwing shoulder occurs (Glousman et al, 1992). By the end of the cocking phase, the shoulder can obtain a nearly horizontal position of 180 degrees of external rotation. This amount of rotation, however, is combined with scapulothoracic and

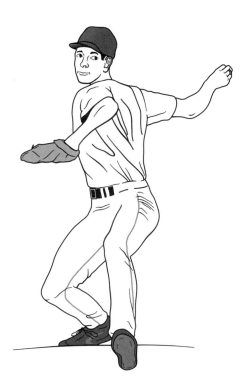

Figure **17-10** Abnormal body position at foot contact: note the increased elbow extension and hyperangulation (excessive shoulder horizontal abduction), increasing stress to the shoulder.

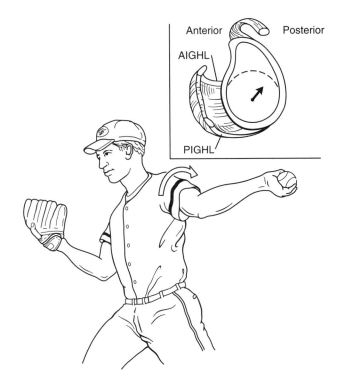

Figure **17-11** In abduction and external rotation (late cocking), the posterior band of the inferior glenohumeral ligament (IGHL) is bowstrung beneath the humeral head, causing a posterosuperior shift in the glenohumeral rotation point. Also in late cocking, the biceps vector shifts in a posterior direction and twists at its base, maximizing peel-back forces. As a result of the tight posteroinferior capsule, this pitcher shows classic derangements of pitching mechanics: hyperexternal rotation, hyperhorizontal abduction (out of the scapular plane), dropped elbow, and premature trunk rotation. (From Burkhart SS, Morgan CD, Kibler WB: The disabled throwing shoulder: spectrum of pathology. Part I. Pathoanatomy and biomechanics, *Arthroscopy* 19(4):416, 2003.)

trunk articulation and gives the appearance of the artificially high external rotation value at the shoulder joint (Fleisig et al, 1989).

At the time of maximal external rotation in the throwing arm, it is important to note that the scapulothoracic joint must be in a retracted position (Kibler, 1998a, 1998b; Burkhart et al, 2003). The scapula actually translates 15 to 18 cm during the throwing motion (Kibler, 1998a, 1998b). Failure to retract the scapula leads to an increase in the antetilting of the glenoid as a result of a protracted scapular position and can exacerbate the instability continuum and create anterior instability and suboptimal performance leading to injury (Kibler, 1998; Burkhart et al, 2003). Research has shown that in late cocking, the abduction and external rotation position places the posterior band of the inferior glenohumeral ligament in a "bowstrung" position under the humeral head such that tightness in this structure can lead to a posterosuperior shift in the humeral head, which can lead to rotator cuff and labral pathology (Burkhart et al, 2003) (Figure 17-11). Improper scapular positioning coupled with increases in horizontal abduction during late cocking and the transition into the acceleration phase has been termed *hyperangulation* and leads to aggravation of undersurface

rotator cuff impingement and labral injury derangement (see Figures 17-6 and 17-11).

The acceleration phase begins after maximal external rotation and ends with ball release. During the delivery phase, the arm initially starts in −30 degrees of horizontal abduction (30 degrees behind the coronal plane) (Dillman et al, 1991). As acceleration of the arm continues, the glenohumeral joint is moved forward to a position of 10 degrees of horizontal adduction (anterior to the coronal plane) (Dillman et al, 1991). During acceleration, the arm moves from a position of 175 to 180 degrees of composite external rotation to a position of nearly vertical (105) degrees of external rotation at release. This is another point at which the video can be paused or a digital image generated for analysis. When viewed from the side, the forearm is in an almost vertical position; however, the arm

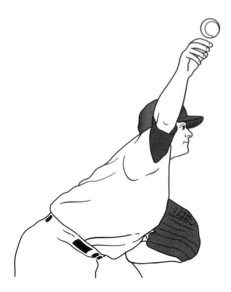

Figure 17-12 Ball release position. Note the vertical position of the forearm and the forward flexed position of the trunk.

appears to be 10 to 15 degrees behind the trunk because the trunk is flexed forward at ball release (Figure 17-12). This internal rotation movement after maximal external rotation is difficult to capture on video and with digital images because it occurs at more than 7000 degrees per second (Dillman et al, 1991; Fleisig et al, 1989).

Another important variable to monitor during arm cocking and acceleration is the abduction angle of the glenohumeral joint. Research has consistently shown that the abduction angle for the throwing motion ranges between 90 and 110 degrees (Dillman et al, 1991; Atwater, 1979). It is important to note that this angle is relative to the trunk, with varying amounts of trunk lateral flexion changing the actual release position while keeping the abduction angle remarkably consistent among individuals and major pitching styles (Dillman et al, 1991; Fleisig et al, 1989; Atwater, 1979). Elevation of the glenohumeral abduction angle to more than 110 degrees can subject the rotator cuff to impingement stresses from the overlying acromion. Careful monitoring of this abduction angle during the throwing motion is recommended using digital still images or video.

Follow-through is the stage after ball release and contains high levels of eccentric muscular activity in the posterior rotator cuff and scapular region (Fleisig et al, 2000). Additional movements of the entire body are necessary to help dissipate the energy of the arm. Close monitoring during this stage of the throwing motion is also recommended to ensure that an abrupt upright posture is not assumed by the pitcher and that a continuation of the for-

ward momentum is gradually dissipated by wrapping the arm across the body with trunk rotation. Also, the rear leg should come forward to assist in this process, leaving the pitcher in a balanced finish position.

Failure at any one of these stages in the throwing motion can have profound implications on the throwing shoulder. As mentioned throughout this section, use of digital still photography from multiple sides of the throwing athlete, as well as the use of video, can enhance the evaluation process and clearly improve biofeedback and education with the injured athlete, parent, and coach. Removal of the shirt when applicable for men and use of a sports bra or sleeveless shirt for women will enhance the ability to estimate arm-trunk relationships. Even with careful clinical monitoring at this level, more extensive biomechanical analysis may be needed to better identify deviations from normal movement patterning. Referral to a biomechanist who has access to three-dimensional motion analysis programs is indicated in many cases.

TENNIS SERVE

The tennis serving motion can be classified into four primary phases: wind-up, cocking, acceleration, and follow-through (Rhu et al, 1988) (Figure 17-13). These phases are used to scientifically break down the movement and do not occur as separate individual stages or phases during actual performance.

The wind-up phase of the tennis serve is similarly quiet with respect to muscular activity, but it does require a balanced position to provide a stable base for optimal performance. Also, the stance should be aligned such that if a long board were placed along the tips of the feet, it would point in the direction the serve is intended. An excessively closed stance leads to blocking the pelvis and would potentially keep the hips from rotating during later stages of the serve, whereas an excessively open stance leads to early opening of the hips and would likely produce nonoptimal transfer of energy from the lower extremities and trunk.

Arm cocking occurs as the hands separate and the ball toss is initiated (Rhu et al, 1988). Initially, the racquet arm classically pursues a downward path followed by an upward motion toward maximal external rotation similar to throwing. Dillman et al (1991) reported a composite maximal external rotation angle of the dominant arm of 154 degrees during serving in elite-level players. During arm cocking, when the elbow is in a position of 90 degrees of elbow flexion, dominant arm abduction angles have been reported at 83 degrees in elite Australian players (Elliott et al, 1986). A digital photo or video footage of the tennis player from multiple angles at the stage of maximal external rotation can be useful to identify significant

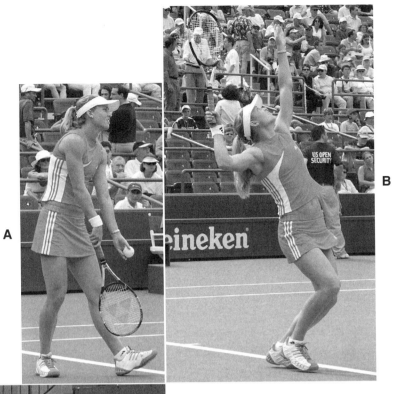

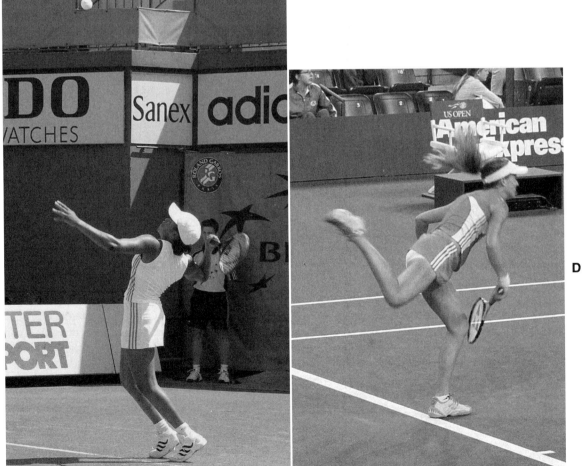

Figure 17-13 Phases of the tennis serve. **A,** Wind-up. **B,** Cocking. **C,** Acceleration. **D,** Follow-through.

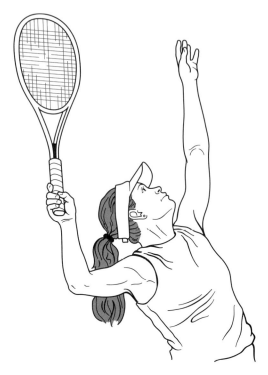

Figure **17-14** Arm cocking. Note the position of glenohumeral joint abduction during this phase.

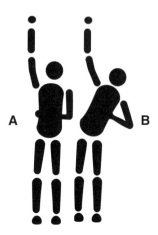

Figure **17-15** Contact positions of the tennis serve. **A,** Improper. **B,** Proper. (Adapted from *Tennis Pro*, Sept/Oct 13:2000.)

alterations in elbow flexion angles, as well as glenohumeral joint abduction angles during maximal apparent composite external rotation (Figure 17-14). Inappropriate abduction angles greater than 90 degrees during arm cocking and acceleration may lead to impingement of the rotator cuff tendons under the coracoacromial arch.

After maximal external rotation, the dominant shoulder undergoes rapid concentric internal rotation. This movement is termed the *acceleration phase* and it occurs between maximal external rotation and ball contact. Angular velocities of 1074 to 1514 degrees per second have been measured during the acceleration phase of the tennis serve in elite players (Shapiro & Stine, 1992). During the acceleration phase, proper evaluation and monitoring are indicated as the hips, trunk, and shoulders rotate segmentally. Premature opening of the hips and trunk can lead to "arm lag," in which the shoulder is placed in extremes of horizontal abduction. This has also been termed *hyperangulation* (Burkart et al, 2003). (see Figures 17-6, 17-10, and 17-11), where the humerus lags behind the scapular plane of the body during internal rotation of the glenohumeral joint. This hyperangulation can lead to rotator cuff and labral injury and has been implicated as a major factor in overuse injury in overhead athletes, including tennis players (Burkart et al, 2003).

For the purpose of analysis, the acceleration phase terminates at ball contact. This is another time point at which a digital photo or "stop/pause" in video is recommended. Specific analysis of the glenohumeral joint abduction angle has considerable relevance for the patient with glenohumeral joint dysfunction. The initial appearance of glenohumeral joint position during ball contact often reveals a nearly vertical humeral position (Figure 17-15, *A*). On closer analysis, however, the contribution from the trunk via lateral flexion allows the glenohumeral joint to be positioned between 90 and 100 degrees (Figure 17-15, *B*). This position is crucial to allow for forceful rotational movements with the glenohumeral joint below positions with inherent subacromial impingement or compression (Ellenbecker, 1995). Frequently, tennis players with nonoptimal trunk control or stabilization or those who are unable to laterally flex their trunk to allow for this important alignment use inappropriate amounts of glenohumeral abduction during their serve. Identification of this important alignment using feedback for the patient is another excellent example of how technique/sport analysis can provide a tremendous advantage in the examination and rehabilitation process.

Another important facet in ball contact is the location of the toss by the contralateral arm. Placement of the ball in the 12 o'clock position (directly overhead) leads to ball contact positions with greater inherent abduction than a ball toss that is placed to the side of the player. A common biomechanical correction for players with pain during the acceleration and follow-through phases of the serving motion is to toss the ball farther laterally to allow for a contact point that reduces the amount of glenohumeral joint abduction and subacromial compression.

After ball contact, the follow-through phase begins and terminates at the end of the serving motion. This phase is characterized by significant eccentric muscular activity (Rhu et al, 1988; Ellenbecker, 1995). A common biomechanical fault found in players with shoulder dysfunction is rapid abbreviation of the follow-through phase after ball contact. Recommended technique includes a full motion, including trunk flexion and rotation, shoulder extension adduction, cross-arm adduction, and internal rotation. Abnormally abbreviated follow-through movement patterns require greater amounts of muscular work (eccentric overload) and must occur over a shorter period of time and motion. Also, reduced internal rotation range of motion in the dominant shoulder of the elite tennis player (Ellenbecker et al, 1996, 2002b; Kibler et al, 1996) may lead to abbreviated patterns of movement and an increase in scapular upward rotation and protraction. This finding can be compared with the clinical examination findings of total rotation range of motion to determine whether abbreviated follow-through patterns are being applied as a result of a true loss of glenohumeral joint internal rotation.

TENNIS GROUNDSTROKES

Tennis groundstrokes consist of the forehand and backhand and can be divided into three primary phases. These phases are termed *preparation, acceleration,* and *follow-through*. The discrimination between the acceleration and follow-through phases is based on ball contact. Most consequences for the tennis playing shoulder occur during acceleration and follow-through, with the preparation phase showing minimal muscular activity in the shoulder region (Rhu et al, 1988). One factor regarding the forehand groundstroke preparation phase is the importance of scapular retraction. Placement of the arm behind the body requires horizontal abduction with trunk rotation. Failure to achieve this position with a scapular protracted position may lead to increased anterior shoulder stress, particularly as forward trunk rotation is imposed on this protracted position with the glenohumeral joint horizontally abducted.

An important concept for analysis of the forehand and backhand groundstroke is the position or stance that the player takes during execution. Three primary stances are prevalent: square, closed, and open (Roetert & Groppel, 2001; Segal, 2002). The traditional position is the square stance, whereby the player stands perpendicular to the net (sideways), with the tips of one foot aligned with the tips of the other foot (Figure 17-16). The shoulders are also perpendicular to the net and baseline such that upper body and trunk rotation can occur. Players using this type

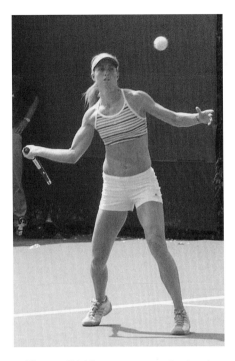

Figure **17-16** Square stance forehand.

of stance rely primarily on linear momentum to gain power, which is initiated as the player steps forward toward the oncoming ball (Roetert & Groppel, 2001). Although this classic stance has been used for a long time, one limitation occurs during follow-through when the pelvis can block further rotation of the trunk and pelvis as a result of the square stance alignment. This blocking phenomenon is particularly prevalent when the player uses a truly closed stance in which the front foot is placed in a position where it crosses over the back foot. This stance is rarely used and is not recommended for forehand groundstrokes because it limits the effective transfer of kinetic energy from the lower body and trunk to the upper body for power generation.

In the modern game of tennis played today (2004), nearly all top players use an open or partially open stance on the forehand, with many top players using the open stance for the two-handed backhand as well. The open stance involves placing the feet parallel to the net or baseline. What is crucially important and the most common error regarding the open stance is that the upper body (shoulders) must be rotated or closed so that they are placed perpendicular to the pelvis and lower body position and perpendicular to the net or baseline (Figure 17-17). This positioning allows for greater generation and utiliza-

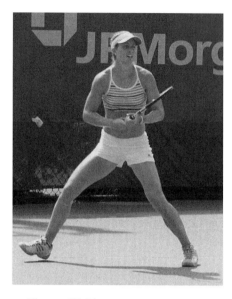

Figure 17-17 Open stance forehand.

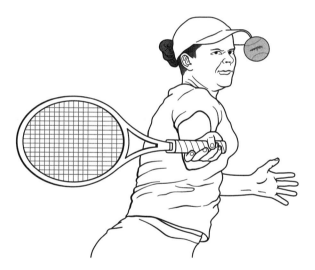

Figure **17-18** Improper open stance forehand demonstrating ball contact behind the body with shoulder in or behind the coronal plane.

tion of angular momentum as a result of the large angle of separation between the pelvis and shoulders. Also, the relationship of the lower extremities in the open stance does not "block" the pelvis and allows for a more optimal rotation pattern as the upper extremity is accelerated toward the ball and continues through the follow-through phase (Roetert & Groppel, 2001).

A common error associated with the open stance forehand that can lead to anterior shoulder pain and rotator cuff dysfunction occurs during early rotation of the pelvis,

where the lower body and trunk rotate too quickly ahead of the arm. This improper sequential rotation leaves power generation to the upper body, as the trunk and pelvis rotate too early so that the optimal transfer of power from the lower extremities and trunk cannot occur (Figure 17-18). Also, this poorly timed rotation places the glenohumeral joint in a position in the coronal plane during ball contact, or in many cases ball contact occurs with even greater amounts of horizontal abduction behind the coronal plane of the body. This creates a position similar to that described during the serving motion of hyperabduction, and when coupled with scapular protraction and imbalanced muscle function can lead to injury (Ellenbecker, 1995). The digital camera should be used to show both an anterior and side view of the acceleration phase of the forehand groundstroke to identify this suboptimal segmental rotation and convey this information to the player, parent, and coach.

One final area of analysis on the forehand groundstroke is the follow-through. This occurs after ball impact and should involve a continued pattern that ultimately ends up with the racquet and racquet hand being placed on the opposite side of the head. Some players use an abbreviated follow-through pattern that leads to a greater amount of eccentric muscular work, shorter follow-through time, and movement arcs that can create injury. Finally, most players generate tremendous topspin on the forehand groundstroke by using a low to high racquet path and grips that enable the generation of topspin (Roetert & Groppel, 2001). However, some players use excessive grips (extreme western grips) and excessive forearm pronation during the acceleration and follow-through phases of the forehand groundstroke. This distal pronation leads to increased upper arm internal rotation and requires greater eccentric deceleration by the posterior rotator cuff (Rhu et al, 1988). This greater load placed on the shoulder by a distal movement is another example of the application of the kinetic link principle to upper extremity sport movement patterns.

BACKHAND GROUNDSTROKE

The backhand groundstroke can be executed both with one and two hands. Research has shown that muscular activity during the one- and two-handed backhands are statistically similar (Giangarra et al, 1993); however, the use of both hands on the racquet can allow for greater facilitation of trunk rotation and more optimal transfer of energy via the kinetic chain theory. Stances used for the backhand are similar to those discussed for the forehand; however, the closed stance is used with more frequency on the backhand side because of the tremendous shoulder rotation that is required for proper execution. Use of digital photography or video should identify tremendous shoulder rotation whereby the player's dominant arm scapula should be pointing at the oncoming ball. Again, a low to high motion should be used to generate topspin on the ball regardless of whether one or two hands are used. Ball contact should occur slightly in front of the body to allow for forward progression of the momentum generated. One common error inherent in many players who report pain during the backhand groundstroke is what is referred to as a *late ball contact*. This occurs when the ball is contacted either in line with the body or actually behind the midline (umbilicus) of the body. This results in a nonoptimal transfer of energy from the lower body and trunk and a reliance on concentric shoulder external rotation for power generation.

During the one- and two-handed backhands, the dominant arm is initially brought into some degree of cross-arm adduction during preparation. If the player does not rotate the pelvis and trunk and merely cross-arm adducts (horizontally adducts) the arm, pain may be reported over either the anterior or superior aspect of the shoulder from primary impingement or compression of the rotator cuff under the coracoacromial arch. Careful monitoring of body position and a reliance on rotation of the pelvis and trunk ensure a clear path for arm movement during this important stroke.

The mechanics developed in this chapter, as well as the simple, straightforward use of either a digital camera or video camcorder, can be clinically applied to allow the clinician greater insight into the possible causes of shoulder dysfunction. The reader is urged to gain further biomechanical information on sport-specific activities inherent in the patients commonly treated to allow for the comprehensive evaluation and treatment of shoulder dysfunction.

CHAPTER 18

Putting It All Together: Using Clinical Tests to Formulate a Clinical Diagnosis for the Patient with Shoulder Dysfunction

INTRODUCTION

In reviewing the previous chapters, clinicians will find no shortage of tests to assess the integrity of specific structures around the shoulder. Methods to test muscular strength and endurance, joint range of motion, and proprioception are also included. This chapter summarizes the evaluation process by discussing several studies that reviewed the differences between the way advanced master clinicians and novice clinicians perform and interpret the evaluation process. A summary of common patterns or clusters of signs and symptoms occurring with common shoulder injuries is presented to provide examples of how the information in the previous chapters can be combined and formulated to achieve a clinical diagnosis.

Clinical evaluations in physical therapy are performed for several reasons. They determine the involved structures, assess the severity of the injury, develop and initiate a treatment program based on the examination data and resultant database, and continually reassess the patient's progress based on the database from the initial examination (Davies, 1995). Several differences in the performance and interpretation of the clinical examination have been researched and reported and deserve mention here (Jensen et al, 1990, 1992).

One of the first main areas identified by Jensen et al (1990, 1992) was the master clinician's recall of meaningful relationships or patterns. Master clinicians performed the examination with a strong tie between information gathered and the clustering of signs and symptoms. Master clinicians not only collected disease data (findings that helped to validate or invalidate a diagnosis) but also gathered illness data regarding the patient's perception of how the disease affected their lives. The main emphasis by the novice clinician was to obtain enough information to complete the evaluation form (Jensen et al, 1992). In addition, the master clinician showed an intense focus on the patient to achieve a connection with the patient, whereas the novice clinician was focused on filling out the evaluation form, which dominated the interaction with

patients (Jensen et al, 1992). Finally, the master clinician described the examination process as achieving a working diagnosis by performing a selective tissue examination to identify the structure or structures at fault (Davies, 1995; Jensen et al, 1992).

DAVIES FUNCTIONAL TESTING ALGORITHM

Davies (1995) developed a functional testing algorithm, using a combination of information gained in the examination and in subjective reports and incorporating the mechanism of injury data with clinical tests. The shoulder examination algorithm is presented in this chapter to provide an example of how clusters of signs and symptoms can be used to formulate a diagnosis on which an objectively based treatment program can be developed. Table 18-1 shows the Davies Functional Testing Algorithm, which includes the test category, critical pathways that represent the types of patients to be considered for the condition being tested for, the special tests used, and the tissues implicated. This table does not contain all of the special tests contained in this text, nor does it include an exhaustive list of possible shoulder injuries. It is meant to serve as a guide to assist the clinician in putting some of the contents of the previous chapters together in a clinically referenced manner for some of the most common shoulder injuries typically presenting to clinicians working in orthopedics and sports medicine.

APPLICATION OF CLINICAL TESTS TO CLASSIFY ROTATOR CUFF IMPINGEMENT

Using a similar format to the Davies Functional Testing Algorithm, the main types of rotator cuff impingement can be identified and differentiated using a summary of the special tests and examination procedures presented in this book. Table 18-2 summarizes this information for rotator cuff impingement.

TABLE 18-1   Davies Modified Functional Testing Algorithm

TEST CATEGORY	CRITICAL PATHWAYS	SPECIAL TESTS	TISSUE(S) IMPLICATED
MDI	All patients	Sulcus sign (neutral)	SGHL, CHL, rotator interval
MDI	All patients	Sulcus sign (90 ABD)	IGHL, anterior inferior capsule
Anterior instability	All patients	Anterior load and shift	Anterior capsule, SGHL, MGHL, IGHL
		Anterior drawer	
		Subluxation relocation test	
		Anterior release test	
	Macrotraumatic injury	Apprehension test	
Posterior instability	All patients	Posterior load and shift	Posterior capsule
		Posterior drawer	
Long-head biceps	MOI: eccentric deceleration	Speeds test	Long-head biceps
	Pain on palpation	Yergason's test	
	C/O anterior shoulder pain	Ludington's test	
AC joint	Age >40 years	AC joint shear test	AC joint and intrinsic and extrinsic ligaments
	MOI: macrotraumatic injury (i.e., fall on lateral side or blow to lateral aspect of shoulder)	Cross-arm adduction	
	C/O pain top of shoulder		
	Pain with AC joint palpation	Impingement test	
	C/O pain with crossover activities	O'Brien's active compression test	
	Asymmetric deformity of AC		
Labral injury	MOI: macrotraumatic injury	Compression rotation test	SLAP
	MOI: eccentric deceleration	Anterior slide test	SLAP
	C/O pain "deep" in shoulder	O'Brien's active compression test	SLAP
	Sensation of locking or pseudolocking	Speed's test	SLAP
	Repetitive clicking/clunking	Clunk test	Labrum nonspecific
	MOI: FOOSH	Circumduction test	Labrum nonspecific
		Crank test	Labrum nonspecific
Rotator cuff tears	Age >40 years	Drop arm test	Supraspinatus
	Macrotraumatic injury with functional disability	Full can/empty can MMT	Supraspinatus
	Idiopathic onset of functional disability	Hornblower's sign	Teres minor
	C/O pain in lateral aspect of arm	Dropping sign	Infraspinatus
	C/O dull constant pain in shoulder	Gerber lift-off test	Subscapularis
	Compensatory shoulder shrug sign	Napoleon test	Subscapularis

ADDITIONAL CONCEPTS FOR CLINICAL EXAMINATION OF THE SHOULDER

As stated earlier, special tests are applied to the uninjured shoulder first to enhance relaxation and gain patient confidence. The exact ordering of clinical testing for shoulder examination, however, has not been clinically tested and at this time remains at the discretion of the examiner. I recommend that special tests be applied first to rule out shoulder instability before using other examination techniques. For example, establishing whether a patient has a positive sulcus sign early in the examination can guide or alert the clinician as to the expected outcome of other examination maneuvers where humeral head translation is measured. A patient with a positive sulcus sign often has increases in anterior and/or posterior translation because of the underlying hypermobility of the glenohumeral joint capsule. After the mobility status and presence of instabil-

TABLE 18-2   Differentiation of Rotator Cuff Impingement Using Clinical Testing

IMPINGEMENT TYPE	SPECIAL TEST/CLINICAL MEASURES	CLINICAL FINDINGS/STATUS
Primary impingement		Anterior/anterolateral shoulder pain, particularly with overhead repetitive activities
	Neer, Hawkins, cross-arm, Coracoid, and Yocum's	Positive traditional impingement testing
	MDI sulcus sign, A/P humeral head translation testing	General joint hypomobility Grade I translation (Altchek et al, 1992)
	Reduced glenohumeral joint range of motion	Loss of internal rotation (IR) common; restricted elevation
	Rotator cuff weakness	Manual muscle testing (MMT) shows <5/5 strength of rotator cuff (RTC) and scapular stabilizers
Secondary impingement		Anterior/anterolateral shoulder pain, particularly with overhead repetitive activities
	Neer, Hawkins, cross-arm, coracoid, and Yocum's	Positive traditional impingement testing
	MDI sulcus sign, anterior/posterior (A/P) humeral head translation testing	General joint hypermobility Grade II or greater translation (Altchek et al, 1992)
	Subluxation relocation test	Positive subluxation relocation test with reproduction of anteriorly based shoulder pain
	Altered glenohumeral joint range of motion	Loss of IR common; increased external rotation (ER) common
	Rotator cuff weakness	MMT shows <5/5 strength of rotator cuff (RTC) and scapular stabilizers
Internal or posterior impingement		Posterior shoulder pain most notable with shoulder in 90/90 position (arm cocking)
	Neer, Hawkins, cross-arm, coracoid, and Yocum's	Negative traditional impingement testing
	MDI sulcus sign, A/P humeral head translation testing	General joint hypermobility Grade II or greater translation (Altchek et al, 1992)
	Subluxation relocation test	Positive subluxation relocation test with reproduction of posteriorly based shoulder pain
	Altered glenohumeral joint range of motion	Loss of IR; increased ER
	Rotator cuff weakness	MMT shows <5/5 strength of RTC and scapular stabilizers

ity have been ruled out, additional testing to determine the status of additional structures in and around the glenohumeral joint can be carried out.

It is also important to point out that all clinical tests are not performed on every patient. Based on patient presentation, subjective history, and clinical experience, an orderly flow of clinical tests is recommended. Every chapter containing special tests reviews not only how to perform the test but the research behind the test and its proven or unproven effectiveness. The use of several tests within a particular category (i.e., labral tests, impingement tests) has been shown to increase the effectiveness and likelihood that a positive test result will be found. For example, the author of this text frequently uses a combination of impingement signs such as the Neer, Hawkins, coracoid, cross-arm, and Yocum's to evaluate the patient's response to movement and possible encroachment of the rotator cuff and biceps long-head tendons against the coracoacromial arch. Greater confidence can be gleaned from the finding of a negative response to five impingement signs than from findings of a negative response on just one maneuver. Repetitive practice with these examination maneuvers allows for the performance of a core group of examination maneuvers in a clinically efficient time frame to optimize clinical interpretation and minimize trauma or exacerbation of symptoms from the patient.

The final chapter of this text contains several case studies that demonstrate one manner in which the clinical examination process can be performed. It is hoped that the combination of the detailed and scientific description and discussion of these clinical tests and examination techniques will lead the clinician to successful identification of shoulder pathology and provide objective assistance for the development of evidence-based treatment plans.

CASE STUDIES

EXAMINATION: SUBJECTIVE HISTORY

Meghan is a 16-year-old right-handed elite junior tennis player with a 3-week history of anterior shoulder pain after increases in training and competitive tennis play. She reports no pain at rest and 9/10 level pain during serving and forehands. The pain is localized to the right dominant shoulder, and she denies any neural symptoms radiating down the arm or numbness or tingling in the distal aspect of her right upper extremity. She does have pain at night (6/10) if she has trained earlier in the day, and she is unable to lie on her affected arm while sleeping. She denies any significant past medical history of right shoulder injury and has no history of neck or back injury. She reports a brief history of medial elbow pain 2 years ago that was treated successfully with physical therapy, allowing a full return to tennis activity. She has no significant medical history and is not taking any medications. She plays with a Prince Graphite midsize tennis racquet strung with synthetic gut at 64 pounds, and denies any change in technique or equipment. She uses a semi-western forehand grip. Her goal is to return to training and compete in tennis as soon as possible.

OBSERVATION/POSTURE

Meghan stands with the right dominant shoulder approximately 1 inch lower than the nondominant left extremity. Mild scoliosis is noted with a right thoracic rib hump noted in the Adams position in 45 degrees of trunk forward flexion. Noted atrophy is present in the hands on hips position in the infraspinous fossa of the right scapula, and a type II Kibler scapula is present, with increased prominence of the entire medial border of the right scapula as compared with the left.

SCAPULAR EXAMINATION

Scapular provocation tests increase the prominence of the entire medial border of the right scapula with waist-level pressure via the extremities against the wall, and similarly with pressure exerted to the upper extremities in 90 degrees of shoulder flexion. In addition, a medial type II Kibler scapula is evident during active scapular plane elevation with loss of scapular control noted at approximately 60 degrees of elevation during arm lowering. This is significantly more visually evident on the right side. Symmetric scapular control is noted during concentric arm elevation in the scapular plane bilaterally. Full pain-free active shoulder elevation in the scapular plane is present; therefore scapular assistance and retraction tests are deferred. Documentation of scapular position is assessed using the Kibler lateral scapular slide test with results listed below.

Position	Left Uninjured	Right Injured
1	9 cm	11 cm
2	8 cm	10.5 cm
3	8 cm	9.5 cm

RELATED REFERRAL JOINT TESTING

A negative Spurling's maneuver was present to both sides, negative acromioclavicular (AC) joint shear test, and bilaterally increased elbow valgus stress and valgus stress test physiologic laxity without pain provocation.

NEUROVASCULAR TESTING

Meghan is intact to light touch sensation from C5 to T1 and has normal biceps, triceps, and brachioradialis reflexes bilaterally; 40 kg of right distal grip strength is measured, with 28 kg on the left. Additional neurovascular testing is deferred at this time based on patient history and presentation.

RANGE OF MOTION MEASUREMENT

Active range of motion was measured in the standing position for forward flexion and abduction, and in the supine position for internal and external rotation with 90 degrees of glenohumeral joint abduction.

Active Range of Motion	Left Uninjured	Right Injured
Forward flexion	0-170	0-170
Abduction	0-175	0-175
External rotation with 90 degrees abduction	0-95	0-100
Internal rotation with 90 degrees abduction	0-55	0-35
Total rotation range of motion with 90 degrees abduction	150	135

MUSCULAR STRENGTH TESTING

Manual muscle testing was performed bilaterally; 5/5 strength was found in the left upper extremity for all tests, with 5/5 flexion/extension, abduction/adduction, and horizontal abduction/adduction, and internal rotation strength in the right shoulder, and 4/5 strength in external rotation tested in both neutral and 90 degrees of glenohumeral joint abduction, which reproduced the patient's pain. Supraspinatus strength of 4+/5 was measured using the empty can test position (scapular plane elevation with internal rotation).

SPECIAL TESTS

A 2 degree multidirectional instability (MDI) sulcus sign was noted on the right shoulder; 1 degree was noted on the left. Impingement testing revealed positive traditional impingement tests of Neer, Hawkins, and Yocum's, with a negative coracoid and cross-arm impingement test. The Speed's, Yergason's, O'Brien's, clunk, circumduction, and compression rotation tests were all negative. Supine humeral head translation testing revealed 2 degree anterior translation at 60 and 90 degrees of abduction in the right shoulder, with 1 degree translation on the left. One degree posterior translation testing was noted bilaterally, tested at 90 degrees of abduction. A positive subluxation/relocation test was present in the right shoulder, which reproduced the patient's anterior symptoms with subluxation and abated the symptoms during posterior humeral head relocation.

CLINICAL IMPRESSION

Secondary impingement of the right shoulder with underlying multidirectional instability and isolated rotator cuff muscular weakness and strength imbalance, scapular dysfunction, and loss of glenohumeral joint internal rotation range of motion.

Case Study 19-2

EXAMINATION: SUBJECTIVE HISTORY

Betty is a 78-year-old right-handed retired female who reports falling on her left outstretched arm 6 months ago while walking her golden retriever. She reports having an immediate onset of anterior and posterior shoulder pain that radiated down the lateral aspect of her left upper arm to a level just below the insertion of her deltoid. Initial pain levels were 10/10 with movement and 4/10 at rest. She tried icing and not using her left arm, but the pain and weakness had worsened. She now presents to the clinic with a primary complaint of 6/10 pain at rest, and 8/10 pain at night. She also reports extreme weakness in the left shoulder and an inability to perform basic functions. Past medical history includes right shoulder bursitis 45 years ago that was treated with a cortisone shot and two right knee surgeries. Medical history is unremarkable with the exception of high blood pressure and high cholesterol, for which she is presently taking medications. No other medications are being used except for Tylenol at night for pain and Advil during the day. She is seeking an evaluation today because her pain levels at night have prevented her from sleeping. Betty's goals are to continue to care for her home and backyard landscaping, as well as to remain active and able to walk her dog every day. Her pain and range of motion presently limit her from walking the dog because even gentle repetitive arm swinging irritates her condition. Betty completed a modified American Shoulder Elbow Surgeons (ASES) shoulder rating scale and scored 22/45 points on the self-report section.

OBSERVATION/POSTURE

Betty stands holding her left injured shoulder in internal rotation and clutching her belt line in front of her. Her left nondominant shoulder is higher than the right dominant shoulder, with obvious guarding noted in the left upper trapezius. Betty has a very forward head posture and significantly increased thoracic kyphosis. Bilateral scapular protraction is noted. Severe atrophy is present in the supraspinous fossa and infraspinous fossa of the left scapula compared with muscular size and resting tone over the right scapula. Betty is unable to achieve the hands-on-hips posture with her left shoulder, most likely because of loss of internal rotation range of motion.

SCAPULAR EVALUATION

No significant increase in either medial or inferior scapular prominence is noted. Betty is unable to elevate her left shoulder more than approximately 70 degrees against gravity. She shows extensive superior movement of the left scapula ("shrug sign") and is classified as having a Kibler type III scapula. The scapular assistance test is positive and increases her left shoulder elevation to 95 degrees, but pain is elicited as she lowers her arm back to the neutral starting position, even with scapular assistance. The Kibler lateral scapular slide test shows relative symmetry between sides, with testing in position 1 measuring 10 cm for both the involved left and uninjured right arm. Kibler positions 2 and 3 could not be assessed because of the patient's inability to assume those positions.

RELATED REFERRAL JOINT TESTING

Spurling's maneuver is negative for shoulder symptom reproduction but is painful at the base of the cervical spine, with both left and right directional testing. The AC shear test is negative, as are the elbow varus and valgus stress tests.

NEUROVASCULAR TESTING

Betty is fully intact to light touch sensation between levels C5 and T1, and has symmetric reflexes of the biceps, triceps, and brachioradialis. Additional neurovascular testing is deferred at this time.

RANGE OF MOTION MEASUREMENT

Active range of motion for forward flexion and abduction was measured in the standing position, with passive flexion and abduction and active glenohumeral joint internal and external rotation range of motion measured in the supine position.

Range of Motion	Left Involved	Right Uninvolved
Active forward flexion	0-70	0-165
Active abduction	0-50	0-155
Passive forward flexion	0-135	0-155
Passive abduction	0-120	0-155
Active external rotation	0-40 with 45 degrees abduction	0-80 with 90 degrees abduction
Active internal rotation	0-40 with 45 degrees abduction	0-45 with 90 degrees abduction

MUSCULAR STRENGTH TESTING

The right shoulder tested 5/5 for all movements, with left shoulder 3-/5 for flexion and abduction, 4-/5 for external rotation in neutral adduction, 5-/5 for internal rotation, and 4/5 adduction and extension; 2/5 strength was measured in the empty can and full can testing positions. Betty has 5/5 biceps and triceps strength bilaterally, with no evidence of a "Popeye" deformity in the left shoulder.

SPECIAL TESTS

Betty has a trace left shoulder sulcus sign, with virtually no motion available in the inferior direction. Pain is reproduced with impingement testing in both the Neer and Hawkins tests, with the other tests deferred because of patient discomfort levels encountered with testing. A positive drop arm test and empty and full can test (positive for both pain reproduction and weakness) are present in the left shoulder. A negative Napoleon sign is present in the left shoulder. Labral testing is deferred because of significant range of motion limitations and baseline pain levels. Trace anterior/posterior humeral head translation is measured in the left shoulder with 1 degree of translation on the right.

CLINICAL IMPRESSION

Full-thickness rotator cuff tear of the left shoulder with secondary adhesive capsulitis and a classic capsular pattern of limited range of motion.

Case Study 19-3

EXAMINATION: SUBJECTIVE HISTORY

Tony is a 55-year-old right-handed male who presents for evaluation of his left shoulder 2 weeks after an episode in which he felt his left shoulder "slip and pop" while unloading a large 4 × 8 sheet of plywood from an overhead position at a Home Depot store at which he works. Tony manages the lumber department and loads and unloads new stock and assists customers; he reports that his arm was in an abducted and externally rotated position when the incident occurred. He denies feeling his shoulder dislocate and did not initially report to the emergency department or industrial medicine center after the injury and was able to continue working. He reports the pain to be 3/10 at rest and 5/10 after a shift at work. He believes he has lost some strength in his shoulder and that his arm occasionally feels "heavy and out of place." Tony reports some occasional tingling in the fourth and fifth digit of his left hand, but this tingling is intermittent and does not appear to have a pattern. His past medical history includes a left clavicle fracture and shoulder separation that he suffered playing high school football more than 30 years ago. He has no other medical history and is not taking any medications. His goal is to increase the strength and function of his left shoulder to continue working in his physical environment in the lumber department. Tony completed the self-report section of the modified ASES rating scale and scored 38 of 45 points.

OBSERVATION/POSTURE

Tony stands with level shoulders. He has excellent overall muscular development and no signs of visible atrophy at rest or in the hands-on-hips position. He has a characteristic step-down sign over the left AC joint, and mild misalignment of the left clavicle with palpable bone formation along the inferior surface of the distal third of the clavicle. Tony has a slightly forward head posture and holds his left scapula in what appears to be greater protraction than his right.

SCAPULAR EXAMINATION

The borders of Tony's scapulae are well concealed with a normal (type IV) scapula and no evidence of a loss of scapular control on bilateral arm elevation and lowering in the scapular plane.

RELATED REFERRAL JOINT TESTING

Spurling's maneuver is negative; AC joint shear test is positive with general hypomobility noted compared with the other side and mild pain provocation directly over the AC joint of the left shoulder. Negative elbow varus and valgus stress tests are noted bilaterally; a negative Tinel's test also occurred bilaterally.

NEUROVASCULAR TESTING

Tony is fully intact to light touch sensation from C5 to T1, shows normal vascular filling, and has bilaterally symmetric upper extremity reflexes. A negative Adson's and costoclavicular test were also encountered.

RANGE OF MOTION MEASUREMENT

Active range of motion was measured in the standing position for forward flexion and abduction and in the supine position for internal and external rotation.

Motion	Left Injured	Right Uninjured
Forward flexion	0-160	0-175
Abduction	0-150	0-175
External rotation with 90 degrees abduction	0-65*	0-90
Internal rotation with 90 degrees abduction	0-45	0-45

MUSCULAR STRENGTH TESTING

The right upper extremity is 5/5 for all tests, with left shoulder manual muscle testing (MMT) revealing 4/5 external and internal rotation tests. Flexion, abduction, and supraspinatus testing were 5-/5 for the left shoulder.

SPECIAL TESTS

Tests revealed 1 degree sulcus sign bilaterally, a positive apprehension sign in approximately 70 degrees of external rotation, and 90 degrees of abduction. Negative impingement signs (Neer, Hawkins, coracoid, cross-arm, and Yocum's) and negative Speed's and Yergason's tests were also noted. Humeral head translation testing showed 2+ anterior humeral head translation at 30, 60, and 90 degrees of abduction and 1 degree posterior translation left shoulder. The right shoulder had 1 degree anterior and posterior translation. The seated load and shift test also showed 2+ anterior and 1 degree posterior translation of the left shoulder and 1 degree translation anteriorly and posteriorly of the right shoulder. Labral testing produced a positive circumduction and crank test with both catching in the shoulder and symptom reproduction. A negative O'Brien's test and negative compression rotation test were noted in both shoulders.

CLINICAL IMPRESSION

Anterior instability of the left shoulder with possible labral tear.

References

Abbott LC, Saunders LB de CM: Acute traumatic dislocation of the tendon of the long head of the biceps brachii: report of 6 cases with operative findings, *Surgery* 6:817-840, 1939.

Adams RD: Pain in the back, neck and extremities. In *Principles of neurology,* New York, 1977, McGraw-Hill.

Adams RD, Victor M, Ropper AH: *Principles of neurology,* ed 6, New York, 1997, McGraw-Hill Health Professions Division.

Aitkens S, Lord J, Bernauer E, et al: Relationship of manual muscle testing to objective strength measurements, *Muscle Nerve* 12:173-177, 1989.

Alderink GJ, Kluck DJ: Isokinetic shoulder strength of high school- and college-aged pitchers, *J Orthop Sports Phys Ther* 7:163-172, 1986.

Allegrucci M, Whitney SL, Lephart SM, et al: Shoulder kinesthesia in healthy unilateral athletes participating in upper extremity sports, *J Orthop Sports Phys Ther* 21(4):220-226, 1995.

Altchek DW, Dines DW: The surgical treatment of anterior instability: selective capsular repair, *Operative Techniques Sports Med* 1:285-292, 1993.

Altchek DW, Warren RF, Wickiewicz TL, et al: Arthroscopic acromioplasty: technique and results, *J Bone Joint Surg* 72A:1198-1207, 1990.

Altchek DW, Warren RF, Wickiewicz TL, et al: Arthroscopic labral debridement: a three year follow-up study, *Am J Sports Med* 20(6):702-706, 1992.

American Academy of Orthopaedic Surgeons: *Clinical measures of joint motion,* Rosemont, IL, 1994, American Academy of Orthopaedic Surgeons.

American Academy of Orthopaedic Surgeons: *School screening programs for the early detection of scoliosis: a position statement,* Rosemont, IL, 1992, American Academy of Orthopaedic Surgeons.

Andrews JA, Wilk KE: *The athletes shoulder,* New York, 1994, Churchill Livingstone.

Andrews JR, Alexander EJ: Rotator cuff injury in throwing and racquet sports, *Sports Med Arthrosc Rev* 3:30, 1995.

Andrews JR, Gillogly S: Physical examination of the shoulder in throwing athletes. In Zarins B, Andrews JR, Carson WG, editors: *Injuries to the throwing arm,* Philadelphia, 1985, WB Saunders.

Andrews JR, Wilk KE, Satterwhite YE, Tedder JL: Physical examination of the throwers elbow, *J Orthop Sports Phys Ther* 6:296-304, 1993.

Arthuis M: Obstetrical paralysis of the brachial plexus I. Diagnosis: clinical study of the initial period, *Rev Chir Orthop Reparatrice Appar Mot* 58(suppl I):124-136, 1972.

Atwater AE: Biomechanics of overarm throwing movements and of throwing injuries, *Exerc Sport Sci Rev* 7:43-85, 1979.

Bagg SD, Forrest WJ: A biomechanical analysis of scapular rotation during arm abduction in the scapular plane, *Arch Phys Med Rehabil* 238-245, 1988.

Bak K, Fauno P: Clinical findings in competitive swimmers with shoulder pain, *Am J Sports Med* 25:254-260, 1997.

Bankart ASB: Recurrent or habitual dislocation of the shoulder joint, *BMJ* 2:1132-1133, 1923.

Bankart ASB: The pathology and treatment of recurrent dislocation of the shoulder joint, *BMJ* 26:23-29, 1938.

Barker D, Banks RW, Harker DW, et al: Studies of the histochemistry, ultrastructure, motor innervation, and regeneration of mammalian intrafusal muscle fibers, *Exp Brain Res* 44:67-88, 1976.

Barrett WP, Franklin JL, Jackins SE, et al: Total shoulder arthroplasty, *J Bone Joint Surg* 69A:865-872, 1987.

Bartlett LR, Storey MD, Simons BD: Measurement of upper extremity torque production and its relationship to throwing speed in the competitive athlete, *Am J Sports Med* 17:89-91, 1989.

Basmajian JV, Bazant FJ: Factors preventing downward dislocation of the adducted shoulder joint, *J Bone Joint Surg* 41A:1182, 1959.

Bassett RW, Browne AO, Morrey BF, et al: Glenohumeral muscle force and moment mechanics in a position of shoulder instability, *J Biomech* 23:405-415, 1994.

Beach ML, Whittney SL, Hoffman SA: Relationship of shoulder flexibility, strength and endurance to shoulder pain in competitive swimmers, *J Orthop Sports Phys Ther* 16:262-268, 1992.

Beaton D, Richards RR: Assessing the reliability and responsiveness of 5 shoulder questionnaires, *J Shoulder Elbow Surg* 7:565-572, 1998.

Beighton P, Horan F: Orthopaedic aspects of the Ehlers-Danlos syndrome, *J Bone Joint Surg* 51(B)3:444-453, 1969.

Bennett WF: Specificity of the speeds test: arthroscopic technique for evaluating the biceps tendon at the level of the bicipital groove, *Arthroscopy* 14(8):789-796, 1998.

Berryman-Reese N, Bandy WD: *Joint range of motion and muscle length testing,* Philadelphia, 2002, WB Saunders.

Bigliani LU, Codd TP, Connor PM, et al: Shoulder motion and laxity in the professional baseball player, *Am J Sports Med* 25(6):609-613, 1997.

Bigliani LU, Ticker JB, Flatow EL, et al: The relationship of acromial architecture to rotator cuff disease, *Clin Sports Med* 10:823, 1991.

Blaiser RB, Carpenter JE, Huston LJ: Shoulder proprioception: effect of joint laxity, joint position, and direction of motion, *Orthop Rev* 23:45-50, 1994.

Boissonnault WG: *Examination in physical therapy practice: screening for medical disease,* ed 2, Philadelphia, 1995, Churchill Livingstone.

Borsa PA, Sauers EL, Herling DE: In vivo assessment of AP laxity in healthy shoulders using an instrumented arthrometer, *J Sports Rehabil* 8:157-170, 1999.

Borsa PA, Sauers EL, Herling DE: Patterns of glenohumeral joint laxity and stiffness in healthy men and women, *Med Sci Sports Exerc* 32:1685-1690, 2000.

Borsa PA, Sauers EL, Herling DE, et al: In vivo quantification of capsular end-point in the nonimpaired glenohumeral joint using an instrumented measurement system, *J Orthop Sports Phys Ther* 31(8):419-431, 2001.

Brown LP, Neihues SL, Harrah A, et al: Upper extremity range of motion and isokinetic strength of the internal and external shoulder rotators in major league baseball players, *Am J Sports Med* 16:577-585, 1988.

Buckley JP, Kerwin DG: The role of the biceps and triceps brachii during tennis serving, *Ergonomics* 31(11):1621-1629, 1988.

Bunn J: *Scientific principles of coaching*, Englewood Cliffs, NJ, 1972, Prentice Hall.

Burkhart SS, Morgan CD: The peel-back mechanism: its role in producing and extending posterior type II SLAP lesions and its effect on SLAP repair rehabilitation, *Arthroscopy* 14:637-640, 1998.

Burkhart SS, Morgan CD, Kibler WB: The disabled throwing shoulder: spectrum of pathology. Part I: pathoanatomy and biomechanics, *Arthroscopy* 19(4):404-420, 2003.

Burkhart SS, Tehrany AM: Arthroscopic subscapularis tendon repair: technique and preliminary results, *Arthroscopy* 18(5):454-463, 2002.

Burkhead WZ, Jr: The biceps tendon. In Rockwood CA, Jr, Matsen FA III, eds: *The shoulder*, Philadelphia, 1990, WB Saunders.

Burkhead WZ, Jr, Arcand MA, Zeman C, et al: The biceps tendon. In Rockwood CA, Jr, Matsen FA III, eds: *The shoulder*, ed 2, Philadelphia, 1998, WB Saunders.

Cain PR, Mutschler TA, Fu F, et al: Anterior stability of the glenohumeral joint: a dynamic model, *Am J Sports Med* 15:144-148, 1987.

Caldron PH: Screening for rheumatic disease. In Boissonnault WG, ed: *Examination in physical therapy practice*, ed 2, Philadelphia, 1995, Churchill Livingstone.

Calis M, Akgun K, Birtane M, et al: Diagnostic values of clinical diagnostic tests in subacromial impingement syndrome, *Ann Rheum Dis* 59:44-47, 2000.

Carpenter JE, Blaiser RB, Pellizon GG: The effects of muscle fatigue on shoulder joint position sense, *Am J Sports Med* 26(2):262-265, 1998.

Cave EF, Burke JF, Boyd RJ: *Trauma management*, Chicago, 1974, Year Book Medical Publishers.

Chandler TJ, Kibler WB, Stracener EC, et al: Shoulder strength, power, and endurance in college tennis players, *Am J Sports Med* 20:455-458, 1992.

Cheng JC, Karzel RP: Superior labrum anterior posterior lesions of the shoulder: operative techniques of management, *Operative Techniques Sports Med* 5(4):249-256, 1997.

Clark JM, Harryman DT: Tendons, ligaments, and capsule of the rotator cuff, *J Bone Joint Surg* 74(A):713-725, 1992.

Clark WA: A protractor for measuring rotation of joints, *J Orthop Surg* 2:154-155, 1921.

Codman EA: *The shoulder*, Boston, 1934, Author.

Constant CR, Murley AHG: A clinical method of functional assessment of the shoulder, *Clin Orthop Rel Res* 214:160-164, 1987.

Cook EE, Gray VL, Savinor-Nogue E, et al: Shoulder antagonistic strength ratios: a comparison between college-level baseball pitchers, *J Orthop Sports Phys Ther* 8:451-461, 1987.

Cotton RE, Rideout DF: Tears of the humeral rotator cuff: a radiological and pathological necropsy survey, *J Bone Joint Surg* 46B:314, 1964.

Curtis AS, Snyder SJ: Evaluation and treatment of biceps tendon pathology, *Orthop Clin North Am* 24(1):33-43, 1993.

Cyriax JH, Cyriax PJ: *Illustrated manual of orthopaedic medicine*, London, 1983, Butterworth.

Cyriax JH, Cyriax PJ: *Cyriax's Illustrated manual of orthopaedic medicine*, ed 2, Oxford England, 1993, Butterworth Heinemann.

Daniels L, Worthingham C: *Muscle testing: techniques of manual examination*, ed 4, Philadelphia, 1980, WB Saunders.

Davidson PA, El Attrache NA, Jobe CM, et al: Rotator cuff and posterior superior glenoid labrum injury associated with increased glenohumeral motion: a new site of impingement, *J Shoulder Elbow Surg* 4:384-390, 1995.

Davies GJ: *A compendium of isokinetics in clinical usage and rehabilitation techniques*, ed 4, Onalaska, WI, 1992, S&S Publishing.

Davies GJ: The need for critical thinking in rehabilitation, *J Sport Rehabil* 4:1-22, 1995.

Davies GJ, DeCarlo MS: *Examination of the shoulder complex: current concepts in rehabilitation of the shoulder*, LaCrosse, WI, 1995, Sports Physical Therapy Association Home Study Course.

Davies GJ, Ellenbecker TS: Eccentric isokinetics, *Orthop Phys Ther Clin North Am* 1:297 336, 1992.

Davies GJ, Ellenbecker TS: *Scientific and clinical rationale for utilization of a total arm strength rehabilitation program for shoulder and elbow overuse injuries*, LaCrosse, WI, 1993, APTA Orthopaedic Section Home Study Course.

Davies GJ, Gould JA, Larson RL: Functional examination of the shoulder girdle, *Physician Sports Med* 9(6):82-104, 1981.

Davies GJ, Hoffman SD: Neuromuscular testing and rehabilitation of the shoulder complex, *J Orthop Sports Phys Ther* 18:449-458, 1993.

Dillman CJ, Fleisig GS, Werner SL, et al: *Biomechanics of the shoulder in sports: throwing activities. Postgraduate studies in sports physical therapy*, Berryville, VA, 1991, Forum Medicum.

DiVeta J, Walker ML, Skibinski B: Relationship between performance of selected scapular muscles and scapular abduction in standing subjects, *Phys Ther* 70(8):470-476, 1990.

Djupsjobacka M, Johansson H, Bergenheim M: Influences on the gamma muscle spindle system from muscle afferents stimulated by increased intramuscular concentrations of arachidonic acid, *Brain Res* 663:293-302, 1994.

Djupsjobacka M, Johansson H, Berenheim M, et al: Influences on the gamma muscle spindle system from muscle afferents stimulated by increased intramuscular concentrations of bradykinin and 5-HT, *Neurosci Res* 22:325-333, 1995a.

Djupsjobacka M, Johansson H, Bergenheim M, et al: Influences on the gamma muscle spindle system from contralateral muscle afferents stimulated by KCl and lactic acid, *Neurosci Res* 21:301-309, 1995b.

Doody SG, Freedman L, Waterland JC: Shoulder movements during abduction in the scapular plane, *Arch Phys Med Rehabil* 595-604, Oct 1970.

Eakin CL, Faber KJ, Hawkins RJ, et al: Biceps tendon disorders in athletes, *J Am Acad Orthop Surg* 7(5):300-310, 1999.

Edwards TB, Bostick RD, Greene CG, et al: Interobserver and intraobserver reliability of the measurement of shoulder internal rotation by vertebral level, *J Shoulder Elbow Surg* 11:40-42, 2002.

Eklund G: Position sense and state of contraction; the effects of vibration, *J Neurol Neurosurg Psychiatry* 35:606-611, 1972.

Ellenbecker TS: A total arm strength isokinetic profile of highly skilled tennis players, *Isok Exerc Sci* 1:9-21, 1991.

Ellenbecker TS: Shoulder internal and external rotation strength and range of motion in highly skilled tennis players, *Isok Exerc Sci* 2:1-8, 1992.

Ellenbecker TS: Rehabilitation of shoulder and elbow injuries in tennis players, *Clin Sports Med* 14(1):87-110, 1995.

Ellenbecker TS: Muscular strength relationship between normal grade manual muscle testing and isokinetic measurement of the shoulder internal and external rotators, *Isok Exerc Sci* 6:51-56, 1996.

Ellenbecker TS, Bailie DS, Andraka J: Subjective and objective follow-up of patients following arthroscopic thermal capsulorrhaphy, 2004.

Ellenbecker TS, Bailie DS, Mattalino AJ, et al: Intrarater and interrater reliability of a manual technique to assess anterior humeral head translation of the glenohumeral joint, *J Shoulder Elbow Surg* 11:470-475, 2002a.

Ellenbecker TS, Bleacher J: A descriptive profile of bilateral glenohumeral joint internal and external rotation strength in uninjured females using the Cybex NORM dynamometer, *Phys Ther* 79:S80, 1999.

Ellenbecker TS, Davies GJ: The application of isokinetics in testing and rehabilitation of the shoulder complex, *J Athletic Training* 35(3):338-350, 2000.

Ellenbecker TS, Davies GJ: *Closed kinetic chain exercise: a comprehensive guide to multiple joint exercises*, Champaign, IL, 2001, Human Kinetics Publishers.

Ellenbecker TS, Davies GJ: *A comparison of three methods for measuring glenohumeral joint internal rotation*, unpublished research, Physiotherapy Associates Scottsdale Sports Clinic Scottsdale Arizona, and Gunderson Lutheran Sports Medicine, LaCrosse, WI, 1997.

Ellenbecker TS, Davies GJ, Rowinski MJ: Concentric versus eccentric isokinetic strengthening of the rotator cuff: objective data versus functional test, *Am J Sports Med* 16:64-69, 1988.

Ellenbecker TS, Manske R, Davies GJ: Closed kinetic chain testing techniques of the upper extremities, *Orthop Phys Ther Clin North Am* 9(2):219-245, 2000b.

Ellenbecker TS, Mattalino AJ: Comparison of open and closed kinetic chain upper extremity tests in patients with rotator cuff pathology and glenohumeral joint instability, *J Orthop Sports Phys Ther* 25:84, 1997.

Ellenbecker TS, Mattalino AJ: Concentric isokinetic shoulder internal and external rotation strength in professional baseball pitchers, *J Orthop Sports Phys Ther* 29:323-328, 1999a.

Ellenbecker TS, Mattalino AJ: *The elbow in sport: injury treatment and rehabilitation*, Champaign, IL, 1996, Human Kinetics Publishers.

Ellenbecker TS, Mattalino AJ: Glenohumeral joint range of motion and rotator cuff strength following arthroscopic anterior stabilization with thermal capsulorrhaphy, *J Orthop Sport Phys Ther* 29(3):160-167, 1999b.

Ellenbecker TS, Mattalino, AJ, Elam EK, et al: Medial elbow joint laxity in professional baseball pitchers: a bilateral comparison using stress radiography, *Am J Sports Med* 26(3):420-424, 1998.

Ellenbecker TS, Mattalino AJ, Elam E, et al: Quantification of anterior translation of the humeral head in the throwing shoulder: manual assessment versus stress radiography, *Am J Sports Med* 28:161-167, 2000a.

Ellenbecker TS, Nazal F, Bailie DS, et al: Subjective rating scales from uninjured unilaterally dominant overhead athletes, 2003a.

Ellenbecker TS, Roetert EP: Age specific isokinetic glenohumeral internal and external rotation strength in elite junior tennis players, *J Sci Med Sport* 6(1):63-70, 2003.

Ellenbecker TS, Roetert EP: A bilateral comparison of upper extremity unilateral closed chain stance stability in elite junior tennis players and professional baseball pitchers, *Med Sci Sports Exerc* 28:S105, 1996.

Ellenbecker TS, Roetert EP: Testing isokinetic muscular fatigue of shoulder internal and external rotation in elite junior tennis players, *J Orthop Sports Phys Ther* 29:275-281, 1999.

Ellenbecker TS, Roetert EP, Bailie DS, et al: Glenohumeral joint total rotation range of motion in elite tennis players and baseball pitchers, *Med Sci Sports Exerc* 34(12):2052-2056, 2002b.

Ellenbecker TS, Roetert EP, Piorkowski PA: Shoulder internal and external range of motion of elite junior tennis players: a comparison of two protocols, *J Orthop Sports Phys Ther* (abstract) 17(1):65, 1993.

Ellenbecker TS, Roetert EP, Piorkowski PA, et al: Glenohumeral joint internal and external rotation range of motion in elite junior tennis players, *J Orthop Sports Phys Ther* 24(6):336-341, 1996.

Elliott B, Marsh T, Blanksby B: A three dimensional cinematographic analysis of the tennis serve, *Int J Sport Biomech* 2:260-271, 1986.

Ellman H, Hander G, Bayer M: Repair of the rotator cuff: end-result study of factors influencing reconstruction, *J Bone Joint Surg* 68A:1136-1144, 1986.

Elmore E, Ellenbecker TS, Bailie DS: Glenohumeral joint range of motion and rotator cuff strength following arthroscopically assisted rotator cuff repair, *J Orthop Sports Phys Ther* 34(Ab1):1, 2003b.

Emery R, Mullaji A: Glenohumeral joint instability in normal adolescents, *J Bone Joint Surg* 73B:406-408, 1991.

Farrally M, Cochran A: *Science and golf III: Proceedings of the World Scientific Congress of Golf*, Champaign, IL, 1999, Human Kinetics Publishers.

Feltner ME, Depena J: Dynamics of the shoulder and elbow joints of the throwing arm during a baseball pitch, *Int J Sport Biomechanics* 2:235-259, 1986.

Fleisig GS, Andrews JR, Dillman CJ, et al: Kinetics of baseball pitching with implications about injury mechanisms, *Am J Sports Med* 23:233, 1995.

Fleisig GS, Dillman CJ, Andrews JR: Proper mechanics for baseball pitching, *Clin Sports Med* 1:151-170, 1989.

Fleisig GS, Jameson EG, Dillman CJ, et al: Biomechanics of overhead sports. In Garrett WE, Kirkendall DT, eds: *Exercise and sport science*, Philadelphia, 2000, Lippincott Williams and Wilkins.

Frese E, Brown M, Norton J: Clinical reliability of manual muscle testing: middle trapezius and gluteus medius muscles, *Phys Ther* 67(7):1072-1076, 1987.

Gartsman GM, Brinker MR, Khan M, et al: Self-assessment of general health status in patients with five common shoulder conditions, *J Shoulder Elbow Surg* 7:228-237, 1998.

Gerber C, Galantay RV, Hersche O: The pattern of pain produced by irritation of the acromioclavicular joint and the subacromial space, *J Shoulder Elbow Surg* 7:352-355, 1998.

Gerber C, Ganz R: Clinical assessment of instability of the shoulder with special reference to anterior and posterior drawer tests, *J Bone Joint Surg* 66B(4):551-556, 1984.

Gerber C, Krushell RJ: Isolated rupture of the tendon of the subscapularis muscle: clinical features in 16 cases, *J Bone Joint Surg* 73B:389-394, 1991.

Gerber C, Werner CML, Macy JC, et al: Effect of selective capsulorrhaphy on the passive range of motion of the glenohumeral joint, *J Bone Joint Surg* 85A(1):48-55, 2003.

Giangarra R, Jobe FW, Tibone JE, et al: Electromyographic and cinematographic analysis of elbow function in tennis players using single- and double-handed backhand strokes, *Am J Sports Med* 21:394-399, 1993.

Gibson MH, Goebel GV, Jordan TM, et al: A reliability study of measurement techniques to determine static scapular position, *J Orthop Sports Phys Ther* 21(2):100-106, 1995.

Gill TJ, Micheli LJ, Gebhard F, et al: Bankart repair for anterior instability of the shoulder, *J Bone Joint Surg* 79A:850-857, 1997.

Glousman RE, Barron J, Jobe FW, et al: An electromyographic analysis of the elbow in normal and injured pitchers with medial collateral ligament insufficiency, *Am J Sports Med* 20(3):311-317, 1992.

Glousman RE, Jobe FW, Tibone JE, et al: Dynamic electromyographic analysis of the throwing shoulder with glenohumeral joint instability, *J Bone Joint Surg* 70A:220-226, 1988.

Goetz CG, Pappert EJ: *Textbook of clinical neurology,* ed 1, Philadelphia, 1999, WB Saunders.

Goldbeck TG, Davies GJ: Test-retest reliability of the closed kinetic chain upper extremity stability test: a clinical field test, *J Sport Rehabil* 9:35-45, 2000.

Golding FC: The shoulder: the forgotten joint, *Br J Radiol* 35:149, 1962.

Goldscheider A: *Gesammelte Abhandlungen.* II. Physiologie des Muskelsinnes, Leipzig, 1898, Barth.

Goodman CC, Snyder TEK: *Differential diagnosis in physical therapy,* ed 3, Philadelphia, 2000, WB Saunders.

Goodwin GM, McCloskey DI, Matthews PBC: The contribution of muscle afferents to kinaesthesia shown by vibration induced illusions of movement and by the effects of paralysing joint afferents, *Brain* 95:705-748, 1972.

Gore DR, Murray MP, Sepic SB, et al: Shoulder muscle strength and range of motion following surgical repair of full thickness rotator cuff tears, *J Bone Joint Surg Am* 68:266-272, 1986.

Gould JA: The spine. In Gould JA, Davies GJ, eds: *Orthopaedic and sports physical therapy,* St Louis, 1985, Mosby.

Greenfield BH, Donatelli R, Wooden MJ, et al: Isokinetic evaluation of shoulder rotational strength between the plane of the scapula and the frontal plane, *Am J Sports Med* 18:124-128, 1990.

Greis PE, Kuhn JE, Schultheis J, et al: Validation of the lift-off test and analysis of subscapularis activity during maximal internal rotation, *Am J Sports Med* 24(5):589-593, 1996.

Grigg P: Peripheral mechanisms in proprioception, *J Sport Rehabil* 3:2-17, 1994.

Grimsby O, Gray JC: Interrelationship of the spine to the shoulder girdle. In Donatelli RA, ed: *Physical therapy of the shoulder,* ed 3, Philadelphia, 1997, Churchill Livingstone.

Groppel JL: *High tech tennis,* ed 2, Champaign, IL, 1992, Human Kinetics Publishers.

Gross ML, Distefano MC: Anterior release test: a new test for occult shoulder instability, *Clin Orthop Rel Res* 339:105-108, 1997.

Grossman TW, Mazur JM, Cummings RJ: An evaluation of the Adams forward bend test and the scoliometer in a scoliosis school screening setting, *J Pediatr Orthop* 15:535-538, 1995.

Guanche CA, Jones DC: Clinical testing for tears of the glenoid labrum, *Arthroscopy* 19(5):517-523, 2003.

Habermeyer P, Kaiser E, Knappe M, et al: Functional anatomy and biomechanics of the long biceps tendon, *Unfallchirurg* 90:319-329, 1987.

Hageman PA, Mason DK, Rydlund KW, et al: Effects of position and speed on eccentric and concentric isokinetic testing of the shoulder rotators, *J Orthop Sports Phys Ther* 11:64-69, 1989.

Halbach JW, Tank RT: The shoulder. In Gould JA, Davies GJ, eds: *Orthopaedic and sports physical therapy,* St Louis, 1985, Mosby.

Halbrecht JL, Tirman P, Atkin D: Internal impingement of the shoulder: comparison of findings between the throwing and nonthrowing shoulders of college baseball players, *Arthroscopy* 15(3):253-258, 1999.

Hamner DL, Pink MM, Jobe FW: A modification of the relocation test: arthroscopic findings associated with a positive test, *J Shoulder Elbow Surg* 9:263-267, 2000.

Hanavan EP: *A mathematical model of the human body,* Dayton, OH, 1964, Wright-Patterson Air Force Base, (AMRL-TR-64-102).

Harryman DT, Sidles JA, Clark MJ, et al: Translation of the humeral head on the glenoid with passive glenohumeral motion, *J Bone Joint Surg* 72A:1334-1343, 1990.

Harryman DT, Sidles JA, Harris SL, et al: Laxity of the normal glenohumeral joint: in-vivo assessment, *J Shoulder Elbow Surg* 1:66-76, 1992.

Hawkins RJ, Bokor DJ: Clinical evaluation of shoulder problems. In Rockwood CA, Matsen FA III, eds: *The shoulder,* Philadelphia, 1990, WB Saunders.

Hawkins RJ, Kennedy JC: Impingement syndrome in athletes, *Am J Sports Med* 8:151-158, 1980.

Hawkins RJ, Mohtadi NGH: Clinical evaluation of shoulder instability, *Clin J Sports Med* 1:59-64, 1991.

Hawkins RJ, Neer CS, Pianta R, et al: Locked posterior dislocation of the shoulder, *J Bone Joint Surg* 69A:9, 1987.

Hawkins RJ, Schulte JP, Janda DH, et al: Translation of the glenohumeral joint with the patient under anesthesia, *J Shoulder Elbow Surg* 5:286-292, 1996.

Hayes KW, Petersen CM: Reliability of assessing end-feel and pain and resistance sequence in subjects with painful shoulders and knees, *J Orthop Sports Phys Ther* 31(8):432-445, 2001.

Heald SL, Riddle DL, Lamb RL: The shoulder pain and disability index: the construct validity and responsiveness of a region specific disability measure, *Phys Ther* 77(10):1079-1089, 1997.

Helmig P, Sojbjerg JE, Kjaersgaaard-Anderson P, et al: Distal humeral migration as a component of multidirectional instability: an anatomical study in autopsy specimens, *Clin Orthop* 252:139-142, 1990.

Hinton RY: Isokinetic evaluation of shoulder rotational strength in high school baseball pitchers, *Am J Sports Med* 16:274-279, 1988.

Holm I, Brox JI, Ludvigsen P, et al: External rotation-best isokinetic movement pattern for evaluation of muscle function in rotator tendonosis. A prospective study with a 2-year follow-up, *Isok Exerc Sci* 5:121-125, 1996.

Hoppenfeld S: *Physical examination of the spine and extremities,* Norwalk, CT, 1976, Appleton-Century-Crofts.

Hsu AT, Chang JH, Chang CH: Determining the resting position of the glenohumeral joint: a cadaver study, *J Orthop Sports Phys Ther* 32(12):605-612, 2002.

Hurley JA, Anderson TE: Shoulder arthroscopy: its role in evaluating shoulder disorders in the athlete, *Am J Sports Med* 18:480-483, 1990.

Ianotti JP, editor: *Rotator cuff disorders,* Chicago, 1991, American Academy of Orthopaedic Surgeons.

Ianotti JP, Bernot MP, Kuhlman JR, et al: Postoperative assessment of shoulder function: a prospective study of full-thickness tears, *J Shoulder Elbow Surg* 5:449-457, 1996.

Ianotti JP, Zlatkin MB, Esterhai JL, et al: Magnetic resonance imaging of the shoulder: sensitivity specificity, and predictive value, *J Bone Joint Surg* 73A:17-29, 1991.

Ide K, Shirai Y, Ito H, et al: Sensory nerve supply in the human subacromial bursa, *J Shoulder Elbow Surg* 5:371-382, 1996.

Inman VT, Saunders JB, Abbott LC: Observations on the function of the shoulder joint, *J Bone Joint Surg* 26(1):1-30, 1944.

Ishii K, Suzuki M, Saito Y, et al: Contribution factors to increase velocity of a distal end in human body: ball throwing. In Adrian M, Deutch H, editors: *Biomechanics, the 1984 Olympic Scientific Congress Proceedings,* Eugene, OR, 1986, Microform Publications.

Itoi E, Kido T, Sano A, et al: Which is more useful the "full can test" or the "empty can test" in detecting the torn supraspinatus tendon? *Am J Sports Med* 27(1):65-68, 1999.

Itoi E, Kuechle DK, Newman SR, et al: Stabilising function of the biceps in stable and unstable shoulders, *J Bone Joint Surg* 75B:546-550, 1993.

Ivey FM, Calhoun JH, Rusche K, et al: Isokinetic testing of shoulder strength: normal values, *Arch Phys Med Rehabil* 66:384-386, 1985.

Jenp YN, Malanga BA, Gowney ES, et al: Activation of the rota`tor cuff in generating isometric shoulder rotation torque, *Am J Sports Med* 24:477-485, 1996.

Jensen GM, Shepard KF, Gwyer J, et al: Attribute dimensions that distinguish master and novice physical therapy clinicians in orthopaedic settings, *Phys Ther* 72:711-722, 1992.

Jensen GM, Shepard KF, Hack LM: The novice versus the experienced clinician: insights into the work of the physical therapist, *Phys Ther* 70:314-323, 1990.

Jerosch JG: Effects of shoulder instability on joint proprioception. In Lephart SM, Fu FH, eds: *Proprioception and neuromuscular control in joint stability*, Champaign, IL, 2000, Human Kinetics Publishers.

Jobe FW, Bradley JP: The diagnosis and nonoperative treatment of shoulder injuries in athletes, *Clin Sports Med* 8:419-437, 1989.

Jobe FW, Kivitne RS: Shoulder pain in the overhand or throwing athlete, *Orthop Rev* 18:963-975, 1989.

Jobe FW, Moynes DR: Delineation and diagnostic criteria and a rehabilitation program for rotator cuff injuries, *Am J Sports Med* 10:336-339, 1982.

Jobe FW, Pink M: The athlete's shoulder, *J Hand Ther* 107, April-June 1994.

Jorgensen K: Force velocity relationships in human elbow flexors and extensors. In Komi PV, ed: *Biomechanics VA*, Baltimore, 1976, University Park Press.

Joris HJJ, Edwards van Muyen AJ, Van Ingen Shenau GJ, et al: Force, velocity and energy flow during the overarm throw in female handball players, *J Biomech* 18:409-414, 1985.

Kaltenborn FM: *Manual mobilization of the extremity joints*, Oslo, Norway, 1989, Olaf Norlis Bokhandel.

Kannus P, Cook L, Alosa D: Absolute and relative endurance parameters in isokinetic tests of muscular performance, *J Sport Rehabil* 1:2-12, 1992.

Kapandji IA: *The physiology of the joints*, New York, 1985, Churchill Livingstone.

Karup Al, Court-Payen M, Skjoldbye B, et al: Ultrasonic measurement of the anterior translation in the shoulder joint, *J Shoulder Elbow Surg* 8:136-141, 1999.

Kazar B, Relovszky E: Prognosis of primary dislocation of the shoulder, *Acta Orthop Scand* 40:216, 1969.

Kebaetse M, McClure P, Pratt NA: Thoracic position effect on shoulder range of motion, strength, and three-dimensional scapular kinematics, *Arch Phys Med Rehabil* 80:945-950, 1999.

Kelly BT, Kadrmas WH, Speer KP: The manual muscle examination for rotator cuff strength: an electromyographic investigation, *Am J Sports Med* 24:581-588, 1996.

Kendall FD, McCreary EK: *Muscle testing and function*, ed 3, Baltimore, 1983, Williams and Wilkins.

Kennedy K, Altchek DW, Glick IV: Concentric and eccentric isokinetic rotator cuff ratios in skilled tennis players, *Isok Exerc Sci* 3:155-159, 1993.

Kibler WB: Evaluation of sports demands as a diagnostic tool in shoulder disorders. In Matsen FA, Fu F, Hawkins RJ, eds: *The shoulder: a balance of mobility and stability*, Rosemont, IL, 1993, American Association of Orthopaedic Surgeons.

Kibler WB: Management of the scapula in glenohumeral instability, *Tech Shoulder Elbow Surg* 4(3):89-98, 2003.

Kibler WB: The role of the scapula in athletic shoulder function, *Am J Sports Med* 26(2):325-337, 1998a.

Kibler WB: Role of the scapula in the overhead throwing motion, *Contemp Orthop* 22(5):525-532, 1991.

Kibler WB: Shoulder rehabilitation: principles and practice, *Med Sci Sports Exerc* 30(4):S40-S50, 1998b.

Kibler WB: Specificity and sensitivity of the anterior slide test in throwing athletes with superior glenoid labral tears, *Arthroscopy* 11(3):296-300, 1995.

Kibler WB, Chandler TJ, Livingston BP, et al: Shoulder range of motion in elite tennis players, *Am J Sports Med* 24(3):279-285, 1996.

Kibler WB, Livingston B, Bruce R: Current concepts in shoulder rehabilitation, *Adv Operative Orthop* 3:249-297, 1995.

Kibler WB, McMullen J: Scapular dyskinesis and its relation to shoulder pain, *J Am Acad Orthop Surg* 11:142-151, 2003.

Kibler WB, Uhl TL, Maddux JWQ, et al: Qualitative clinical evaluation of scapular dysfunction: a reliability study, *J Shoulder Elbow Surg* 11:550-556, 2002.

Kikuchi T: Histological studies on the sensory innervation of the shoulder joint, *J Iwate Med Assoc* 20(5):554-567, 1968.

Kim SH, Ha KI, Ahn JH, et al: Biceps load test II: a clinical test for SLAP lesions of the shoulder, *Arthroscopy* 17(2):160-164, 2001.

Kim SH, Ha KI, Han KY: Biceps load test: a clinical test for superior labrum anterior and posterior lesions in shoulders with recurrent anterior dislocations, *Am J Sports Med* 27(3):300-303, 1999.

Kim TK, Queale WS, Cosqarea AJ, et al: Clinical features of the different types of slap lesions, *J Bone Joint Surg* 85A:66-71, 2003.

Kirschenbaum D, Coyle MP, Leddy JP, et al: Shoulder strength with rotator cuff tears: pre and post-operative analysis, *Clin Orthop Rel Res* 288:174-178, 1993.

Klafs CE, Arnheim DD: *Modern principles of athletic training*, St Louis, 1981, Mosby.

Knops JE, Meiners TK, Davies GJ, et al: *Isokinetic test retest reliability of the modified neutral shoulder test position*, unpublished research, LaCrosse, WI, 1998, University of LaCrosse.

Koffler KM, Bader D, Eager M, et al: *The effect of posterior capsular tightness on glenohumeral translation in the late-cocking phase of pitching: a cadaveric study*, Abstract (SS-15) presented at Arthroscopy Association of North America Annual Meeting, Washington, DC, 2001.

Koslow PA, Prosser LA, Strony GA, et al: Specificity of the lateral scapular slide test in asymptomatic competitive athletes, *J Orthop Sports Phys Ther* 33(6):331-336, 2003.

Kraushaar BS, Nirschl RP: Tendonosis of the elbow (tennis elbow): clinical features and findings of histological, immunohistochemical, and electron microscopy studies, *J Bone Joint Surg* 81A(2):259-278, 1999.

Kreighbaum E, Barthels KM: *Biomechanics: a qualitative approach for studying human movement*, Minneapolis, MN, 1985, Burgess.

Kuhn JE, Lindholm SR, Huston LJ, et al: *Failure of biceps superior labral complex in the throwing athlete: a biomechanical model comparing maximal cocking to early deceleration*, Presented at the Annual Meeting of the American Academy of Orthopaedic Surgeons, AANA Specialty Day, Anaheim, CA, February 1999.

Kumar VP, Satku K, Balasubramaniam P: The role of the long head of the biceps brachii in the stabilization of the head of the humerus, *Clin Orthop* 244:172-175, 1989.

Kvitne KS, Jobe FW, Jobe CM: Shoulder instability in the overhead or throwing athlete, *Clin Sports Med* 14(4):917, 1995.

Lephart SM, Fu FH: *Proprioception and neuromuscular control in joint stability,* Champaign, IL, 2000, Human Kinetics Publishers.

Lephart SM, Myers JB, Bradley JP, et al: Shoulder proprioception and function following thermal capsulorrhaphy, *J Shoulder Elbow Surg* 18(7):770-778, 2002.

Lephart SM, Warner JJP, Borsa PA, et al: Proprioception of the shoulder joint in healthy, unstable, and surgically repaired shoulders, *J Shoulder Elbow Surg* 3:371-380, 1994.

Leroux JL, Codine P, Thomas E, et al: Isokinetic evaluation of rotational strength in normal shoulders and shoulders with impingement syndrome, *Clin Orthop Rel Res* 304:108-115, 1994.

Leroux JL, Thomas E, Bonnel F, et al: Diagnostic value of clinical tests for shoulder impingement syndrome, *Rev Rheum* 62(6):423-428, 1995.

Levy AS, Kelly BT, Lintner SA, et al: Function of the long head of the biceps at the shoulder: electromyographic analysis, *J Shoulder Elbow Surg* 10(3):250-255, 2001.

Levy AS, Lintner S, Kenter K, et al: Intra- and interobserver reproducibility of shoulder laxity examination, *Am J Sports Med* 27(4):460-463, 1999.

Lilienfeld AM, Jacobs M, Willis M: A study of the reproducibility of muscle testing and certain other aspects of muscle scoring, *Phys Ther Rev* 34:279-289, 1954.

Lintner SA, Levy A, Kenter K, et al: Glenohumeral translation in the asymptomatic athlete's shoulder and its relationship to other clinically measurable anthropometric variables, *Am J Sports Med* 24(6):716-720, 1996.

Lippman RK: Frozen shoulder: periarthritis, bicipital tenosynovitis, *Arch Surg* 47:283-296, 1943.

Litchfield DG, Jeno S, Mabey R: The lateral scapular slide test: is it valid in detecting glenohumeral impingement syndrome? *Phys Ther* 78(5):S29, 1998.

Liu SH, Henry MH, Nuccion S, et al: Diagnosis of glenoid labrum tears. A comparison between magnetic resonance imaging and clinical examinations, *Am J Sports Med* 24(2):149-154, 1996a.

Liu SH, Henry MH, Nuccion S: A prospective evaluation of a new physical examination in predicting glenoid labrum tears, *Am J Sports Med* 24(6):721-725, 1996b.

Lucas DB: Biomechanics of the shoulder joint, *Arch Surg* 107:425, 1973.

Ludington NA: Rupture of the long head of the biceps flexor cubiti muscle, *Ann Surg* 77:358-363, 1923.

Lukasiewicz AC, McClure P, Michener L, et al: Comparison of 3-dimensional scapular position and orientation between subjects with and without shoulder impingement, *J Orthop Sports Phys Ther* 29(10):574-586, 1999.

Lyons AR, Tomlinson JE: Clinical diagnosis of tears of the rotator cuff, *J Bone Joint Surg (Br)* 74:41-45, 1993.

MacDonald PB, Clark P, Sutherland K: An analysis of the diagnostic accuracy of the Hawkins and Neer subacromial impingement signs, *J Shoulder Elbow Surg* 9(4):299-301, 2000.

Magarey ME, Hayes MG, Trott PH: The accuracy of manipulative physiotherapy diagnosis of shoulder complex dysfunction: a pilot study. In *Proceedings of the Sixth Biennial Conference,* Adelaide, Australia, 1989, Manipulative Physiotherapists Association of Australia.

Magee DJ: *Orthopaedic physical assessment,* ed 3, Philadelphia, 1997, WB Saunders.

Malanga GA, Jemp YN, Growney ES, et al: EMG analysis of shoulder positioning in testing and strengthening the supraspinatus, *Med Sci Sports Exerc* 28(6): 661, 1996.

Mallon WJ, Herring CL, Sallay PI, et al: Use of vertebral levels to measure presumed internal rotation at the shoulder: a radiographic analysis, *J Shoulder Elbow Surg* 5:299-306, 1996.

Mallon W, Speer K: Multidirectional instability: current concepts, *J Shoulder Elbow Surg* 4:55-64, 1995.

Marshall RN, Elliott BC: Long-axis rotation: the missing link in proximal to distal sequencing, *J Sports Sci* 18:247-254, 2000.

Marshall RN, Noffal GJ, Legnani G: *Simulation of the tennis serve: factors affecting elbow torques related to medial epicondylitis,* Paris, 1993, ISB.

Matsen FA, Fu FH, Hawkins RJ: *The shoulder: a balance of mobility and stability,* Park Ridge, IL, 1992, American Academy of Orthopaedic Surgeons.

Matsen FA, Harryman DT, Sidles JA: Mechanics of glenohumeral instability, *Clin Sports Med* 10:783, 1991.

Matsen FA, Lippitt SB, Sidles JA, et al: *Practical evaluation and management of the shoulder,* Philadelphia, 1994, WB Saunders.

Matsen FA, Thomas SC, Rockwood CA, et al: Glenohumeral instability. In Rockwood CA, Matsen FA, eds: *The shoulder,* Philadelphia, 1998, WB Saunders.

Matsen FA III, Artnz CT: Subacromial impingement. In Rockwood CA, Jr, Matsen FA III, eds: *The shoulder,* Philadelphia, 1990, WB Saunders.

Mattingly GE, Mackarey PJ: Optimal methods for shoulder tendon palpation: a cadaver study, *Phys Ther* 76(2):166-174, 1996.

Maughon TS, Andrews JR: The subjective evaluation of the shoulder in the athlete. In Andrews JR, Wilk KE, eds: *The athlete's shoulder,* New York, 1994, Churchill Livingstone.

McFarland E, Campbell G, McDowell J: Posterior shoulder laxity in asymptomatic adolescent athletes, *Am J Sports Med* 24:460-471, 1991.

McFarland EG, Campbell G, McDowell J: Posterior shoulder laxity in asymptomatic athletes, *Am J Sports Med* 24(4):468-471, 1996a.

McFarland EG, Kim TK, Savino RM: Clinical assessment of three common tests for superior labral anterior-posterior lesions, *Am J Sports Med* 30(6):810-815, 2002.

McFarland EG, Torpey BM, Carl LA: Evaluation of shoulder laxity, *Sports Med* 22:264-272, 1996b.

McMahon PJ, Jobe FW, Pink MM, et al: Comparative electromyographic analysis of shoulder muscles during planar motions: anterior glenohumeral joint instability versus normal, *J Shoulder Elbow Surg* 5:118, 1996.

McQuade JK, Shelley I, Cvitkovic J: Patterns of stiffness during clinical examination of the glenohumeral joint, *Clin Biomech* 14:620-627, 1999.

Mennell JM: *Joint pain: diagnosis and treatment using manipulative techniques,* Boston 1964, Little, Brown.

Mimori K, Muneta T, Nakagawa T, et al: A new pain provocation test for superior labral tears of the shoulder, *Am J Sports Med* 27(2):137-142, 1999.

Moffroid M, Whipple R, Hofkosh J, et al: A study of isokinetic exercise, *Phys Ther* 49:735-747, 1969.

Mont MA, Cohen DB, Campbell KR, et al: Isokinetic concentric versus eccentric training of the shoulder rotators with functional evaluation of performance enhancement in elite tennis players, *Am J Sports Med* 22:513-517, 1994.

Moore ML: The measurement of joint motion. Part I: Introductory review of the literature, *Phys Ther* 29:195-205, 1949.

Morgan CD, Burkhart SS, Palmeri M, et al: Type II SLAP lesions: three subtypes and their relationships to superior instability and rotator cuff tears, *Arthroscopy* 14:553-565, 1998.

Morisawa Y, Kawakami T, Uermura H, et al: Mechanoreceptors in the coraco-acromial ligament: a study of the aging process, *J Shoulder Elbow Surg* 3:S45, 1994.

Morrey BF: *The elbow and its disorders,* ed 2, Philadelphia, 1993, WB Saunders.

Morrey BF, An KN: Articular and ligamentous contributions to the stability of the elbow joint, *Am J Sports Med* 11:315, 1983.

Myers JB, Guskiewicz KM, Schneider RA, et al: Proprioception and neuromuscular control of the shoulder after muscle fatigue, *J Athletic Training* 34(4):362-367, 1999.

Myers JB, Lephart SM: The role of the sensorimotor system in the athletic shoulder, *J Athletic Training* 35(3):351-363, 2000.

Naredo E, Aguado P, DeMiguel E, et al: Painful shoulder: comparison of physical examination and ultrasonographic findings, *Ann Rheum Dis* 61:132-136, 2002.

Neer CS: Anterior acromioplasty for the chronic impingement syndrome in the shoulder, *J Bone Joint Surg* 54A:41-50, 1972.

Neer CS: Cuff tears, biceps lesions, and impingement. In Neer CS, ed: *Shoulder reconstruction,* Philadelphia, 1990, WB Saunders.

Neer CS: Impingement lesions, *Clin Orthop* 173:70-77, 1983.

Neer CS, Foster CR: Inferior capsular shift for involuntary inferior and multidirectional instability of the shoulder: a preliminary report, *J Bone Joint Surg* 62A:897, 1980.

Neer CS, Watson KC, Stanton FJ: Recent experience in total shoulder replacement, *J Bone Joint Surg* 64A:319-337, 1982.

Neer CS, Welsh RP: The shoulder in sports, *Clin Orthop Rel Res* 8:583, 1977.

Nirschl RP: Prevention and treatment of elbow and shoulder injuries in the tennis player, *Clin Sports Med* 7:289-308, 1988a.

Nirschl RP: Shoulder tendonitis. In Pettrone FP, ed: *Upper extremity injuries in athletes, American Academy of Orthopaedic Surgeons Symposium,* Washington, DC, 1988b, Mosby.

Norkin CC, White DJ: *Measurement of joint motion: a guide to goniometry,* ed 2, Philadelphia, 1995, FA Davis.

Norwood LA, Terry GC: Shoulder posterior and subluxation, *Am J Sports Med* 12:25-30, 1984.

Nyland JA, Caborn DNM, Johnson DL: The human glenohumeral joint: a proprioceptive and stability alliance, *Knee Surg Sports Traumatol Arthrosc* 6:50-61, 1998.

O'Brien SJ, Beves MC, Arnoczky SJ, et al: The anatomy and histology of the inferior glenohumeral ligament complex of the shoulder, *Am J Sports Med* 18:449-456, 1990.

O'Brien SJ, Pagnani MJ, Fealy S, et al: The active compression test: a new and effective test for diagnosing labral tears and acromioclavicular joint abnormality, *Am J Sports Med* 26(5):610-613, 1998.

Odem CJ, Taylor AB, Hurd CE, et al: Measurement of scapular asymmetry and assessment of shoulder dysfunction using the lateral scapular slide test: a reliability and validity study, *Phys Ther* 81(2):799-809, 2001.

Osbahr DC, Diamond AB, Speer KP: The cosmetic appearance of the biceps muscle after long-head tenotomy versus tenodesis, *Arthroscopy* 18(5):483-487, 2002.

Paavolainen P, Bjorkenheim JM, Slatis P, et al: Operative treatment of severe proximal humeral fractures, *Acta Orthop Scand* 54:374-379, 1983.

Pagnani MJ, Deng XH, Warren RF, et al: Role of the long head of the biceps brachii in glenohumeral stability. A biomechanical study in cadavers, *J Shoulder Elbow Surg* 5:255-262, 1996.

Pagnani MJ, Warren RF: Stabilizers of the glenohumeral joint, *J Shoulder Elbow Surg* 3:73-90, 1994.

Paley KJ, Jobe FW, Pink MM, et al: Arthroscopic findings in the overhand throwing athlete: evidence for posterior internal impingement of the rotator cuff, *Arthroscopy* 16(1):35-40, 2000.

Patte D, Goutallier D, Monpierre H, et al: Over-extension lesions, *Rev Chir Orthop* 74:314-318, 1988.

Pedegana LR, Elsner RC, Roberts D, et al: The relationship of upper extremity strength to throwing speed, *Am J Sports Med* 10:352-354, 1982.

Pedersen J, Lönn J, Hellström F, et al: Localized muscle fatigue decreases the movement sense in the human shoulder, *Med Sci Sports Exerc* 31:1047, 1999.

Penny JN, Welsh RP: Shoulder impingement syndrome in athletes and their surgical management, *Am J Sports Med* 9:11-15, 1981.

Perthes G: Ueber Operationen der habituellen Schulterluxation, *Deutsche Ztschr Chir* 85:199, 1906.

Piatt BE, Hawkins RJ, Fritz RC, et al: Clinical evaluation and treatment of spinoglenoid notch ganglion cysts, *J Shoulder Elbow Surg* 11:600-604, 2002.

Plafcan DM, Truczany PJ, Guenin BA, et al: An objective measurement technique for posterior scapular displacement, *J Orthop Sports Phys Ther* 25(5):336-341, 1997.

Plagenhoef S: *Patterns of human movement,* Englewood Cliffs, NJ, 1971, Prentice Hall.

Poppen NK, Walker PS: Forces at the glenohumeral joint in abduction, *Clin Orthop* 135:165, 1978.

Portney LG, Watkins MP: *Foundations of clinical research applications to practice,* Stamford, CT, 1993, Appleton & Lange.

Post M, Cohen J: Impingement syndrome: a review of late stage II and early stage III lesions, *Clin Orthop Rel Res* 207:127-132, 1986.

Priest JD, Nagel DA: Tennis shoulder, *Am J Sports Med* 4(1):28-42, 1976.

Putnam CA: Sequential motions of the body segments in striking and throwing skills: descriptions and explanations, *J Biomechan* 26(suppl 1):125-136, 1993.

Quanbury AO, Winter DA, Reimer GD: Instantaneous power and power flow in body segments during walking, *J Human Movement Studies* 1:59-67, 1975.

Quincy R, Davies GJ, Kolbeck K, et al: Isokinetic exercise: the effects of training specificity on shoulder power, *J Athletic Training* 35:5, 2000.

Rabin SJ, Post MP: A comparative study of clinical muscle testing and Cybex evaluation after shoulder operations, *Clin Orthop Rel Res* 258:147-156, 1990.

Rathbun JB, MacNab I: The microvascular pattern of the rotator cuff, *JBJJ (Br)* 52-B:540, 1970.

Rayan GM: Thoracic outlet syndrome, *J Shoulder Elbow Surg* 7(4):440-451, 1998.

Rayan GM, Jensen C: Thoracic outlet syndrome: provocative examination maneuvers in a typical population, *J Shoulder Elbow Surg* 4:113-117, 1995.

Reider B: *The orthopaedic physical examination,* Philadelphia, 1999, WB Saunders.

Rhu KN, McCormick J, Jobe FW, et al: An electromyographic analysis of shoulder function in tennis players, *Am J Sports Med* 16:481-485, 1988.

Richards RR, An KN, Bigliani LU, et al: A standardized method for the assessment of shoulder function, *J Shoulder Elbow Surg* 3:347-352, 1994.

Riddle DL, Rothstein JM, Lamb RL: Goniometric reliability in a clinical setting: shoulder measurements, *Phys Ther* 67:668-673, 1987.

Roach KE, Budiman-Mak E, Songsiridez N, et al: Development of a shoulder pain and disability index, *Arthritis Care Res* 4:143-149, 1991.

Robertson DGE, Winter DA: Mechanical energy generation, absorption, and transfer amongst segments during walking, *J Biomechanics* 13:845-854, 1980.

Rockwood CA: Subluxations and dislocations about the shoulder. In Rockwood CA, Green DP, eds: *Fractures in adults*, Philadelphia, 1984, JB Lippincott.

Roddey TS, Olson SL, Cook KF, et al: Comparison of the University of California-Los Angeles shoulder scale and the Simple Shoulder Test with the Shoulder Pain and Disability Index: Single-Administration reliability and validity, *Phys Ther* 80(8):759-768, 2000.

Rodosky MW, Harner CD, Fu F: The role of the long head of the biceps muscle and superior glenoid labrum in anterior stability of the shoulder, *Am J Sports Med* 22:121-130, 1994.

Roetert EP, Ellenbecker TS: *Complete conditioning for tennis*, Champaign IL, 1998, Human Kinetics.

Roetert EP, Ellenbecker TS, Brown SW: Shoulder internal and external range of motion in nationally ranked junior tennis players: a longitudinal analysis, *J Strength Conditioning Res* 14(2):140-143, 2000.

Roetert EP, Groppel J: *World class tennis technique*, Champaign IL, 2001, Human Kinetics Publishers.

Roland PE, Ladegaard-Pedersen H: A quantitative analysis of sensations of tension and of kinaesthesia in man: evidence for a peripherally originating muscular sense and for a sense of effort, *Brain* 100:671-692, 1977.

Roos D: Transaxillary for first rib resection to relieve thoracic outlet syndrome, *Ann Surg* 163:354-358, 1966.

Rowe CR: Acute and recurrent dislocations of the shoulder, *J Bone Joint Surg* 44A:998, 1962.

Rowe CR: Dislocations of the shoulder. In Rowe CR, ed: *The shoulder*, Edinburgh, 1988, Churchill Livingstone.

Rowe CR, Patel D, Southmayd WW: The Bankart procedure: a long term end-result study, *J Bone Joint Surg* 60A:1-16, 1978.

Rowe CR, Zarins B: Recurrent transient subluxation of the shoulder, *J Bone Joint Surg* 63A:863-871, 1981.

Rubin BD, Kibler WB: Fundamental principles of shoulder rehabilitation: conservative to postoperative management, *Arthroscopy* 18(9)(suppl 2):29-39, 2002.

Rupp S, Berninger K, Hopf T: Shoulder problems in high level swimmers: impingement, anterior instability, muscular imbalance? *Int J Sports Med* 16:557-562, 1995.

Saha AK: Mechanism of shoulder movements and a plea for the recognition of "zero position" of glenohumeral joint, *Clin Orthop* 173:3-10, 1983.

Sauers EL, Borsa PA, Herling DE, et al: Instrumented measurement of glenohumeral joint laxity and its relationship to passive range of motion and generalized joint laxity, *Am J Sports Med* 29:143-150, 2001a.

Sauers EL, Borsa PA, Herling DE, et al: Instrumented measurement of glenohumeral joint laxity: reliability and normative data, *Knee Surg Sports Traumatol Arthrosc* 9:34-41, 2001b.

Segal DK: *Tennis sistema biodinamico*, Buenos Aires, Argentina, 2002, Tenis Club Argentino.

Shapiro R, Stine RL: *Shoulder rotation velocities*, technical report submitted to the Lexington Clinic, Lexington, KY, 1992.

Sher JS, Uribe J, Posada A, et al: Abnormal findings on magnetic resonance images of asymptomatic shoulders, *J Bone Joint Surg* 77(1):10-15, 1995.

Sherrington C: *The integrative action of the nervous system*, New York, 1906, Scribner's Son.

Shimoda F: Innervation, especially sensory innervation of the knee joint and motor organs around it in early stage of human embryo, *Arch Histol Japan* 9:91-108, 1955.

Slobounov SM, Poole ST, Simon RF, et al: The efficacy of modern technology to improve healthy and injured shoulder joint position sense, *J Sport Rehabil* 8:10-23, 1999.

Smith RL, Brunoli J: Shoulder kinesthesia after anterior glenohumeral joint dislocation, *Phys Ther* 69(2):106-112, 1989.

Snyder SJ, Banas MP, Karzel RP: An analysis of 140 injuries to the superior glenoid labrum, *J Shoulder Elbow Surg* 4:243-248, 1995.

Snyder SJ, Karzel RP, Del Pizzo W, et al: SLAP lesions of the shoulder, *Arthroscopy* 6:274-279, 1990.

Sobush DC, Simoneau GG, Dietz KE, et al: The Lennie test for measuring scapular position in healthy young adult females: a reliability and validity study, *J Orthop Sports Phys Ther* 23(1):39-50, 1996.

Soderberg GJ, Blaschak MJ: Shoulder internal and external rotation peak torque production through a velocity spectrum in differing positions, *J Orthop Sports Phys Ther* 8:518-524, 1987.

Soldatis JJ, Moseley JB, Etminan M: Shoulder symptoms in healthy athletes: a comparison of outcome scoring systems, *J Shoulder Elbow Surg* 6:265-271, 1997.

Solem-Bertoft E, Thuomas K, Westerberg C: The influence of scapula retraction and protraction on the width of the subacromial space, *Clin Orthop* 266:99-103, 1993.

Speer KP: Anatomy and pathomechanics of shoulder instability, *Clin Sports Med* 14(4):751-760, 1995.

Speer KP, Deng X, Borrero S, et al: Biomechanical evaluation of a simulated Bankart lesion, *J Bone Joint Surg* 76-A(12):1819-1826, 1994b.

Speer KP, Hannafin JA, Altchek DW, et al: An evaluation of the shoulder relocation test, *Am J Sports Med* 22(2):177-183, 1994a.

Sprigings E, Marshall R, Elliott B, et al: A three-dimensional kinematic method for determining the effectiveness of arm segment rotations in producing racquet head speed, *J Biomechan* 27:245-254, 1994.

Stefko JM, Jobe FW, VanderWilde RS, et al: Electromyographic and nerve block analysis of the subscapularis liftoff test, *J Shoulder Elbow Surg* 6:347-355, 1997.

Stetson WB, Templin K: The crank test, the O'Brien test, and routine magnetic resonance imaging scans in the diagnosis of labral tears, *Am J Sports Med* 30(6):806-809, 2002.

Struhl S: Anterior internal impingement: an arthroscopic observation, *Arthroscopy* 18(1):2-7, 2002.

Telford E, Mottershead S: Pressure at the cervical brachial junction: an operative and anatomical study, *J Bone Joint Surg* 30B:249-265, 1948.

Terry GC, Friedman SJ, Uhl TL: Arthroscopically treated tears of the glenoid labrum. Factors influencing outcome, *Am J Sports Med* 22(4)504-512, 1994.

Tibone JE, Bradley JP: Evaluation of treatment outcomes for the athletes shoulder. In Matsen FA, Fu FH, Hawkins RJ, eds: *The shoulder: a balance of mobility and stability*, Rosemont, IL, 1993, American Academy of Orthopaedic Surgeons.

T'Jonck L, Lysens R, Gunther G: Measurement of scapular position and rotation: a reliability study, *Physiother Res Int* 1(3):148-158, 1996.

Tohyama H, Yasuda K, Ohkoshi Y, et al: Anterior drawer test for acute anterior talofibular ligament injuries in the ankle: how much load should be applied during the test? *Am J Sports Med* 31(2):226-232, 2003.

Tomberlin J: *Physical diagnostic tests of the shoulder. An evidence based perspective,* LaCrosse, WI, 2001, Orthopaedic Section of the APTA, Home Study Course 11.1.2.

Toussaint HM, de Hollander P, van den Berg C, et al: Biomechanics of swimming. In Garrett WE, Kirkendall DT, eds: *Exercise and sport science,* Philadelphia, 2000, Lippincott Willians and Wilkins.

Treiber FA, Lott J, Duncan J, et al: Effects of Theraband and light weight dumbbell training on shoulder rotation torque and serve performance in college tennis players, *Am J Sports Med* 26:510-515, 1998.

Tyler TF, Nicholas SJ, Roy T, et al: Quantification of posterior capsular tightness and motion loss in patients with shoulder impingement, *Am J Sports Med* 28(5):668-673, 2000.

Tyler TF, Roy T, Nicholas SJ, et al: Reliability and validity of a new method of measuring posterior shoulder tightness, *J Orthop Sports Phys Ther* 29(5):262-274, 1999.

Tzannes A, Murrell GAC: Clinical examination of the unstable shoulder, *Sports Med* 32(7):447-457, 2002.

Valadie AL, Jobe CM, Pink MM, et al: Anatomy of provocative tests for impingement syndrome of the shoulder, *J Shoulder Elbow Surg* 9(1):36-46, 2000.

VanGheluwe B, Hebbelinck M: The kinematics of the service movement in tennis: a three dimensional cinematographical approach. In Winter DA, Norman RW, Wells RP, et al, eds: *Biomechanics IX-B,* Champaign IL, 1985, Human Kinetics Publishers.

Vangsness CT, Ennis M, Taylor JG, et al: Neural anatomy of the glenohumeral ligaments, labrum, and subacromial bursa, *Arthroscopy* 11(2):180-184, 1995.

Van Moppes FI, Veldkamp O, Roorda J: Role of ultrasonography in the evaluation of the painful shoulder, *Eur J Radiol* 19:142-146, 1995.

Vaughan RE: An algorithm for determining arm action during overarm baseball pitches. In Winter DA, Norman RW, Wells RP, et al, eds: *Biomechanics IX-B,* Champaign, IL, 1985, Human Kinetics Publishers.

Voight ML, Hardin JA, Blackburn TA, et al: The effects of muscle fatigue on and the relationship of arm dominance to shoulder proprioception, *J Orthop Sports Phys Ther* 23(6):348-352, 1996.

Voss H: Tabelle der absoluten und relativen Muskel-spindelzahlen der menschlichen Skelettmuskulatur, *Anat Anz* 129:562-572, 1971.

Waddell G, McCulloch JA, Kummer E, et al: Nonorganic physical signs in low back pain, *Spine* 5(2):117-125, 1980.

Walch F, Boulahia A, Calderone S, et al: The "dropping" and 'Hornblower's signs in evaluation of rotator cuff tears, *J Bone Joint Surg* 80B:(4):624-628, 1998.

Walch G, Boileau P, Noel E, et al: Impingement of the deep surface of the supraspinatus tendon on the posterosuperior glenoid rim: an arthroscopic study, *J Shoulder Elbow Surg* 1:238, 1992.

Walch G, Nove-Josserand L, Levigne C, et al: Tears of the supraspinatus tendon associated with "hidden" lesions of the rotator interval, *J Shoulder Elbow Surg* 3:353-360, 1994.

Walker SW, Couch WH, Boester GA, et al: Isokinetic strength of the shoulder after repair of a torn rotator cuff, *J Bone Joint Surg Am* 69:1041-1044, 1987.

Walmsley RP, Hartsell H: Shoulder strength following surgical rotator cuff repair: a comparative analysis using isokinetic testing, *J Orthop Sports Phys Ther* 15:215-222, 1992.

Walmsley RP, Szybbo C: A comparative study of the torque generated by the shoulder internal and external rotator muscles in different positions and at varying speeds, *J Orthop Sports Phys Ther* 9:217-222, 1987.

Ware JE, Jr, Snow KK, Kosinski M, et al: *SF-36 health survey manual and interpretation guide,* Boston, 1993, The Health Institute.

Warner JP, Micheli LJ, Arslanian LE, et al: Patterns of flexibility, laxity, and strength in normal shoulders and shoulders with instability and impingement, *Am J Sports Med* 18:366-375, 1990.

Warner JP, Micheli LJ, Arslanian LE, et al: Scapulothoracic motion in normal shoulders and shoulders with glenohumeral instability and impingement syndrome: a study using Moiré topographic analysis, *Clin Orthop Rel Res* 285:191-199, 1991.

Warner JJP, Lephart S, Fu FH: Role of proprioception in pathoetiology of shoulder instability, *Clin Orthop Rel Res* 330:35-39, 1996.

Warner JJP, McMahon PJ: The role of the long head of the biceps brachii in superior stability of the glenohumeral joint, *J Bone Joint Surg* 77a:366-373, 1995.

Wilk KE, Andrews JR, Arrigo CA, et al: The strength characteristics of internal and external rotator muscles in professional baseball pitchers, *Am J Sports Med* 21:61-66, 1993.

Wilk KE, Arrigo CA: Current concepts in the rehabilitation of the athletic shoulder, *J Orthop Sports Phys Ther* 18:335, 1993.

Wilk KE, Arrigo CA, Andrews JR: Isokinetic testing of the shoulder abductors and adductors: windowed vs nonwindowed data collection, *J Orthop Sports Phys Ther* 15:107-112, 1992.

Wilk KE, Arrigo CA, Andrews JR: Standardized isokinetic testing protocol for the throwing shoulder: the throwers series, *Isok Exerc Sci* 1:63-71, 1991.

Williams GN, Gangel TJ, Arciero RA, et al: Comparison of the single assessment numeric evaluation method and two shoulder rating scales: outcomes measures after shoulder surgery, *Am J Sports Med* 27(2):214-221, 1999.

Williams JW, Holleman DR, Simel DL: Measuring shoulder function with the shoulder pain and disability index, *J Rheumatol* 22:727-732, 1995.

Wolf EM, Agrawal V: Trandeltoid palpation (the rent test) in the diagnosis of rotator cuff tears, *J Shoulder Elbow Surg* 10:470-473, 2001.

Wuelker N, Plitz W, Roetman B: Biomechanical data concerning the shoulder impingement syndrome, *Clin Orthop* 303:242, 1994.

Wyke B: Articular neurology: a review, *Physiotherapy* 58:94-99, 1972.

Wyke BD: The neurology of joints, *Ann R Coll Surg Engl* 41:25, 1967.

Yamaguchi K, Riew BK, Galatz LM, et al: Biceps activity during shoulder motion: an electromyographic analysis, *Clin Orthop* 336:122-129, 1997.

Yergason RM: Supination sign, *J Bone Joint Surg* 13:160, 1931.

Yocum LA: Assessing the shoulder, *Clin Sports Med* 2:281-289, 1983.

Zaslav KR: Internal rotation resistance strength test: a new diagnostic test to differentiate intra-articular pathology from outlet (Neer) impingement syndrome in the shoulder, *J Shoulder Elbow Surg* 10:23-27, 2001.

Zeier FG: The treatment of winged scapula, *Clin Orthop Rel Res* 91:128-133, 1973.

Zemek MJ, Magee DJ: Comparison of glenohumeral joint laxity in elite and recreational swimmers, *Clin J Sports Med* 6:40-47, 1996.

Zuckerman JD, Gallagher MA, Cuomo F, et al: The effect of instability and subsequent anterior shoulder repair on proprioceptive ability, *J Shoulder Elbow Surg* 12:105-109, 2003.

Zuckerman JD, Gallagher MA, Lehman C, et al: Normal shoulder proprioception and the effect of lidocaine injection, *J Shoulder Elbow Surg* 8(1):11-16, 1999.

Zuckerman JD, Kummer FJ, Cuomo, et al: The influence of coracoacromial arch anatomy on rotator cuff tears, *J Shoulder Elbow Surg* 1:4, 1992.

Index*

---

*Page numbers followed by *f* indicate figures; *t*, tables; *b*, boxes.

197